T0184649

Issues in the developmental approach to mental retardation

Issues in the developmental approach to mental retardation

Edited by
ROBERT M. HODAPP
JACOB A. BURACK
and
EDWARD ZIGLER
Yale University

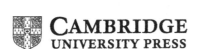

CAMBRIDGE
UNIVERSITY PRESS

CAMBRIDGE
UNIVERSITY PRESS

32 Avenue of the Americas, New York NY 10013-2473, USA

Cambridge University Press is part of the University of Cambridge.

It furthers the University's mission by disseminating knowledge in the pursuit of education, learning and research at the highest international levels of excellence.

www.cambridge.org
Information on this title: www.cambridge.org/9780521467575

First published 1990
First paperback edition 1995

A catalogue record for this publication is available from the British Library

ISBN 978-0-521-34619-1 Hardback
ISBN 978-0-521-46757-5 Paperback

....

Every effort has been made in preparing this book to provide accurate and up-to-date information which is in accord with accepted standards and practice at the time of publication. Although case histories are drawn from actual cases, every effort has been made to disguise the identities of the individuals involved. Nevertheless, the authors, editors and publishers can make no warranties that the information contained herein is totally free from error, not least because clinical standards are constantly changing through research and regulation. The authors, editors and publishers therefore disclaim all liability for direct or consequential damages resulting from the use of material contained in this book. Readers are strongly advised to pay careful attention to information provided by the manufacturer of any drugs or equipment that they plan to use.

This book honors and commemorates Emily Fraser Beede, 1869–1964. With courage and love rising above sorrow she enriched and made happy the life of her retarded daughter.

Contents

vii

Preface

The timing of a book is a curious thing. Sometimes the book appears as a herald to a field, the first inkling that a new theory or new approach has arrived. It points the way, outlines the territory, and energizes workers who may be interested but not quite know how to proceed. Or a book may serve as a capstone to a discipline, the last word (and work) of an over-mature area.

More often, however, books appear in a middle position, somewhere between the beginning and the ending of research in an area. Books of this sort attempt to make explicit or to redirect theoretical and empirical efforts, explaining what the authors do for the benefit of other workers in the field. These workers, in turn, usually have some sense of the growing enterprise, but desire to know more, to understand the limits and tensions, the ways in which the particular theory or new approach fits in or contrasts with more widely accepted approaches.

Although we are not certain that all will agree, we envision this volume as a book of the middle variety – an explication, reexamination, and elaboration of an area that has existed for some time. Granted, a hardy band of developmentally oriented workers has for 20 plus years pursued issues such as similar sequences and structures in retarded individuals, the two-group approach, and motivational–personality functioning in retarded individuals. But these researchers have for the most part remained iconoclastic, and their interest in understanding retarded functioning through the lens of normal development has not been accepted in the field at large. In mental retardation, these developmentally oriented workers have been outnumbered by the various defect or difference theorists, whereas in developmental psychology the focus on normal development has relegated those interested in mental retardation to a peripheral status.

But recently, changes have occurred both inside and outside the field of mental retardation to justify an interest in the developmental approach. Within the mental retardation field itself, a renewed interest in etiology has made it clear that one or another defect will not account for all retarded functioning, and that simple defect theories will always remain inadequate. The inadequacy of defect theories also threatens to diminish the hopes of mental retardation workers that their findings might have a broader impact than in the mental retardation field alone. In essence, one needs to think in terms of different types of mental retardation, and in terms of development within these different etiological groups, to make the link between work with mentally retarded and nonretarded individuals more effective.

At the same time, there are broader currents within psychology at large that are affecting mental retardation work. Specifically, Dante Cicchetti, Michael Rutter, and others have begun examining a host of problems in terms of "developmental psychopathology." This field, although itself very new, attempts to apply developmental principles, theories, findings, and approaches to the study of atypical development. The approach stresses the interplay between typical and atypical development and uses so-called experiments of nature to tell us more about normal processes.

This volume is very much a mental retardation work in the developmental psychopathology line. It endeavors to explain the developmental approach and expand it beyond more conventional notions of sequences and stages. Issues such as homologies and limits in cross-domain relations, biology versus culture in the sequencing of achievements, the differences between micro and macro levels of development, and the nature and impact of the environment all attest to the desire to expand developmental theory among those interested in the developmental approach to mental retardation. Complementary expansions are occurring as well in the mental retardation area, such that more explicit attention must be paid to different etiological groups and how such groups differ one from another. Finally, a cross-fertilization of the developmental and mental retardation literatures allows one to assess which aspects of normal development can be profitably applied to retarded individuals of different etiologies and which constants holding across various etiological groups allow for statements of true developmental findings for all groups, both retarded and nonretarded.

In line with this emphasis on both developmental theory and its application to different etiological groups, the book is divided into two parts. Part 1 discusses the important theoretical issues in development. Beginning with an overview of the developmental approach, chapters in this section discuss the history and practice of differentiating by etiology; similar sequences; similar structures; environmental effects on development; and motivational–personality factors in the functioning of retarded individuals. In every instance, contributors have been encouraged to, in had inspected schools in London as part of the present research project, Dr H. Hollenstein (Deputy Director of the Centre for Research of Economic Activity at the Swiss Federal Institute of Technology in Zürich) who had previously spent a year with us at the National Institute on associated research, Mr R. Bernheim (for many decades, London correspondent of the *Neue Zürischer Zeitung*) and an anonymous referee. Frau Trudi Sprock allowed us to include in Appendix C a translated version of an article by her on the socialisation of pupils in Swiss secondary schools. We are indebted to them all, as to colleagues in our team at the Institute – Geoff Mason, Valerie Jarvis and Julia Whitburn – and to the Institute's Director, Martin Weale, for general advice, encouragement, and detailed improvements. Needless to say, remaining errors of fact or judgement must be blamed solely on the authors.

The Institute is glad to acknowledge the generous financial support for this research provided by the Leverhulme Foundation and by the Gatsby Charitable Foundation.

H.B., S.J.P.
London
April 1996

Contributors

Jacob A. Burack
Department of Psychology
Yale University
New Haven, CT

Dante Cicchetti
Departments of Psychology and
   Psychiatry
University of Rochester
Rochester, NY

Donald J. Cohen
Child Study Center
Yale University
New Haven, CT

Elisabeth Dykens
Child Study Center
Yale University
New Haven, CT

Mark Edison
Department of Psychology
Yale University
New Haven, CT

Jody Ganiban
Department of Psychology
University of Rochester
Rochester, NY

Robert M. Hodapp
Department of Psychology
Yale University
New Haven, CT

Connie Kasari
Department of Psychiatry
University of California at
   Los Angeles
Los Angeles, CA

Claire B. Kopp
Department of Psychology
University of California at
   Los Angeles
Los Angeles, CA

James Leckman
Child Study Center
Yale University
New Haven, CT

Joseph Merighi
Department of Psychology
Yale University
New Haven, CT

Peter Mundy
Department of Psychiatry
University of California at
   Los Angeles
Los Angeles, CA

Susan L. Recchia
Department of Psychology
University of California at
  Los Angeles
Los Angeles, CA

Arnold J. Sameroff
Departments of Psychiatry and
  Human Behavior
Brown University
Providence, RI

Fred R. Volkmar
Child Study Center
Yale University
New Haven, CT

John R. Weisz
Department of Psychology
University of North Carolina
Chapel Hill, NC

Edward Zigler
Department of Psychology
Yale University
New Haven, CT

Part 1

Developmental theory

1 The developmental perspective in the field of mental retardation

Robert M. Hodapp, Jacob A. Burack, and Edward Zigler

The late 20th century is a challenging period for those concerned about development and developmental approaches to pathological populations. On the one hand, influential workers in the field of developmental psychology are questioning the very foundations of the discipline itself (Bronfenbrenner, Kessel, Kessen, & White, 1986). They question whether progressive development (i.e., change that leads to a specified end point) can be documented in any or all domains, and, if so, whether developmental progressions hold across all children in all contexts. Similarly, these workers raise issues about whether achievements are universal or are specific to one culture, and note that many changes that occur during childhood seem regressive in nature (e.g., Bever, 1982). All of these concerns, voiced by major figures in developmental psychology, throw into disarray long-held views about the very nature of human development.

On the other hand, there is a broad movement toward the developmental camp, as many people working with different groups purportedly employ "developmentally based" approaches. In the mental retardation (MR) field, we note the ubiquity of group homes, leisure-activity training, and even behavior-modification programs that are supposedly based on the principles of normal development. The term "development" here implies that the program promotes positive change over time or better adaptation to the environment. Given the imprecision in terminology, it is understandable that those who do not consider themselves to be developmentally oriented (e.g., Switzky, Rotatori, Miller, & Freagon, 1979) decry the use of the term at all. With many workers questioning classical views of development, and others using the term in superficial ways, now is an exciting, albeit confusing, time for developmental theorists and developmental approaches to mental retardation.

It is our contention – and of the book itself – that there is such a phenomenon as development, and that a developmental perspective is a useful way to understand and intervene with retarded individuals. This is

3

not to say that the developmental perspective is unidimensional or that it applies to all areas of change, in all societies, and throughout the life span. On the contrary, our view is that there are universal principles of development from which we can inform work on mentally retarded and otherwise handicapped populations. Such principles pertain to the nature of the organism itself, organismic change, the environment and its effects, and even to methodologies, research paradigms, and ways of thinking about functioning in mentally retarded and nonretarded populations.

Although adherents of the developmental perspective, then, disagree about a variety of issues, they generally agree that normal development can inform work with retarded populations. At the same time, they believe that data from mentally retarded individuals help to provide a fuller understanding of nonretarded development. To quote Cicchetti (1984), "We can learn more about the normal functioning of an organism by studying its pathology, more about its pathology by studying its normal condition" (p. 1). The exploration and application of this reciprocal relationship serves as the basis for the developmental approach to mental retardation.

Classical and expanded developmental theory

Although there is no single developmental approach, all developmental theories share several common themes. These themes set them off from other, nondevelopmental theories and help provide the rationale for different intervention or research strategies. Recent developmental theorists have added to, refined, and extended classical developmental theory into new areas, but these extensions continue to use the basic themes of the classical approach. The discussion that follows details six principles of classical developmental theory; subsequent sections will describe some of the modifications, revisions, and elaborations found in expanded developmental theory.

Principles of classical developmental theory

Active versus passive organism. To developmentally oriented theorists, the organism is considered to be active and involved in dynamic change. This change is self-propelled; it does not occur as a result of external forces, rewards, or contingencies. Langer (1969) has used as his metaphor the "organic lamp," a self-starting, self-continuing being.

Conceptualizing the child as an active organism leads to certain specific approaches toward human behavior and intervention. Children are seen as experimenting with, manipulating, and actively participating in their environments. Developmentally based programs of early childhood education, for example, emphasize the need to structure the environment to foster the child's own internal mechanisms for development. Considering early education programs based on the work of Piaget and Montessori, Elkind (1970) notes that in both theories, "environment provides nourishment for the growth of mental structures just as it does for the growth of physical organs" (p. 107). Programs of early intervention for retarded children, while more directive, still provide opportunities for children to experience and learn from a structured environment. The role of the interventionist is primarily to facilitate developmental achievements by structuring and guiding tendencies the child already possesses; for the most part, the interventionist does not "teach" per se.

In contrast, consider the view of the child in mechanistic theories, of which behaviorism is a good example. In behaviorist theories, the child is conceptualized as a passive organism (Overton & Reese, 1973; Reese & Overton, 1970) whose behavior is the result of contingent reinforcements from the external environment. Judicious application of these external contingencies controls and forces behavior to occur. Even the development of the nonretarded child is seen as resulting from the proper application of contingent reinforcement over time (e.g., Bijou & Baer, 1967). The view throughout behaviorism is that all change is caused by the external environment, not by the child's own intrinsic activity.

These conflicting views of the child also dictate different practices of intervention. According to behaviorists, intervention involves the teaching or instruction of the child from the outside, not the facilitation or even enhancement of already occurring internal schemes. In contrast, developmentally oriented workers suspect that externally imposed reinforcements may even be counterproductive, lessening the child's own internally generated attempts to develop (e.g., Lepper, Greene, & Nisbett, 1973; Seibert & Oller, 1981). To use (and mix) two metaphors, developmentally oriented interventionists see themselves as facilitating the flow and removing barriers from an already moving stream, whereas interventionists who espouse behaviorism are essentially kick-starting an inert motor on a cold day.

Directed change. Intrinsic to all developmental theories is the view that change is directed toward a specifiable end point, as opposed to occurring in a random fashion. Thus the developmentalist's interest in progressive stages, each of which occurs in an invariant order. Piaget's progression from sensorimotor, to preoperational, to concrete, to formal operational thought is an example of such an invariant stage theory, but examples can be found in moral development (Kohlberg, 1969), early language development (Lenneberg, 1967), perspective-taking (Selman, 1976), and in other domains as well. Although more will be discussed in this chapter and in chapter 3 on similar sequences, developmentalists generally hold to the view that development proceeds in an invariant, orderly fashion.

The roots of this belief in invariant sequences come from the original developmental metaphor – the "unfolding" or "unwrapping" implied in the etymology of the very word "development" (from the Old French *developer* or "un" + "wrap-up"). A teleological flavor therefore pervades developmental theories: Piaget's endpoint of "formal operational thought," Kohlberg's "postconventional or autonomous level" of moral reasoning, even Freud's "genital" stage of psychosexual development. In every area, the highest stage is thought to be characterized by more adaptive, more flexible, and more abstract understanding. The higher-level child can perform more and more sophisticated behavior, in more situations, and understands the rationale behind the behavior. Kessen (1984) notes that "In the strong form of the end-point argument, development is measured as a discrepancy from the values of the goal" and "all observations and evidence are gathered with an eye on the horizon that represents finished forms" (p. 5). Whether such a characteristic is harmful (as Kessen believes) to the study of children is unclear, but developmental theories do tend to be teleological in nature.

Again, the developmental view can be most easily contrasted with the behaviorist concept of change. To the behaviorist, there are many roads to travel, not one preferred or mandatory route. Watson's prediction that he could take any child and make him or her into a success in any profession exemplifies this view, but there are other examples as well. Behaviorists either deny or pay lip service to the biological constraints of the organism, including the possibility of invariant sequences of development. In essence, where the behaviorist sees many paths to the attainment of a particular behavior, the developmentalist, examining normal development to glean a sense of how it "unwraps," often sees one or a small number of either preferred or mandatory pathways.

Behavior as evidence of underlying schemes. To developmentally oriented workers, behavior is important mainly because it reflects underlying mental schemes, or concepts. These concepts may manifest themselves in behavior, but they consist of more than the behaviors themselves.

This does not imply that developmentally oriented psychologists are not interested in behavior, only that behavior is examined in an attempt to understand the mind. In the most famous example, Piaget (1952; 1954) continually tested his three children to examine their behavior; his goal, however, was not to see if Jacqueline, Lucienne, or Laurent could uncover an object hidden behind a cloth, or discover their father when he played peek-a-boo. Instead, Piaget used their behavior as evidence of whether his children possessed a certain concept, in this case, object permanence. He and other developmentalists are therefore behavioral psychologists – because they examine behavior – although they are not behaviorists (behavior as behavior is not their concern).

Although seemingly an esoteric point, the developmentalist's understanding of behavior has important implications when conceptualizing functioning or intervening with retarded children. The developmentalist's concern for underlying concepts, for example, gives importance to Kopp and Shaperman's (1973) search for evidence of sensorimotor schemes in children without limbs (or newly introduced to limbs through prostheses). Even if children cannot perform or have little experience with motor activities involved in sensorimotor tasks, their understanding of underlying sensorimotor concepts will eventually permit more advanced and flexible functioning in higher-level tasks (see Kopp & Recchia, chapter 10).

In intervention work as well, the developmentalist's concern for underlying schemes leads to the fostering of behaviors that might seem on the surface to be very different indeed. The early interventionist hoping to foster the concept of object permanence will hide objects under cloths, have the mother loudly and obviously leave the room (going out of the child's sight), and play peek-a-boo with the child. The interventionist will then accept as evidence of object-permanence three very different behaviors: uncovering the object, crying when the mother departs, and laughing when the adult reappears in peek-a-boo. Focusing on behavior alone would not obviously lead to an intervention approach that so clearly fosters the concept of the permanent object by using three such diverse tasks.

Qualitative and quantitative change. The developmentally oriented worker believes in change in children that is both qualitative and quantitative in nature. Each stage theory – be it Piaget's, or Kohlberg's, or Selman's – involves a qualitative restructuring of internal mental schemes at each successive level. Whereas the sensorimotor infant has only action schemes, the preoperational child can represent events in language and other symbol systems. Similarly, the individual with the highest levels of moral reasoning can perform abstract, principled thought on moral problems, just as Selman's high-level children can simultaneously understand both their own and the other's perspective in the interactive setting.

The idea of higher stages that restructure previous schemes, that incorporate but go beyond prior understandings, is a central tenet in developmental thought. Developmentalists conceptualize stage transformations as major events that are akin to Kuhn's (1962) "paradigm shifts" in the history of science. The world is never again the same once the child is able to think symbolically, perform formal operational thought, or apply principles of justice to moral problems. Even if some of these stage transformations have been challenged in developmental work, the idea of qualitative – even revolutionary – changes across development remains.

This is not to say that developmentalists fail to appreciate quantitative change, or that quantitative and qualitative change are not both important. From the earliest years of the study of children, workers were preoccupied with documenting such quantitative achievements as the increasing size of the child's spoken vocabulary at various ages (McCarthy, 1954), or what the child at each of several ages can do in any number of areas (Gesell, 1934). Relationships between qualitative and quantitative changes have also received attention (Wohlwill, 1973). But whereas the behaviorist sees change as predominantly quantitative, the developmentalist, while acknowledging quantitative changes in children, is most fascinated by those qualitative shifts that seem to mark new understandings in any number of areas.

The role of time. Related to the issue of qualitative versus quantitative change is the common misconception that development equals time, that once one knows how old the child is, one knows those particular behaviors that the child is able to perform. Such views were first made popular by maturationists such as Gesell (1934), and are held even today.

Although there is a complicated relationship between a child's level of development and its chronological age, most modern developmentalists would agree that development is not a synonym for the amount of time the child has lived. Granted, greater chronological age is usually associated with higher-level abilities in many areas, but time and development are not synonymous (Wohlwill, 1973; Zigler, 1963). Instead, it is the experiences that occur over time – and their incorporation into the child's schemes – that are important for development. In chapter 5, Sameroff elaborates on the nature and uses of ongoing transactions between the organism and the environment; suffice it to say here that time does not equal development, that the nature and effects of what happens over time are more important for the acquisition of higher-level skills than the passage of time per se.

Orthogenetic principle. A final principle of classical developmental theories is the implicit or explicit adherence to the orthogenetic principle.

As defined by Werner (1948; 1957), the orthogenetic principle states that development "proceeds from a state of relative globality and lack of differentiation to a state of increasing differentiation, articulation, and hierarchic integration" (Werner, 1957, p. 126).

This emphasis on differentiation and integration at higher levels arises from the original developmental metaphor, and can be seen in many domains. Thus, the original focus on development of the embryo – the progression from a state in which all cells are similar to one in which cells are differentiated in both structure and function – has been transferred from biological to psychological development. Children's increasing ability to distinguish between means and ends (and coordinate the two) in sensorimotor development, to move from uttering single-word sentences to organized multiword utterances in communicative development, and to distinguish and coordinate ideas of self and other in social development – all are examples of the process of differentiation and reintegration at a higher level. Although the orthogenetic principle, like any "world view" (Pepper, 1942) or "frame of reference" (Zigler, 1963), is not falsifiable, it is noteworthy how often and in how many domains this model has proven to be a useful way to conceptualize development in children.

Extending and expanding classical developmental theory

The six principles just described apply to what has been termed "classical developmental theory." This approach was originated by workers such as Piaget and Werner and remains the general orientation followed by most developmentally oriented workers. Some of these principles – active organism, behavior reflecting underlying structures, the distinction between time and development, and qualitative change – have become so accepted as to be almost second nature to developmentalists. Other principles – end points, orthogenetics – are more controversial, although they too are generally accepted.

But while the tenets of classical developmental theory continue to provide general guides to those studying children's development, there is a growing feeling that these principles are not all-inclusive, that there needs to be an extension of the classical model. This extension has characterized much work in the 1970s and 1980s, and can be clustered around four areas – the environment, noncognitive changes, individual differences, and the interplay between biology and the environment.

Considering the environment first, we note that classical developmental theory pays little attention to the child's environment. Werner (1948) wrote of the organism's *Umwelt*, or the environment in the organism's terms (e.g., smell to a dog), but did not elaborate on the concept.

Similarly, Piaget (1977) occasionally noted the child's environment, but usually confined himself to the object world and its use as "aliment" to the child's developing schemes. Even when focusing on the interpersonal environment, his emphasis was on the child, because "there can be no effect of social or linguistic experience unless the child is ready to assimilate and integrate this experience into his own structures" (Piaget, 1977, p. 9). For both Werner and Piaget, the exact nature and effects of the environment – especially the interpersonal environment – remain unexplored.

The first extension of the classical model, then, involves greater specification of what can be called the length, breadth, and nature of the environment. In terms of length, Sameroff (1975; Sameroff & Chandler, 1975) has proposed that children and their parents engage in a series of continuing transactions over time. To quote Sameroff:

> If developmental processes are to be understood, it will not be through continuous assessment of the child alone, but through a continuous assessment of the transactions between the child and his environment to determine how these transactions facilitate or hinder adaptive integration as both the child and his surroundings change and evolve. (1975, p. 283)

Children thus develop within an interpersonal environment that is itself changing, thereby providing a developing environment to the developing child (see chapter 5).

Another aspect of the environment concerns its breadth – the extensiveness of the (interpersonal) environment. Children live in a world populated by parents, siblings, friends, schools, and houses of worship; they are therefore influenced by individuals other than their mothers (as often assumed by earlier environmentally oriented theorists). In this light, we note the recent inclusion of family systems theory (Kaye & Furstenburg, 1985; Minuchin, 1985) into developmental work, and its understanding that children are developing within a family system, of which they themselves are but one part. Bronfenbrenner (1979) has further expanded this idea to include the multiple effects of various systems, some of which directly influence the child (e.g., family itself, individual family members, friends), others of which indirectly affect the child (e.g., the economic system, which affects parental employment opportunities). In short, there is a breadth to the child's interpersonal environment at any one time, and this breadth affects children's development.

But what exactly *is* the environment, and what is the nature of its influences? There is no simple answer to this question, as we continue to have no agreed-upon theory of the environment (Kessen, 1968). At the very least, however, the environment consists of the object world with which the child experiments (in a Piagetian sense), and an interpersonal world of mothers, fathers, siblings, and others. This interpersonal world has received attention in the past several decades, in particular in the areas of mother–infant interaction (Hodapp & Mueller, 1982; Lewis & Rosenblum, 1974; Tronick, 1982) and in input language from adults to children (Phillips, 1973; Snow, 1972). In these and other domains, the interpersonal environment is thought to guide development by providing contextual support, easier-to-assimilate language, and other stimulation that is appropriate to the child's developmental level. This emphasis on the adult as aiding development mirrors Vygotsky's ideas on adult mediation of the child's development (Vygotsky, 1978; Wertsch, 1985) and can be seen in a variety of situations. More importantly, adult mediation is thought to foster children's own internal developmental processes; both "other" and "self" regulation may be occurring simultaneously (Hodapp & Goldfield, 1985; Kaye, 1982).

A second area in which classical developmental theory has been expanded involves extracognitive factors. Historically, developmental theory has concerned itself primarily with the development of abilities related to cognition or to tasks in which there is a major cognitive component – thus, Piaget's interest in cognitive development, Kohlberg's in moral reasoning, Selman's in interpersonal understandings. Some have gone so far as to call classical theory "cognitive developmental theory" (Kohlberg, 1969; Zigler, Lamb, & Child, 1982), although some developmentalists (e.g., Werner, 1948; Werner & Kaplan, 1963) have addressed noncognitive areas. Still, for the most part, developmental theory has featured a heavy emphasis on children's development of thought.

Recent work has added noncognitive areas to child development, expanding our view of children and the important areas of children's functioning. The work of Zigler (1971; see also Merighi, Edison, & Zigler, chapter 6) and others has shown that a complete understanding of children and their development includes some appreciation of children's changing self-concept, and of the degree to which children solve problems on their own or look to others for solutions (outerdirectedness) and are dependent on – or wary of – surrounding adults (positive- and negative-reaction tendencies). The entire idea of social adaptation – of how one succeeds socially in the world – might also be considered among the extracognitive domains of child development (Doll, 1953; Sparrow, Balla, & Cicchetti, 1984). In short, children are more than thinking organisms, and a complete understanding of the child must not be limited to examinations of cognitive or linguistic development.

A third extension of classical developmental theory involves the study of individual differences. Earlier theorists such as Piaget were little interested in how one child differs from another; indeed, Kessen (1962) has noted that "Piaget has little interest in individual variation among children in the rate at which they achieve a stage ...; he is a student of the development of thinking more than he is a student of children" (p. 77). Although the usual modal patterns of development continue to interest developmentally oriented workers, the issue of individual differences and individual styles of development is increasingly being studied in nonretarded children. As the various chapters in this book show, workers interested in the development of mentally retarded children have also become fascinated by the nature and causes of individual differences.

A final extension of classical developmental theory involves the interplay between biological and environmental factors, the so-called biology–culture question. In all children there is an interplay between the biological organism and the surrounding environment. But the degree to which biological and environmental factors affect functioning differs at different periods of the child's life, and may be specific for different domains. McCall (1981; also Scarr-Salapatek, 1975) has shown, for example, that genetic and environmental factors differentially influence variation in children's IQ at different ages. When development in mentally retarded individuals is examined, the relationship between biological and environmental factors becomes particularly important, as retarded children are delayed compared with nonretarded children. At the same time, even within the mentally retarded population, different etiological groups may perform differently because of syndrome-specific differences in genetic, neurological, and/or biochemical properties. For both retarded and nonretarded children, different learning environments, different parental expectations, even different cultural values and practices will then influence aspects of both the child's biology and behavior, which will in turn affect how individuals in the environment respond, and so on. Some domains (e.g., those that are more social or culturally based) may be very open to environmental influences, whereas others (e.g., motor development and physical changes such as puberty) seem much more maturationally determined. More and more, developmentalists are becoming aware of this complicated, dynamic interplay between the child's biology and the child's environment.

Combined with the six tenets of classical developmental theory, recent emphases on the environment, noncognitive determinants of behavior, individual differences, and the ongoing interaction between biology and the environment help to round out developmental theory. Each of these ideas, in one guise or another, will be dealt with in this volume. We now move to a preliminary discussion of mental retardation and the application of developmental models to the retarded population.

Applying the developmental perspective to mental retardation

The two-group approach

Before discussing the uses of the developmental approach within the field of mental retardation, it is first necessary to provide some historical background. Indeed, developmental approaches have had a checkered history with regard to studying and understanding the functioning of retarded individuals, and there are at least three schools of thought on the subject. In the first, "defect" or "difference" theorists argue that mentally retarded persons are qualitatively different from nonretarded persons. All retarded persons are thought to suffer from one or several specific defects that are biological and/or cognitive in nature; retarded individuals cannot therefore be studied within more traditional developmental perspectives (e.g., Ellis, 1963; Ellis & Cavalier, 1982; Spitz, 1963, 1979; Zeaman & House, 1963, 1979). In the second school, "conservative" developmental psychologists show that traditional developmental approaches apply to familial, or nonorganically, retarded persons, but not to those mentally retarded persons with organic insult (Zigler, 1967, 1969; Zigler & Balla, 1982). In the third school, "liberal" developmental psychologists argue that developmental approaches can be applied to individuals with organic etiologies as well as to nonorganically retarded persons (Cicchetti & Pogge-Hesse, 1982).

The disagreement among advocates of each of the three schools essentially reduces to a debate over the necessity and consequences of differentiating among retarded individuals on the basis of etiology. Difference or defect theorists generally take an undifferentiated approach to mental retardation: Mentally retarded persons are thought to comprise a homogeneous population with regard to behavioral functioning, and can be studied as a single group that differs only in its level of functioning. In contrast, developmental theorists (both conservative and liberal) have traditionally been concerned with etiological differences within this population. They have distinguished between two groups of retarded individuals: familial, or nonorganically, retarded, and organically retarded individuals. The first group consists of persons with no known organic etiology. Their IQs are generally in the mild range of retardation, and they are usually indistinguishable from persons whose IQs fall within the low–normal range with regard to appearance, socioeconomic background, and education. The second group consists of those whose retardation involves some type of recognizable organic damage. Organic mental retardation may be a consequence of a dominant gene (e.g., epiloia), a single recessive gene (PKU), chromosomal abnormalities (Down syndrome, fragile X syndrome), or infections (encephalitis; rubella in the mother), toxic agents (intrauterine radiation; lead poisoning), cerebral trauma, or other agents that may cause brain damage (Zigler & Cascione, 1984). Persons with organic retardation often appear much different than their nonretarded peers, and have IQs that are typically below 50. Thus, whereas defect theorists see all retarded persons as suffering from organic damage, developmentalists distinguish familial and organic retardation as the two basic groups of retarded individuals.

At this point, workers within the developmental camp can themselves be distinguished. Conservative proponents of the developmental approach have historically focused on familial retarded persons, emphasizing the similarities between familial retarded and nonretarded individuals (Zigler, 1967; 1969). Familial retarded individuals are viewed as normal in that they possess the same basic cognitive equipment as persons with higher IQs. They differ from the normal population only in their rate of development and, ultimately, in the highest levels attained. Thus, the same principles of cognitive development that apply throughout the normal ranges of intelligence should also describe familial retarded persons.

In emphasizing the similarities of nonorganically retarded individuals to nonretarded persons, conservative developmentalists also note the differences between organically retarded individuals and nonorganically retarded (and nonretarded) persons, especially with regard to development. For example, Zigler (1969) noted that "if the etiology of the phenotypic intelligence (as measured by IQ) of two groups differs, it is far from logical to assert that the course of development is the same, or that even similar contents in their behaviors are mediated by exactly the same processes" (p. 533). In fact, differences between the two groups of retarded persons have been found on intelligence profiles (Beck & Lam, 1955); on levels of performance across different Piagetian (for a review, see Weisz and Yeates, 1981), moral, and cognitive reasoning tasks (Kahn, 1985); and on socioeconomic and familial backgrounds (Broman, Nichols, Shaughnessy, & Kennedy, 1987). Thus, conservative developmentalists have emphasized the behavioral consequences of different etiologies, noting that the developmental approach might not apply to those individuals who are organically retarded.

In contrast, liberal developmentalists, while acknowledging differences between the two retarded groups, have countered that developmental approaches can also be applied to organically retarded persons. They argue that all organisms, even if biologically damaged, demonstrate certain principles that guide their growth and maturation. For example, Cicchetti and Pogge-Hesse (1982) assert that systems in organically retarded persons are similar enough to those of persons without organic insult that certain developmental properties will be consistent across both groups. In examining these principles of developmental organization across groups, researchers such as Cicchetti (Cicchetti & Pogge-Hesse, 1982; Cicchetti & Sroufe, 1976) and Kopp (1983) have extended the two-group approach by studying specific etiological groups such as Down syndrome. In so doing, they have been able to provide a more precise understanding of the manner in which development is affected by specific defects. The value of differentiating among specific etiological groups is discussed further by Burack in chapter 2.

Among developmental approaches, then, there are two schools of thought. Proponents of the conservative school feel that only familial retarded individuals develop as do nonretarded children; liberal develop-mentalists feel that both organically and familial retarded individuals can be included within a developmental perspective. The discussion that follows, then, will examine both the hypotheses derived from the developmental perspective, and whether such predictions hold true for familial retarded persons only or for both familial and organically retarded persons.

The similar-sequence hypothesis

In considering development in retarded individuals, one must first examine the sequences through which development occurs. A basic tenet of developmental thought is that there are regular and invariant sequences of development, all leading to a clear end point. Within a given sequence, there are several stages, each of which is based on a preceding stage and in turn lays the groundwork for subsequent stages. This ordering of stages within a given domain of functioning is thought to apply to all individuals regardless of cultural, intellectual, or neurological characteristics (e.g., Kohlberg, 1969; Piaget, 1956). In summarizing this view, Zigler (1963) refers to the "orderliness, sequentiality, and apparent lawfulness of the transition taking place from birth to the attainment of maturity" (p. 344). This position is probably best exemplified in Piagetian theory, in which it is hypothesized that the child traverses cognitive stages in invariant order, beginning with sensorimotor modes of thinking and ending with the acquisition of formal operational thought.

The strongest evidence for universal sequences of development has been observed in the study of skills attained early in life. Many researchers have suggested that the development of early behaviors is biologically determined. For example, in her discussion of the development of sensorimotor behaviors such as social smiling, laughter, and play, Kopp (1983) notes that "these sensorimotor behaviors have a firm biological basis that reflects strong evolutionary pressures and are distorted only in the wake of profound organic damage" (p. 1119). These behaviors are therefore thought to occur in invariant order in all children, even those with organic impairments.

In formulating the developmental framework for the study of familial mental retardation, Zigler (1969) argued that mentally retarded individuals proceed through the various stages of development in much the same manner as do nonretarded individuals. This position was clearly supported by Weisz and Zigler's review (1979; Weisz, Yeates, & Zigler, 1982) of 3 longitudinal and 28 cross-sectional studies. Such support for universal sequences of development occurred for both familial retarded persons (the conservative developmental approach) and for mentally retarded persons who showed evidence of organic impairment (the liberal developmental approach). The only possible exception to the finding of similar sequences of development for all retarded children – those with and without organic impairment – occurred with children who showed pronounced EEG abnormalities, especially dysrhythmias or a history of seizures (Wohlhueter & Sindberg, 1975).

Evidence for the similar-sequence hypothesis within both familial and organic mentally retarded individuals has been found consistently across domains of functioning. Such evidence has been reported in studies of sensorimotor stages, many types of conservation, seriation, transitivity, moral reasoning, comparison processes, time, space, relative thinking, role-taking, classification, class inclusion, and geometry (see Weisz & Zigler, 1979; Weisz, Yeates, & Zigler, 1982). Further discussion of the similar-sequence approach and its role within developmental theory will be provided by Hodapp in chapter 3.

Similar-structure hypothesis

The second hypothesis of the developmental approach involves what have been called similar structures of development. Retarded children, when matched on overall measures of cognitive functioning such as mental age (MA, first used by Kounin, 1941), are predicted to perform at similar levels on tasks in a second domain.

In the original, conservative version of the developmental approach,

Zigler (1967; 1969) predicted that only familial retarded children would show similar structures of intelligence compared with groups of non-retarded, MA-matched children. As in nonretarded children, MA should provide a general guide to performance on other cognitive–linguistic tasks. Conversely, organically retarded children, who did suffer from one or another set of organic defects, were predicted to demonstrate lowered performance compared with MA-matched nonretarded children.

Although this issue is covered in more detail by Mundy and Kasari in chapter 4 and Weisz in chapter 7, we note here that groups of familial retarded children have been shown to perform similarly to MA-matched nonretarded children on a host of Piagetian tasks. Reviewing studies using a wide variety of Piagetian tasks, Weisz and Zigler (1979) found that for the large majority of these comparisons (35 of 39), familial mentally retarded and MA-matched nonretarded children performed at identical levels. In contrast, on tasks involving such information-processing skills as attention, retrieval, and memory, Weiss, Weisz, and Bromfield (1986) found that familial retarded children often performed at lower levels than did MA-matched nonretarded children. Thus, it appears that familial retarded children may be deficient on information-processing tasks but not on Piagetian tasks, but more work is needed in this area.

If the issue of similar structures of intelligence is unclear in the familial group, it seems apparent that organically retarded children do not show similar structures. Unlike groups of nonretarded and familial retarded individuals, organically retarded children often perform lower on Piagetian tasks compared with MA-matched groups of nonretarded children (Weisz & Zigler, 1979). Thus, whereas the similar-structure hypothesis seems to hold true for nonorganically retarded children – at least for Piagetian tasks (evidence is less clear about information processing tasks) – organically retarded groups definitely show deficient performance compared with their nonretarded, MA-matched peers.

The issue of cross-domain relationships

Related to the concept of similar structures is the larger issue of the organization of development across domains for any individual child. In stage theories such as Piaget's, all areas of cognitive development are thought to occur at similar levels in any one child. The child able to perform at a certain substage within a major stage (e.g., at sensorimotor stage IV) will be at the same stage in all sensorimotor tasks. This child will be able to uncover an object hidden behind one screen (level IV of object permanence), imitate familiar words (level IV of vocal imitation; Dunst,

1980), and perform at sensorimotor level IV on other sensorimotor tasks as well. The child will be "even" in development across different domains.

As in the case of classical developmental theory, new research and thinking have led to several modifications of the classical stage model. Specifically, examinations of nonretarded children have led to the realization that development may not be even across domains for many individual children. From one domain to another, each child demonstrates his or her own idiosyncratic strengths and weaknesses. To continue our earlier example, any one child might be at a particular level in object permanence but at another level in imitation, means–ends, or causality. The finding of uneven development for any one child seems to hold true for nonretarded children (Flavell, 1982) as well as for retarded children (Curcio & Houlihan, 1987). Thus, although different *groups* of children may be even across domains, *individuals* show varying patterns of strengths and weaknesses. This position is probably best summed up in Fischer's dictum (1980) that "unevenness is the rule of development."

A first solution to the problem of even versus uneven development involves what have been called "local homologies through shared origins" (Bates, Benigni, Bretherton, Camaioni, & Volterra, 1979; Mundy, Seibert, & Hogan, 1984). Local homologies refers to individual behaviors that are manifestations of a single underlying scheme. Thus, uncovering a hidden object in the object permanence scale of the Ordinal Scales of Infant Development (Uzgiris & Hunt, 1975), crying when mother leaves the room, and uncovering the mother and laughing during peek-a-boo all seem to indicate that the child is developing a concept of the permanent object. Similarly, the ability to use one object as a means to retrieve another (e.g., using a stick as a rake) is similar to using a person as a means to attain goals that are either social (e.g., adult attention) or nonsocial (e.g., desired object) (Bates, Camaioni, & Volterra, 1975). In both examples, a single underlying concept seems to be manifested by very different behaviors; individual children should therefore be able to perform each of the behaviors that reflect the underlying concept.

The idea of local homologies is shown graphically for Down syndrome children in Figure 1.1 (from Hodapp & Zigler, in press). Down syndrome children have particular difficulties with linguistic tasks (Gibson, 1978), several of which might constitute homology C. Behaviors that reflect each homology constitute small (i.e., "local") areas of organization, even within a picture of disorganized development across the three domains.

One should not, however, overemphasize the lack of identical-level functioning across different domains. Granted, Sachs (1987), Gardner (1983), and others have identified so-called idiot savant individuals – those

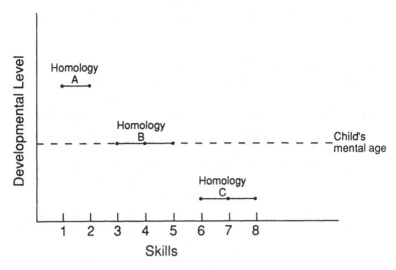

Figure 1.1. Local homologies. From Hodapp & Zigler, in press.

who seem to have particular, high-level skills in some areas while being deficient in all other domains – but this phenomenon is exceedingly rare. For the most part, even children with particular etiologies of retardation (e.g., Down syndrome, Cicchetti & Ganiban, chapter 8; fragile X syndrome, Dykens & Leckman, chapter 9) do not show high-level abilities in some areas and very low-level abilities in others.

Furthermore, the extent to which behaviors in two areas can differ seems constricted by both organismic and intertask relationships. Cicchetti and Pogge-Hesse (1982) emphasize the first of these relationships, the various intraorganismic factors limiting discrepancies among domains. Employing systems concepts of Bertalannfy (1968), they note that parts of systems (e.g., domains) work together and that systems have feedback mechanisms whereby one system "knows" what the other is doing. These systems' features ensure that while different domains might be more or less advanced compared with other domains, there is a limit to interdomain variation. Similarly, Bates et al. (1979) note that some skills serve as prerequisite skills for later behaviors, again constraining the amount of interdomain differences. Higher-level adaptive behavior, for example, seems to be dependent on certain levels of linguistic ability. These relationships between tasks in different domains, like intraorganismic relationships, serve to limit the size of differences between performance levels in any two domains. This issue will be discussed further in relation to various etiological groups in chapter 12 (Hodapp, Burack, & Zigler).

Benefits of using the developmental approach in intervention with retarded individuals

Our discussion so far has highlighted ways in which the functioning of retarded individuals fits within the developmental formulation. Yet similar sequences, structures, homologies, and prerequisites are not simply theoretical issues, devoid of practical application. Indeed, developmental knowledge is essential in intervention with retarded individuals. For example, the finding that similar sequences of development hold across all types of retarded individuals is particularly helpful in forming curricula of intervention in many areas. If retarded children proceed in the same order of development in a particular domain as do nonretarded children, the best interventions should be those that take advantage of such "natural orderings."

In the same way, knowledge of the relationships between different domains is useful in intervention work. Prerequisite skills in one area have to be developed before the child can acquire later achievements that are dependent on such skills, and information about local homologies can help identify likely targets of intervention across seemingly disparate domains. In terms of both similar structures and similar sequences, knowledge from nonretarded development can be profitably employed to help intervention efforts with many types of retarded individuals.

Furthermore, intervention efforts for several different etiological groups might be aided by an understanding of the particular profile of abilities of each. Different types of information-processing skills are differentially affected in fragile X syndrome (Dykens, Hodapp, & Leckman, 1987), whereas linguistic and social skills show different degrees of impairment in children with Down syndrome (Cicchetti & Beeghly, in press; Gibson, 1978) compared with autism (Paul, 1987; Volkmar, 1987; Volkmar, Burack, & Cohen, chapter 10). Thus, in addition to gaining useful information about retarded functioning in general, developmental approaches help to focus attention on the particular profiles of abilities in different etiological groups.

Other information from developmental research can also be used in intervention work. Findings from mother–infant interaction have helped identify the content and style of interaction thought best for children at different levels of development in different domains. Interactions between mothers and their retarded children can then be examined to determine if – and with what consequences – interactions differ from those expected from the child's overall levels of ability (Marfo, 1984; Rondal, 1977). Similarly, family systems approaches originally designed for families of nonretarded children have recently been applied to the families of retarded children (Crnic, Friedrich, & Greenberg, 1983; Gallagher, Beckman, & Cross, 1983). Such applications show the ways in which expanded developmental approaches have recently been used in intervention work.

But in line with Cicchetti's dictum, the relationship between nonretarded and retarded development is not unidirectional; indeed, we learn more about normal development through our work in mental retardation. Examinations of retarded and otherwise disabled groups provide rigorous tests of issues such as the presence of universal sequences of development and of unified stages of development across domains. As a result, we are now more confident in designating as universal only certain sequences in certain domains, with other sequences more culturally determined. Concerning the similar-structure hypothesis, research on retarded populations makes clear which behaviors must go together, in contrast to those that may but need not be linked in development.

There is, then, considerable wisdom to the idea of learning about nonretarded development from retarded individuals and learning more about retarded individuals from normal development. This crossing of perspectives from both retarded and nonretarded populations also provides insights into the nature of the environment, the causes of change throughout childhood, and how certain developmental disabilities disrupt both intraorganismic and external systems. These ideas, only touched upon in this chapter, will receive detailed attention throughout this book, as the contributors attempt to further delineate the developmental approach to mental retardation.

References

Bates, E., Benigni, L., Bretherton, I., Camaioni, I., & Volterra, V. (1979). *The emergence of symbols: Cognition and communication in infancy.* New York: Academic Press.

Bates, E., Camaioni, L., & Volterra, V. (1975). The acquisition of performatives prior to speech. *Merrill-Palmer Quarterly, 21*, 205–226.

Beck, H., & Lam, R. (1955). Use of the WISC in predicting organicity. *Journal of Clinical Psychology, 11*, 154–158.

Bertalannfy, L. von (1968). *General systems theory.* New York: Braziller.

Bever, T.G. (Ed.) (1982). *Regression in mental development: Basic phenomena and theories.* Hillsdale, NJ: Erlbaum Associates, Inc.

Bijou, S., & Baer, D. (1967). *Child development: Readings in experimental analysis.* New York: Appleton-Century-Crofts.

Broman, S., Nichols, P., Shaughnessy, P., & Kennedy, W. (1987). *Retardation in young children: A developmental study of cognitive deficit.* Hillsdale, NJ: Erlbaum.

Bronfenbrenner, U. (1979). *The ecology of human development.* Cambridge, MA: Harvard University Press.

Bronfenbrenner, U., Kessel, F., Kessen, W., & White, S. (1986). Toward a critical social history of developmental psychology: A propadeutic discussion. *American Psychologist*, *41*, 1218–1230.

Burack, J.A. (this volume). Differentiating mental retardation: The two-group approach and beyond. Chapter 2.

Cicchetti, D. (1984). The emergence of developmental psychopathology. *Child Development*, *55*, 1–7.

Cicchetti, D., & Beeghly, M. (Eds.) (in press). *Children with Down syndrome: A developmental perspective*. New York: Cambridge University Press.

Cicchetti, D., & Ganiban, J. (this volume). The organization and coherence of developmental processes in infants and children with Down syndrome. Chapter 8.

Cicchetti, D., & Pogge-Hesse, P. (1982). Possible contributions of the study of organically retarded persons to developmental theory. In E. Zigler & D. Balla (Eds.), *Mental retardation: The developmental–difference controversy*. Hillsdale, NJ: Erlbaum.

Cicchetti, D., & Sroufe, L.A. (1976). The relationship between affective and cognitive development in Down syndrome children. *Child Development*, *47*: 920–929.

Crnic, K., Friedrich, W., & Greenberg, M. (1983). Adaptation of families with mentally retarded children: A model of stress, coping, and family ecology. *American Journal of Mental Deficiency*, *88*, 125–138.

Curcio, F., & Houlihan, J. (1987). Varieties of organization between domains of sensorimotor intelligence in normal and atypical populations. In I. Uzgiris & J. Mc.V. Hunt (Eds.), *Infant performance and experience: New findings with the Ordinal Scales*. Urbana, IL: University of Illinois Press.

Doll, E.A. (1953). *Measurement of social competence*. Circle Pines, MN: American Guidance Service.

Dunst, C.J. (1980). *A clinical and educational manual for use with the Uzgiris and Hunt Scales of Infant Psychological Development*. Austin, TX: Pro-Ed Press.

Dykens, E.M., Hodapp, R.M., & Leckman, J.F. (1987). Strengths and weaknesses in the intellectual functioning of males with fragile X syndrome. *American Journal of Mental Deficiency*, *92*, 234–236.

Dykens, E.M., & Leckman, J.F. (this volume). Developmental issues in fragile X syndrome. Chapter 9.

Elkind, D. (1970). Piaget and Montessori. In D. Elkind, *Children and adolescents: Interpretive essays on Jean Piaget* (pp. 104–114). New York: Oxford University Press. (Originally published in the *Harvard Educational Review*, 1967, *37*, 535–545.)

Ellis, N.R. (1963). The stimulus trace and behavioral inadequacy. In N.R. Ellis (Ed.), *Handbook of mental deficiency*. New York: McGraw-Hill.

Ellis, N.R., & Cavalier, A.R. (1982). Research perspectives in mental retardation. In E. Zigler & D. Balla (Eds.), *Mental retardation: The developmental–difference controversy*. Hillsdale, NJ: Erlbaum.

Fischer, K. (1980). A theory of cognitive development: The control and construction of a hierarchy of skills. *Psychological Review*, *87*, 477–531.

Flavell, J. (1982). Structures, stages, and sequences in cognitive development. In W.A. Collins (Ed.), *The concept of development: The Minnesota symposia on child psychology*. Vol. 15. Hillsdale, NJ: Erlbaum.

Gallagher, J., Beckman, P., & Cross, A. (1983). Families of handicapped children: Sources of stress and its amelioration. *Exceptional Children*, *50*, 1–19.

Gardner, H. (1983). *Frames of mind: The theory of multiple intelligences*. New York: Basic Books.

Gesell, A. (1934). *Infant behavior: Its genesis and growth*. New York: McGraw-Hill.

Gibson, D. (1978). *Down's Syndrome: The psychology of mongolism*. Cambridge, England: Cambridge University Press.

Hodapp, R.M. (this volume). One road or many? Issues in the similar-sequence hypothesis. Chapter 3.

Hodapp, R.M., Burack, J.A., & Zigler, E. (this volume). Summing up and going forward: New directions in the developmental approach to mental retardation. Chapter 12.

Hodapp, R.M., & Goldfield, E.C. (1985). Self and other regulation in the infancy period. *Development Review, 5,* 274–288.

Hodapp, R.M., & Mueller, E. (1982). Early social development. In B. Wolman (Ed.), *Handbook of developmental psychology.* Englewood Cliffs, NJ: Prentice-Hall.

Hodapp, R.M., & Zigler, E. (in press). Applying the developmental perspective to individuals with Down syndrome. In D. Cicchetti & M. Beeghly (Eds.), *Children with Down syndrome: A developmental perspective.* New York: Cambridge University Press.

Kahn, J.V. (1985). Evidence of the similar structure hypothesis controlling for organicity. *American Journal of Mental Deficiency, 89,* 372–378.

Kaye, K. (1982). *The mental and social life of babies.* Chicago: University of Chicago Press.

Kaye, K., & Furstenburg, F. (Eds.). (1985). Family development and the child [Special issue]. *Child Development, 56*(2).

Kessen, W. (1962). Stage and structure in the study of young children. In W. Kessen & C. Kuhlman (Eds.), *Thought in the young child. Monographs of the Society for Research in Child Development, 27,* 53–70.

Kessen, W. (1968). The construction and selection of environments: Discussion of Richard H. Walter's paper on social isolation and social interaction. In D.C. Glass (Ed.), *Environmental influences.* New York: Rockefeller University Press and Russell Sage Foundation.

Kessen, W. (1984). Introduction: The end of the age of development. In R. Sternberg (Ed.), *Mechanisms of cognitive development.* New York: Freeman.

Kohlberg, L. (1969). Stage and sequence: The cognitive–developmental approach to socialization. In D. Goslin (Ed.), *Handbook of socialization theory and research.* Chicago: Rand McNally.

Kopp, C. (1983). Risk factors in development. In P. Mussen (Ed.), *Handbook of Child Psychology,* Vol. 2, *Infancy and Developmental Psychobiology.* New York: Wiley.

Kopp, C., & Recchia, S.L. (this volume). The issue of multiple pathways in the development of handicapped children. Chapter 11.

Kopp, C., & Shaperman, J. (1973). Cognitive development in the absence of object manipulation during infancy. *Developmental Psychology, 9,* 430.

Kounin, J. (1941). Experimental studies of rigidity: I. The measurement of rigidity and feeblemindedness. *Character and Personality, 9,* 251–272.

Kuhn, T. (1962). *The structure of a scientific revolution.* Chicago: University of Chicago Press.

Langer, J. (1969). *Theories of development.* New York: Holt, Rinehart & Winston.

Lenneberg, E. (1967). *Biological foundations of language.* New York: Wiley.

Lepper, M., Greene, D., & Nisbett, R. (1973). Test of the "overjustification hypothesis." *Journal of Personality and Social Psychology, 28,* 129–137.

Lewis, M., & Rosenblum, L.A. (Eds.). (1974). *The effect of the infant on its caregiver.* New York: Wiley.

Marfo, K. (1984). Interactions between mothers and their mentally retarded children: Integration of research findings. *Journal of Applied Developmental Psychology, 5,* 45–69.

McCall, R.B. (1981). Nature–nurture and the two realms of development: A proposed integration with respect to mental development. *Child Development, 52,* 1–12.

McCarthy, D. (1954). Language development. In L. Carmichael (Ed.), *Manual of child psychology* (2nd ed.). New York: Wiley.

Merighi, J., Edison, M., & Zigler, E. (this volume). The role of motivational factors in the functioning of retarded individuals. Chapter 6.

Minuchin, P. (1985). Families and individual development: Provocations from the field of family therapy. *Child Development, 56*, 289–302.

Mundy, P., & Kasari, C. (this volume). The similar-structure hypothesis and differential rate of development in mental retardation. Chapter 4.

Mundy, P., Seibert, J., & Hogan, A. (1984). Relationship between sensorimotor and early communication abilities in developmentally delayed children. *Merrill-Palmer Quarterly, 30*, 33–48.

Overton, W., & Reese, H. (1973). Models of development: Methodological implications. In J. Nesselroad & H. Reese (Eds.), *Life span developmental psychology*. New York: Academic Press.

Paul, R. (1987). Communication. In D. Cohen & A. Donnellan (Eds.), *Handbook of autism and pervasive developmental disorders*. New York: Wiley.

Pepper, S. (1942). *World hypotheses*. Berkeley, CA: University of California Press.

Phillips, J. (1973). Syntax and vocabulary of mothers' speech to young children: Age and sex comparisons. *Child Development, 44*, 182–185.

Piaget, J. (1952). *Origins of intelligence in children*. New York: International Universities Press.

Piaget, J. (1954). *The construction of reality in the child*. New York: Ballantine.

Piaget, J. (1956). The general problem of the psychobiological development of the child. *Discussions on Child Development, 4*, 3–27.

Piaget, J. (1977). Problems of equilibration. In M.S. Appel & L.S. Goldberg (Eds.), *Topics in cognitive development*. Vol. 1. New York: Plenum.

Reese, H., & Overton, W. (1970). Models of development and theories of development. In L.R. Goulet & P. Baltes (Eds.), *Life span developmental psychology: Research and theory*. New York: Academic Press.

Rondal, J. (1977). Maternal speech to normal and Down syndrome children. In P. Mittler (Ed.), *Research to practice in mental retardation*. Vol. 2. Baltimore: University Park Press.

Sachs, O. (1987). *The man who mistook his wife for a hat*. New York: Harper & Row.

Sameroff, A. (1975). Early influences on development: Fact or fancy? *Merrill-Palmer Quarterly, 21*, 267–294.

Sameroff, A. (this volume). Neo-environmental perspectives in developmental theory. Chapter 5.

Sameroff, A., & Chandler, M. (1975). Reproductive risk and the continuum of caretaker casualty. In F.D. Horowitz, M. Hetherington, S. Scarr-Salapateck, & G. Siegel (Eds.), *Review of child development research*, Vol. 4. Chicago: University of Chicago Press.

Scarr-Salapatek, S. (1975). An evolutionary perspective on infant intelligence: Species patterns and individual variation. In M. Lewis (Ed.), *Origins of intelligence*. New York: Plenum.

Seibert, J., & Oller, D. (1981). Linguistic pragmatics and language intervention strategies. *Journal of Autism and Developmental Disorders, 11*, 75–88.

Selman, R. (1976). Social cognitive understanding: A guide to educational and clinical practice. In T. Lickona (Ed.), *Theory, research, and social issues*. New York: Holt, Rinehart & Winston.

Snow, C. (1972). Mothers' speech to children learning language. *Child Development, 43*, 549–565.

Sparrow, S., Balla, D., & Cicchetti, D. (1984). *Vineland Scales of Adaptive Behavior, Survey Form Manual*. Circle Pines, MN: American Guidance Service.

Spitz, H. (1963). Field theory and mental deficiency. In N.R. Ellis (Ed.), *Handbook of mental deficiency*. New York: McGraw-Hill.

Spitz, H. (1979). Beyond field theory in the study of mental deficiency. In N.R. Ellis (Ed.),

Handbook of mental deficiency, psychological theory and research. Hillsdale, NJ: Erlbaum.

Switsky, H., Rotatori, A., Miller, T., & Freagon, S. (1979). The developmental model and its implications for assessment and instruction for the severely/profoundly handicapped. *Mental Retardation, 17,* 167–170.

Tronick, E.Z. (Ed.). (1982). *Social interchange in infancy: Affect, cognition, and communication.* Baltimore, MD: University Park Press.

Uzgiris, I., & Hunt, J. McV. (1975). *Assessment in infancy: Ordinal scales of psychological development.* Urbana, IL: University of Illinois Press.

Volkmar, F. (1987). Social development. In D. Cohen & A. Donnellan (Eds.), *Handbook of autism and pervasive developmental disorders.* New York: Wiley.

Volkmar, F., Burack, J.A., & Cohen, D. (this volume). Deviance and developmental approaches in the study of autism. Chapter 10.

Vygotsky, L.S. (1978). *Mind in society.* Cambridge, MA: Massachusetts Institute of Technology Press.

Weiss, B., Weisz, J., & Bromfield, R. (1986). Performance of retarded and nonretarded persons on information-processing tasks: Further tests of the similar structure hypothesis. *Psychological Bulletin, 100,* 157–175.

Weisz, J. (this volume). Cultural–familial retardation: A developmental perspective on cognitive performance. Chapter 7.

Weisz, J., & Yeates, K. (1981). Cognitive development in retarded and nonretarded persons: Piagetian tests of the similar structure hypothesis. *Psychological Bulletin, 90,* 153–178.

Weisz, J., Yeates, K., & Zigler, E. (1982). Piagetian evidence and the developmental-difference controversy. In E. Zigler & D. Balla (Eds.), *Mental retardation: The developmental-difference controversy.* Hillsdale, NJ: Erlbaum.

Weisz, J., & Zigler, E. (1979). Cognitive development in retarded and nonretarded persons: Piagetian tests of the similar sequence hypothesis. *Psychological Bulletin, 86,* 831–851.

Werner, H. (1948). *Comparative psychology of mental development* (rev. ed.). New York: Follett.

Werner, H. (1957). The concept of development from a comparative and organismic point of view. In D. Harris (Ed.), *The concept of development.* Minneapolis, MN: University of Minnesota Press.

Werner, H., & Kaplan, B. (1963). *Symbol formation.* New York: Wiley.

Wertsch, J.V. (1985). *Vygotsky and the social formation of mind.* Cambridge, MA: Harvard University Press.

Wohlhueter, M., & Sindberg, R. (1975). Longitudinal development of object permanence in mentally retarded children: An exploratory study. *American Journal of Mental Deficiency, 79,* 513–518.

Wohlwill, J.F. (1973). *The study of behavioral development.* New York: Academic Press.

Zeaman, D., & House, B. (1963). The role of attention in retardate discrimination learning. In N.R. Ellis (Ed.), *Handbook of mental deficiency.* New York: McGraw-Hill.

Zeaman, D. & House, B. (1979). A review of attention theory. In N.R. Ellis (Ed.), *Handbook of mental deficiency* (2nd ed.). Hillsdale, NJ: Erlbaum.

Zigler, E. (1963). Metatheoretical issues in developmental psychology. In M. Marx (Ed.), *Theories in contemporary psychology.* New York: Macmillan.

Zigler, E. (1967). Familial mental retardation: A continuing dilemma. *Science, 155,* 292–298.

Zigler, E. (1969). Developmental versus difference theories of mental retardation and the problem of motivation. *American Journal of Mental Deficiency, 73,* 536–556.

Zigler, E. (1971). The retarded child as a whole person. In H.E. Adams & W.K. Boardman (Eds.), *Advances in experimental clinical psychology.* New York: Pergamon.

Zigler, E., & Balla, D. (Eds.) (1982). *Mental retardation: The developmental–difference controversy.* Hillsdale, NJ: Erlbaum.

Zigler, E., & Cascione, R. (1984). Mental retardation: An overview. In E.S. Gollin (Ed.), *Malformations of development: Biological and psychological sources and consequences.* New York: Academic Press.

Zigler, E., Lamb, M., & Child, I. (1982). Socialization. In E. Zigler, M. Lamb, & I. Child (Eds.), *Socialization and personality development.* New York: Oxford University Press.

2 Differentiating mental retardation: The two-group approach and beyond

Jacob A. Burack

For several centuries, medical workers have been interested in differences in etiology among mentally retarded persons. As early as the 17th century, the Swiss physician Felix Platter differentiated between two general types of mentally retarded persons (Scheerenberger, 1983). Individuals of the first type were characterized by simplicity and foolishness that was evident as early as infancy. Individuals of the second type, referred to as endemic cretins, were considered to be dull from before birth and to be suffering from defects of nature (i.e., physical deformity). In the 19th century, John Langdon Down (1887) classified mentally deficient persons ("idiots" and "feeble-minded") into three etiological groups: congenital, accidental, and developmental. Down also was the first worker to distinguish between mongolism and cretinism. Also at that time, William Wetherspoon Ireland (1877) proposed a 10-category classification of mental retardation that was based primarily on the causes of and the physical differences among the various conditions included in this system. Nine of Ireland's categories were concerned with medical conditions associated with mental retardation; the tenth was "idiocy by deprivation" (Scheerenberger, 1983). These early workers recognized that mentally deficient persons did not comprise a homogeneous population, and could be better understood when the cause of the mental retardation was taken into account.

Medical workers today continue to study disorders associated with mental retardation separately. In these endeavors, they have been successful both in providing information about well-known types of mental retardation (e.g., Down syndrome, PKU) and in identifying formerly unknown conditions related to mental retardation. Fragile X syndrome (Lubbs, 1969) and fetal alcohol (Cooper, 1987) syndrome are examples of two disorders associated with mental retardation that have been identified in the past quarter of a century. By using this increasing precision in differentiating among mentally retarded persons on the basis of etiology, medical workers are better able to understand the physical, social, and cognitive development seen in specific syndromes.

27

Unfortunately, too many workers in the field of mental retardation ignore the advances made by medical workers during the past 100 years. Rather than recognizing the vast etiologically based differences among mentally retarded persons, these researchers choose to focus on the arbitrary diagnostic criteria (e.g., IQ less than 70) that are common to all mentally retarded persons and that unites them as a single-disease entity in today's psychiatric classificatory schemes (APA, 1980, 1987).

The current operational definition of mental retardation is significantly subaverage general intellectual functioning, indicated by a score of 70 or below on a standardized test that results in or is associated with deficits or impairments in adaptive behavior, with onset before the age of 18 years (APA, 1980; Grossman, 1983). However, Zigler, Balla, and Hodapp (1984) have argued that the criterion of impairments of adaptive behavior should be removed from the official classification of mental retardation, because mental health workers generally consider only IQ when making a diagnosis of mental retardation (Junkala, 1977). In any case, it is generally agreed that the diagnosis of mental retardation is usually made on the basis of some set of arbitrarily decided criteria of cognitive functioning; at present, the cutoff is a score of two standard deviations below the mean on a standardized intelligence test. The arbitrary nature of the diagnostic criteria is evidenced by the fact that in recent years the cutoff IQ score for mental retardation has fluctuated between 85 (APA, 1966) and 70 (APA, 1980; Grossman, 1983), thereby affecting the classification of approximately 24 million persons in the United States alone (Zigler & Cascione, 1984).

Researchers of mental retardation who recognize the limitations of these diagnostic guidelines argue both that mental retardation is not a single entity and that there is generally no distinct delineation between the normal and mentally retarded ranges of functioning. In addition, they note that although the diagnosis of mental retardation provides information about an individual's overall level of cognitive functioning, it reveals nothing about that person's various cognitive processes or the specific defects that may hinder his or her development.

These researchers have generally advocated a two-group approach to mental retardation in which organically retarded persons are distinguished from nonorganically retarded individuals. Although the two-group approach has served as an optimal and more fine-tuned framework than the undifferentiated view for understanding and researching mental retardation, it now needs to be further developed so that research in this field can be even more precise. In preliminary efforts to expand the two-group approach, Zigler and Hodapp (1986) attempted to differentiate the category of nonorganic etiology, and Burack, Hodapp, and Zigler (1988) argued for the utility of differentiating among organic etiologies.

The goal of this chapter is to further the case for more differentiated research. I will begin by briefly outlining the argument made by many leading workers in mental retardation that there is no value in differentiating among etiological groups for research purposes. In contrast to this position, the historical development of the two-group approach will then be reviewed. Next, the current need for a research strategy that is even more sophisticated and precise than the two-group approach will be discussed. Finally, I will make the argument that such a fine-grained approach to mental retardation will lead to improved research efforts and a better understanding of the functioning of the many different groups of retarded persons.

The undifferentiated view

During the past quarter of a century, many leading researchers have ignored the fact that the classification of mental retardation provides limited information about mentally retarded persons. They have generally made the assumption that mental retardation is a single disorder, or at least that cognitive and behavioral functioning is similar for all mentally retarded persons. These researchers have failed to acknowledge the relevance of etiological differences to the understanding of the nature, course, and outcome of mental retardation; instead, they have argued against the utility of differentiating mentally retarded persons by etiology. Consequently, their research considers mentally retarded individuals as a homogeneous population that can be studied as a single group, regardless of etiology.

In the late 1960s, Ellis (1969) argued that "in spite of all the possible criticisms of ignoring etiology in behavioral research, it should be strongly emphasized that rarely have behavioral differences characterized different etiological groups" (p. 561). More than a decade later, Ellis and Cavalier (1982) reiterated this point when they asserted that "even easily diagnosed clinical types such as Down's syndrome do not display behavioral characteristics that set them apart" (pp. 126–127). With regard to development, Fisher and Zeaman (1970) stated that "it does not appear to make any difference how one gets to be a retardate, whether through bad genes, brain pathology, or seizures, the maturational results are the same" (p. 164). In summarizing these views, MacMillan (1982) concluded that "there is now considerable skepticism as to the usefulness of classifying mental retardation by form, due primarily to our current inability to separate biological and psychological forces...when dichotomized (cultural–familial versus organic retardation) groups have been compared for behavioral differences, findings have been inconsistent" (p. 60). Other leading researchers in the field of mental retardation have made similar statements, thereby implying a homogeneous nature for mental retardation (Baueister & MacLean, 1979; Leland, 1969; Luria, 1963; Milgram, 1969; Spitz, 1963).

The proposition that mental retardation is a single disorder has given rise to a profusion of theories of specific defects that are presented as primary causes or markers of mental retardation. The proposed defects include cognitive rigidity (Kounin, 1941; Lewin, 1936), memory processes (Detterman, 1979; Ellis, 1963, 1969), discrimination learning (Zeaman & House, 1963), attention–retention capabilities (Fisher & Zeaman, 1973; Mosley, 1980; Zeaman & House, 1979), neural satiation related to cortical conductivity (Spitz, 1963), the verbal system (Luria, 1963; O'Connor & Hermelin, 1959), the orienting response (Heal & Johnson, 1970; Luria 1963), and cross-modal coding (O'Connor & Hermelin, 1959). In addition, researchers attempting to apply knowledge about mentally retarded persons to the understanding of normal intellectual functioning have generally assumed that there is a similar style of intellectual functioning for all mentally retarded persons (e.g., Anderson, 1986; Detterman, 1987).

The origins of the two-group approach

The differentiated view of mental retardation, in which etiology is taken into account, stands in contrast to the conceptualization of mentally retarded persons as a homogeneous group suffering from some common defects. The two-group approach, which distinguishes between cultural–familial (nonorganic) and organic etiologies, represents the most common and basic of the differentiated conceptualizations of mental retardation.

The origins of the two-group approach date back to early researchers of mental retardation such as Ireland (1877), who realized the need to distinguish between mentally retarded persons of differing etiologies. At the beginning of the 20th century, Tredgold (1908) differentiated between "primary" and "secondary" retardation. Primary retardation referred to the product of a damaged germ cell, and secondary retardation to the arrested development of a potentially normal brain arising from environmental factors. During the past half century, several forms of this dichotomous approach to mental retardation have been proposed (Dingman & Tarjan, 1960; Lewis, 1933; Penrose, 1949; Zigler, 1967, 1969; Zigler & Hodapp, 1986).

The argument for the two-group approach is based on the theoretical premise that the majority of retarded persons do not differ qualitatively from the normal population. These retarded persons are individuals who would be expected, by statistical chance, to be significantly below average on intellectual functioning (Dingman & Tarjan, 1960; Lewis, 1933). Similarly to other human characteristics such as height and weight, intelligence can be thought of within the framework of a normally distributed curve, with variation within the population thought to be influenced by genetic and environmental factors (Guilford, 1954; Pearson & Jaederholm, 1914; Penrose, 1949; Zigler, 1967). According to this model, there is a given percentage of persons who deviate *statistically* from the norms for average functioning even though they may not differ *qualitatively* from those persons falling within the normal range of intellectual functioning.

This view was first articulated at the beginning of the 20th century by Pearson and Jaederholm (1914). In comparing Binet scores of children considered to be feeble-minded with those of normal school children, Jaederholm found that the distribution of scores was continuous over the whole range of scores. He found no indication of a natural split between the so-called feeble-minded and normal groups. In fact, there was a great deal of overlap on the Binet scores between the children considered to be feeble-minded and the normal school children.

Lewis (1933) differentiated between the "subcultural" mental defectives, whose deficiency he considered to be an extreme variety of normal variations of cognitive capabilities, and "pathological" mental defectives, whose condition was considered to be associated with and in most cases a result of recognized organic insult. Lewis (1933) concurred with Jaederholm's view that persons in the subcultural group were not readily distinguishable from those in the nonretarded population. He argued that

> the higher grades of subcultural deficiency merge gradually into the lower grades of dullness or of temperamental instability. There seems to be a close biological kinship between the subcultural defective and the main body of normal persons – a kinship which cannot be attributed to the pathological defective. (p. 300)

Furthermore, Lewis contrasted the biological integrity of the subcultural group with the physiological impairments of the pathological group. He asserted that the pathological group included persons whose mental deficiency was attributable to one of the clinical varieties of either "primary" or "secondary amentia." Types of primary amentia included mongolism, amaurotic family idiocy, progressive lenticular degeneration, hypertelorism, and naevoid amentia, while varieties of secondary amentia that often led to mental deficiency included trauma, inflammatory conditions, hydrocephalus, syphilis, epilepsy, cretinism, and nutritional and sensory defects (Lewis, 1933).

Lewis (1933) argued that there are many more subcultural retarded persons than pathological ones, and that these persons tend to be higher-functioning than those in the latter group whom he considered to be "lower-grade defectives." He also suggested that although pathological persons are evenly distributed among all sections of the community, the subcultural mentally retarded persons are concentrated in the section of the community that is associated with "various chronic social evils – pauperism, slumdom and its concomitants" (p. 301). Despite the socially controversial tone of his conclusions, Lewis's work provided a strong theoretical foundation for later advocates of the two-group approach.

Strauss and his colleagues (Kephart & Strauss, 1940; Strauss & Lehtinen, 1947) argued that mentally retarded persons could be divided into two groups – "exogenous" and "endogenous." This differentiation closely resembled Lewis's dichotomy between pathological and subcultural defectives. Similar to Lewis's pathological defectives, the exogenous group consisted of persons with clear indications of physical damage and with no unusual family history of mental deficiency. The endogenous group, which resembled Lewis's subcultural defectives, consisted of persons who showed no signs of brain damage but had a family history of mental deficiency. The two groups differed in that endogenous persons responded positively to favorable changes in the environment, as indicated by a marked acceleration of mental growth, whereas environmental changes had little effect on mental growth in exogenous persons (Kephart & Strauss, 1940). These findings provided early evidence of the contribution of deleterious and impoverished environmental surroundings to the incidence of nonorganic mental retardation. The findings also contradicted the assertions of earlier workers (Goddard, 1912; Lewis, 1933) that genetic heredity played a singularly important role in the familial transmission of mental retardation.

The validity of Lewis's (1933) dichotomous classificatory system was discussed by Penrose (1949) within the context of the Gaussian curve. He showed that there were many more persons whose cognitive abilities were three or four standard deviations below the mean than would be expected by a normal Gaussian distribution. Penrose attributed the relatively high incidence of imbecility and idiocy to the occurrence of organically caused mental retardation resulting from rare genetic processes, accidents, and diseases. Penrose differentiated between this "severe" form of mental retardation, and "mild" retardation, a split that closely mirrored the secondary–primary and exogenous–endogenous dichotomies. According to Penrose, mild retardation resulted from a combination of hereditary and environmental causes. Specifically, Penrose identified common genes and multiple additive genes as hereditary causes, and deprivation and antisocial environments as environmental causes. He argued that the lack of any marked distinction between the cases of mild defect and members of the general population makes it reasonable to assume that the same *genetical* mechanisms which produce variations in intelligence in the general population will be determining factors in the production of mild defects. The genetical factors, as those which cause normal variations in stature, are certainly multiple and possibly additive in their effects. (pp. 58–59; italics in original)

These ideas formed a theoretical base for Zigler and Hodapp's (1986) recent work in differentiating among the various nonorganic etiologies of mental retardation.

Despite Penrose's proposal (1949, 1963) of a dichotomous classificatory scheme, he cautioned that assigning persons to one or the other group is a complex and often imprecise task. In particular, qualities thought to be characteristic of either mildly or severely retarded persons can often be found in the other group, and it is often clinically difficult to accurately determine the existence of an organic causation. Penrose (1949) suggested, however, that as medical technology became more sophisticated, organic bases for retardation would be found in persons previously thought to be endogenously retarded. This prediction has been realized with the discovery of several previously unrecognized forms of organic retardation such as fragile X syndrome (Lubbs, 1969; see chapter 9), while Penrose's concerns about the precision in assigning retarded persons to appropriate etiological groups remains a major concern for researchers of mental retardation (Zigler & Hodapp, 1986).

Similar versions of the two-group approach were proposed by Dingman and Tarjan (1960; Dingman, 1959; Tarjan, 1959, 1960), who utilized epidemiological data on the incidence of mental retardation to demonstrate the existence of two basic types of mental retardation. Dingman (1959) distinguished the group of generally mildly retarded persons – for whom sociocultural factors had interfered with opportunities to acquire educational sophistication – from the group of mentally retarded persons suffering from various pathological conditions. Similarly, Tarjan (1959) differentiated between "physiological" and "pathological" mental retardation. In support of the two-group approach, these researchers cited their own data (Dingman & Tarjan, 1960; Tarjan, 1960) as well as the data of others (Fraser Roberts, Norman, & Griffiths, 1938; Pearson, 1931; Pearson & Jaederholm, 1914; Penrose, 1954; Thomson, 1953) to demonstrate that despite the normal distributions generally produced by intelligence tests, more persons are found at the retarded ranges of functioning than would be predicted by a normal curve. Thus, in addition to the physiologically or socioculturally deprived retarded persons who blend "gradually into the continuum of the general population" (Tarjan, 1960; p. 60), there is the group of the pathologically retarded persons who make up the *excess* cases of mental retardation compared with that expected from a normal – or Gausian – distribution. This group is comprised of persons with moderate to severe handicaps that are associated with organic damage and physical infirmities. IQs in this group are generally below 50, with group means thought to be around 30 (Dingman & Tarjan, 1960; Tarjan, 1960).

Dingman and Tarjan (1960; Tarjan, 1960) noted that the discrepancy between the theoretical distribution of intelligence and epidemiologically based estimates increased at the more severe levels of mental retardation. They found a small excess of persons with IQs between 50 and 70, twice as many persons in the 20 to 50 IQ group as would be expected, and an excess by a factor of nearly 2000 in the group of persons with IQs below 20. Figure 2.1 depicts the type of combined curve presented by Dingman and Tarjan (1960). Two curves are shown – a normal curve based on the general population, and a truncated normal curve based on the excess frequencies. This second distribution originates at 0, reaches a peak at 30, and has a long tail that reaches into the normal and even above-average range of IQs. This graphic illustration of the actual prevalence of mental retardation has been utilized by several researchers (e.g., Penrose, 1963; Zigler, 1967) to depict the existence of two different groups of mentally retarded persons.

Modern era of the two-group approach

The debate over the merits of the two-group approach became a major focus of research in mental retardation during the 1960s. At that time, defect theories (e.g., Ellis, 1963; Leland, 1969; Luria, 1963; Milgram, 1969; Spitz, 1963; Zeaman & House, 1963) began to predominate as the leading researchers in the field sought a single physiological or cognitive cause of mental retardation. These theorists, although in disagreement about the nature of the specific defect, viewed mentally retarded persons as homogeneous because their impaired cognitive functioning resulted from some common deficit. It is evident that the proponents of such an all-encompassing orientation had no use for a fine-grained research strategy such as the two-group approach that differentiated mentally retarded persons by etiology.

In opposition to these defect theorists, Zigler (1967, 1969) argued extensively that both research and intervention efforts would be aided by differentiating between two basic groups of mentally retarded persons (for a review of the basic characteristics of the two groups, see Table 2.1). One

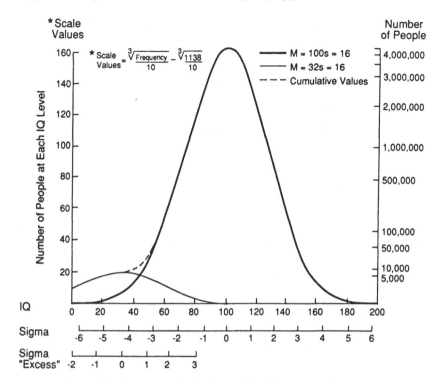

Figure 2.1. Frequency distribution of intelligence quotients assuming a total population of 175,000,000. Figures should be adjusted to reflect current U.S. population (approximately 245,000,000). Taken from Dingman and Tarjan (1960), with permission.

group includes those persons suffering from organic damage arising from inborn or prenatal phenomena (e.g., chromosomal disorders, irradiation, fetal alcohol syndrome, and PKU), or postnatal events (e.g., anoxia and lead poisoning) that can affect the brain's functioning in varying degrees of severity. The second group consists of familial retarded persons – those with no known organic etiology. As implied by the name, this type of mental retardation tends to run in families (Zigler & Hodapp, 1986). There is little consensus among researchers as to the etiology of familial mental retardation, with genetic factors, environmental conditions, unidentified organic damage, and interactions between any or all of these factors being cited as possible causes.

Zigler's (1967) discussion of the two-group approach was framed within a developmental model that considered only the group of familial retarded persons. This model depicts a general developmental delay in familial mentally retarded persons that is global in nature and cannot be attributed

Table 2.1. *A three-group model for the classification of retarded persons*

Organic IQ 0–70	Familial 50...70	Undifferentiated 0...70
Classificatory principle		
Demonstrable organic etiology	No demonstrable organic etiology. Parents have the same type of retardation	Cannot reliably be placed in either of the other two classes
Correlates		
Found at all SES levels	More prevalent at lower SES levels	
IQs most often below 50	IQs rarely below 50	
Siblings usually of normal intelligence	Siblings often at lower levels of intelligence	
Often accompanied by severe health problems	Health within normal range	
Appearance often marred by physical stigmata	Normal appearance	
Mortality rate higher (More likely to die at a younger age than the general population)	Normal mortality rate	
Often dependent on care from others throughout life	With some support can lead an independent existence as adults	
Unlikely to marry and often infertile	Likely to marry and produce children of low intelligence	
Unlikely to experience neglect in their homes	More likely to experience neglect in their homes	
High prevalence of other physical handicaps (e.g., epilepsy, cerebral palsy)	Less likely to have other physical handicaps	

Source: From Zigler, Balla, & Hodapp (1984), with permission.

to one or a few specific cognitive defects. According to this view, familial retarded persons develop in much the same way as nonretarded persons, but at a slower rate and with a lower asymptote. Two specific hypotheses arise from this formulation. One is the similar-sequence hypothesis (see chapter 3) in which familial retarded persons are thought to proceed through the stages of development in the same order as do nonretarded children. Second is the similar-structure hypothesis (see chapters 4 and 7) in which the profiles of cognitive strengths and weaknesses are thought to be the same as those of nonretarded persons with the same mental age.

Zigler (1967, 1969) argued that although the developmental approach could be applied to familial retarded persons, it was not necessarily relevant to the study of organically retarded persons. He asserted that because individuals of various organic etiologies suffer from different types of physiological damage, it is likely that their cognitive development is affected in a variety of different ways. In explaining this, Zigler (1969) stated that "if the etiology of the phenotypic intelligence (as measured by an IQ) of the two groups differs, it is far from logical to assert that the course of development is the same, or that even similar contents in their behaviors are mediated by exactly the same cognitive processes" (p. 533).

Zigler's dichotomization of familial and organic mentally retarded individuals with regard to the developmental approach is supported by much evidence that shows that the similar-structure hypothesis holds true for familial retarded individuals but not for organically retarded persons. In an early study of this type, Beck and Lam (1955) examined the WISC profiles of both organic and nonorganic mentally retarded children. They found that the profiles of the nonorganically retarded were similar to those generally found in the nonretarded population, whereas the profiles of the organically retarded children did not follow the general pattern outlined by Wechsler (1944). In a review of numerous studies relating to the similar-structure issue, Weisz and Yeates (1981) found that the performance of nonorganically retarded individuals was similar to that of MA-matched nonretarded persons on a variety of tasks. However, the performance of the mentally retarded subjects was found to be deficient in studies that included organically retarded individuals.

In a more recent study, Kahn (1985) compared MA-matched socioculturally mildly retarded, organically impaired mildly retarded, organically impaired moderately retarded, and nonretarded children on moral and cognitive reasoning tasks. He found no differences between the sociocultural retarded and nonretarded children or between the two organically retarded groups. However, the performances of both the sociocultural retarded and nonretarded children were found to be at a higher level than those of either of the organically retarded groups. Although Kahn (1985) raises some question as to the interpretation of these findings, they indicate at least that organically retarded children may perform differently than their familial retarded peers.

Although the behavioral implications of the two-group approach will be discussed in other chapters, a recent study by Broman, Nichols, Shaughnessy, and Kennedy (1987) demonstrated the physical and socioeconomic implications of familial and organic retardation. Over a 15-year period, Broman et al. (1987) followed 53,000 pregnancies from gestation to 8 years. Using an IQ of approximately 50 as a cutoff, the authors found numerous differences in the origins of mild and severe mental retardation.

Mildly mentally retarded children tended to come from low socioeconomic status (SES) backgrounds, and generally had mentally retarded relatives. In contrast, most severely retarded children had suffered some organic insult, came from relatively affluent backgrounds, and had no relatives suffering from mental retardation. Furthermore, Broman et al. (1987) found that severely retarded children (IQ below 50) without organic damage came from backgrounds resembling those of the mentally retarded children without organic insult, whereas the mildly retarded children who had suffered some organic damage were closer to the severely retarded group on demographic variables.

Beyond the two-group approach

Zigler and colleagues (Burack, Hodapp, & Zigler, 1988; Zigler & Hodapp, 1986) have recently argued that even the two-group approach is too gross a classificatory system to adequately account for many differences between mentally retarded persons. They note that there are over 200 identified etiologies of organic retardation (Grossman, 1983; Lubs & Maes, 1977) and at least three subtypes of nonorganic retardation (Zigler & Hodapp, 1986). In light of this, and in keeping with the assertion that differences in the etiology of phenotypic intelligence between persons leads to differences in the course of development, Burack, Hodapp, and Zigler (1988) assert that it is simplistic to think that all mentally retarded persons can be viewed as belonging to one of two fairly homogeneous groups. They warn that the consequences of such gross classificatory schemes include imprecise and confounded research resulting in misguided strategies for interventions.

Burack, Hodapp, and Zigler (1988) suggest that one way to improve the current inexact classificatory systems would be with a double-branched "tree structure" of classification, with organic mental retardation forming one main branch and familial mental retardation the other. Descending from each branch would be smaller branches for more precise groupings. These researchers assert that this type of differentiating strategy represents both a conservative and optimal approach to research by maximizing the amount of information that can be gained from a given study. A more detailed discussion of the tree structure and its implications for research will be presented later in this chapter.

Differentiating nonorganic mental retardation

Tarjan (1970) described nonorganic mentally retarded persons as

> those retardates in whom currently available biomedical technology cannot demonstrate significant physical or laboratory pathology; in whom no

specific, single somatic agent can be made significantly accountable for the condition; in whom the diagnosis often disappears at young adult age; who are normal in physical appearance; whose morbidity and mortality rates do not differ greatly from those of the average population; in whom the retardation is usually mild, with the difference between average parental IQ and that of the index case rather small; who generally come from socially, economically, and educationally underprivileged strata of our society. (pp. 745–746)

The comprehensiveness of this description, in its identification of the factors thought to be associated with nonorganic retardation, serves to highlight the difficulty in providing a specific definition of this type of mental retardation; it also sheds light on the long-standing debate concerning the exact nature of its etiology. As seen in the earlier review of the two-group approach, past researchers have suggested various causes of nonorganic retardation, including familial, genetic, social, environmental, undiscovered organic defects, and any number of combinations of these factors. Accordingly, these researchers have employed a variety of terms to describe the etiology of this type of retardation (e.g., unknown, cultural–familial, familial, and sociocultural).

Although researchers have traditionally viewed nonorganically retarded persons as homogeneous, and applied any one or more of these labels to the entire group, it seems likely that this group may in fact be quite heterogeneous. Certainly, as medical technology continues to become more sophisticated, previously unrecognized types of organic impairments will be identified. In this manner, mental retardation of unknown etiology seems an appropriate label for some of the nonorganically retarded persons. As indicated earlier, however, it is generally accepted by many workers that there is a group of nonorganic mentally retarded persons who have no organic impairment that would distinguish them from the average population. Yet, even this group is likely to be a heterogeneous one.

In a first effort to provide a more differentiated approach to the familial branch of the mental retardation tree, Zigler and Hodapp (1986) hypothesized that the group of familial retarded persons is actually comprised of several subgroups. First, there are individuals who are familial-retarded in the traditional sense, in that they have at least one parent who is also mentally retarded. Second, there is a group whose members are referred to as "polygenic isolates." These persons are the polygenically mentally retarded offspring of parents who are themselves not mentally retarded. Persons in this group have received a "poor genetic draw" (MacMillan, 1977) in ways outlined by the Gottesman (1963) and other polygenic models. Third, there is the group of socioculturally retarded persons. These individuals are mentally retarded because of prolonged exposure to an extremely poor environment. In providing a more differentiated approach to familial retardation, a grouping previously thought to represent a homogeneous population, Zigler and Hodapp (1986) illustrated the need for researchers to provide a more precise description of the type of mentally retarded persons with whom they are working.

Differentiating organic mental retardation

The organic branch of the tree is more easily separated into specific etiologies, because the biological causes can usually be readily ascertained. The various causes of organic damage include chromosomal abnormalities, metabolic imbalances, neurological insults, congenital defects, perinatal complications, and infections. The physical manifestations of these types of organic insult are often readily evident to a casual observer, and almost always easily diagnosed by medical workers. Thus, it is surprising that so little work has been done to assess the different ways that the various types of organic damage can affect psychological functioning.

Differences in levels of cognitive functioning among etiological groups

Extensive research with specific etiological groups has shown that individuals of a common etiology often display patterns of behavioral strengths and weaknesses that are unique to that group. The research on children with idiopathic infantile hypercalcemia of the Fanconi type (IIHF) provides an example of such a distinctive psychological profile. IIHF is a rare condition that typically shows itself in infancy (Udwin, Yule, & Martin, 1987) and is characterized by elfin facies (Joseph & Parrott, 1958), cardiovascular and renal abnormalities (Martin, Snodgrass, & Cohen, 1984), and moderate to severe mental retardation (Udwin et al., 1987). In the largest psychological study of children with IIHF, Udwin et al. (1987) found that the verbal abilities of these children were markedly superior to their visual–spatial skills. Performance on reading and spelling tasks showed that these children generally had good phonological and verbal-processing skills. Reports of parents and teachers indicated that IIHF children were talkative and articulate, with good verbal recall and mimicry skills. With regard to social development, these children were found to manifest high rates of emotional and behavioral disturbances, particularly overactivity, poor peer relationships, excessive anxiety, and sleeping and eating difficulties. In summarizing their findings, Udwin et al. (1987) concluded that "the combination of psychological characteristics and cognitive characteristics and cognitive strengths and deficits found overall, clearly differentiates these children as a group from other mentally handicapped groups."

Research with children with Down syndrome shows a psychological profile that is strikingly different than the one seen in children with IIHF. Children with Down syndrome have been found to have particular difficulty with language (Gibson, 1978), visual monitoring (Kopp, 1983; Krakow & Kopp, 1982), and abstract reasoning. In contrast, these children show relative strengths in the areas of visual–motor integration (Pueschel, Gallagher, Zartler, & Pezzullo, 1987), social adaptation (Centerwall & Centerwall, 1960; Cornwell & Birch, 1969), and in the more social aspects of cognitive tasks (e.g., the pragmatics of language; Beeghly & Cicchetti, 1987; Leifer & Lewis, 1984).

The cognitive functioning of children with Down syndrome has also been shown to differ from that of children with fragile X syndrome. As noted earlier, differences between persons with these two syndromes are particularly noteworthy because both are chromosomal disorders. Down syndrome children showed no differences between levels of simultaneous and sequential processing on the Kaufman Assessment Battery for Children (K-ABC; Kaufman & Kaufman, 1983) (Pueschel et al., 1987). The simultaneous processing in fragile X boys, however, was found to be almost two years ahead of their sequential processing (Dykens, Hodapp, Leckman, 1987). Furthermore, in contrast to the Down syndrome children's relative superiority in visual–motor integration, this area was the single most delayed in fragile X boys.

These examples of differing psychological profiles among children with IIHF, Down, and fragile X syndromes provide only brief examples of the type of unique profiles of psychological functioning that can be found when studying persons of a single etiological group. The chapters in part 2 of this volume provide a more thorough discussion of the types of profiles of cognitive and/or social strengths and weaknesses that can be seen in certain etiologically homogeneous groups of mentally retarded individuals.

Methodological issues in the employment of the multigroup approach

The hierarchical tree structure of classification

The type of double-branched tree structure of classification proposed by Burack, Hodapp, and Zigler (1988) helps to illustrate the manner in which mental retardation can be understood within the framework of the multigroup approach. In this model there are two primary branches, one representing organic mental retardation, the other representing familial mental retardation. Descending from these branches are several more levels of branches, with the branches becoming progressively smaller the farther they are from the main branch. The smaller the branches at a given level, the more specific the groupings. The branches on the familial side only descend one level, at which point the three types of familial retardation are specified. The organic side of the tree is much more complex, because there are so many varieties of organic retardation. Types of organic disorders (e.g., chromosomal abnormalities, congenital defects) are represented on the first level of branches down from the primary organic branch. This is followed by specific etiological disorders (e.g., Down syndrome, cerebral palsy) and finally by subtypes of the disorder (e.g., trisomy 21, mosaicism, or chromosomal translocation in Down syndrome; spastic, athetoid, or ataxia in cerebral palsy).

Each lower level of branch represents a more differentiated strategy than the one above. On the organic side, type of disorder provides a natural criterion for differentiating organically retarded individuals, and has been used by some researchers (e.g., Goodman, 1977). In addition, differentiation at this level generally allows for the discrimination between persons whose organicity is the clear cause of their mental retardation, and those whose organicity is related to their mental retardation but is not necessarily the cause of it. For example, chromosomal disorders, such as Down and fragile X syndromes, are clearly implicated as causes of impaired cognitive development, although not always of mental retardation. On the other hand, neurological disorders such as cerebral palsy and epilepsy are related to higher incidences of mental retardation, but do not necessarily result in cognitive impairment. Despite the increase in information available at this level of differentiation, the research just reviewed showing behavioral differences between persons with different types of chromosomal disorders (i.e., Down syndrome and fragile X syndrome) provides an example of the need for differentiation among organically retarded individuals to extend beyond the level of disorder type.

The next, more differentiated level down in the tree structure is the specific etiologies. Burack, Hodapp, and Zigler (1988) suggest that this level is an optimal one for workers to strive for in their research endeavors. Diagnoses at this level are generally easily recognized by workers in the field, and represent the minimum knowledge of the etiology ascertained for both medical and educational purposes. Furthermore, findings of differences between etiological groups can be easily communicated to a wide range of workers, and thereby provide the impetus for comprehensive programming and intervention efforts specific to each etiological group.

Although the level of differentiation by etiological group appears appropriate for much research, there are circumstances when an even more fine-grained approach is necessary. Such situations arise when there are identifiable subgroups within a specific etiological group. These subgroups may differ from each other on one or more of a variety of criteria including: etiological bases that are more precise than those indicated in common etiological groupings; associated physical conditions and their severity; and associated behavioral disorders.

Down syndrome and cerebral palsy are two examples of commonly identified etiological groups that are comprised of persons with different types of organic insult. Down syndrome individuals, for instance, can be suffering from one of three chromosomal abnormalities. Approximately 95 percent of these individuals have an additional chromosome (Jacobs, Baikie, Court-Brown, & Strong, 1959), resulting in the karyotype generally labeled as trisomy 21. Chromosomal translocations – the fusing of an additional chromosome to another chromosome – are responsible for about 3 percent of the cases of Down syndrome. The remaining 2 percent of cases of Down syndrome are of the mosaic type, in which there are two or more different cell types, with one of the cell types having a Down syndrome karyotype (Pueschel, 1983). In cerebral palsy, the various subgroups are identified by differences in physical dysfunction that are the result of damage to different areas of the brain. The largest group (about three quarters) of persons with cerebral palsy have suffered damage to the motor cortex, and are categorized as spastics. Other kinds of cerebral palsy include the athetoid type that is due to impairments of the basal ganglia, and the ataxic type that results from damage to the cerebellum. (For a more complete review of the subgroups within both the Down syndrome and cerebral palsy groups, see Lewis, 1987.) Although little research has been done to investigate possible differences in behavioral and psychological functioning among the different types of Down syndrome persons, some evidence has been cited to show such differences among the subgroups of persons with cerebral palsy (Stephen & Hawks, 1974).

Differences in psychological functioning among subgroups of both Down syndrome and cerebral palsy have also shown to be related to physical development. For example, Cicchetti and Sroufe (1976, 1978) have shown that Down syndrome infants who are most hypotonic (i.e., have the weakest muscle tone) are most delayed. Cullen, Cronk, Pueschel, Schnell, and Reed (1981) later found a parallel relation between hypotonicity in children with Down syndrome and self-help skills. Similarly, researchers have noted a relationship between psychological performance and severity of the physical handicap among persons with cerebral palsy. For example, in children with the spastic type of cerebral palsy, the more limbs that are affected the greater the likelihood of below-average intelligence. For an extensive review of the relationship between psychological functioning and physical handicap see Lewis, 1987, and chapter 11 of this volume.

Finally, subgroups within an etiologically homogeneous group of mentally retarded persons may differ as a result of behavioral disorders. For example, autism is generally found in organically retarded persons, and has been shown to be related to various aspects of psychological functioning (see DeMyer, Hintgen, & Jackson, 1981). Thus, researchers should consider differences between autistic and nonautistic mentally retarded children of a common etiology. This would be especially important in the study of organic etiologies in which autism is not uncommon (e.g., congenital rubella). For a more thorough discussion of the relationship between autism and mental retardation with regard to psychological functioning, see chapter 10 of this volume.

Issues in implementing the multigroup approach

Although the multigroup approach to mental retardation is an optimal one for research, it must be noted that there are certain problems in using this strategy. The first is the difficulty researchers often have in attaining accurate and precise diagnostic information about the mentally retarded persons they are studying. As a result, these workers often are unable to appropriately categorize subjects by etiology. The second problem is that this more precise approach to research generally results in small subject groups. Although both these problems pose concerns for researchers using the multigroup approach, they should not be viewed as insurmountable issues, but rather as challenges for implementing improved research programs.

The problem in differentiating etiology occurs because the official diagnoses found in the medical and educational records of mentally retarded persons are often vague, confusing, and inaccurate. Although some disorders such as Down syndrome are generally easily diagnosed, others are much harder to identify. As medical technology becomes more sophisticated, however, the differentiating process should become more finegrained. Rather than discouraging this type of more precise differentiation, researchers in mental retardation should emphasize the need for it, and stress the value of group-specific information.

The problem of small numbers of subjects that arises from using the multigroup approach necessitates a consistent strategy to which this approach should be applied. As noted earlier, the multigroup approach provides a conservative strategy for researchers because it preserves a maximum amount of knowledge by maintaining information within precise homogeneous groupings of individuals, rather than collapsing across heterogeneous groupings. Thus, differences between these small homogeneous groups will be identified by working within the multigroup approach, whereas they will be obscured by research designs that employ larger, less differentiated groups. In this manner, the emphasis on large numbers of subjects impedes the discovery of new insights. On the other hand, if no differences are found between certain groups, these groups can be combined together for statistical purposes, and nothing would be lost. In those cases where the groups are combined, the statistical analysis would then continue up in the proposed tree structure of mental retardation toward the next less-differentiated level (e.g., from etiological subgroups to etiological groups). Groups that are differentiated at this next higher level, then, are compared. Again, if they differ on a certain measure, that information should be preserved, but if they perform similarly, the data can be collapsed into a single group. Thus, research in mental retardation should begin with a precise approach in which a maximum of information is maintained, and in which large numbers of subjects can be attained when appropriate.

References

American Psychiatric Association (1966). *Diagnostic and statistical manual* (2nd ed.). Washington, DC.

American Psychiatric Association (1980). *Diagnostic and statistical manual* (3rd ed.). Washington, DC.

American Psychiatric Association (1987). *Diagnostic and statistical manual* (3rd ed. rev.). Washington, DC.

Anderson, M. (1986). Understanding the cognitive deficit in mental retardation. *Journal of Child Psychology and Psychiatry, 27*, 297–306.

Baumeister, A., & MacLean, W. (1979). Brain damage and mental retardation. In N.R. Ellis (Ed.), *Handbook of mental deficiency: Psychological theory and research* (2nd ed.). Hillsdale, NJ: Erlbaum.

Beck, H.S., & Lam, R.L. (1955). Use of the WISC in predicting organicity. *Journal of Clinical Psychology, 11*, 154–157.

Beeghly, M., & Cicchetti, D. (1987). An organizational approach to symbolic development in children with Down syndrome. In D. Cicchetti & M. Beeghly (Eds.), *Symbolic development in atypical children. New directions for child development.* San Francisco: Jossey-Bass.

Broman, S., Nichols, P.L., Shaughnessy, P., & Kennedy, W. (1987). *Retardation in young children: A developmental study of cognitive deficit.* Hillsdale, NJ: Erlbaum.

Burack, J.A., Hodapp, R.M., & Zigler, E. (1988). Issues in the classification of mental retardation: Differentiating among organic etiologies. *Journal of Child Psychology and Psychiatry, 29*.

Centerwall, S., & Centerwall, W. (1960). A study of children with mongolism reared in the home versus those reared away from home. *Pediatrics, 25*, 678–685.

Cicchetti, D., & Sroufe, L. (1976). The relationship between affective and cognitive development in Down syndrome infants. *Child Development*, 47, 920–929.

Cicchetti, D., & Sroufe, L. (1978). An organizational view of affect: Illustration from the study of Down syndrome infants. In M. Lewis & L. Rosenblum (Eds.), *The development of affect*. New York: Plenum.

Cooper, S. (1987). The fetal alcohol syndrome. *Journal of Child Psychology and Psychiatry*, 28, 223–227.

Cornwell, A., & Birch, H. (1969). Psychological and social development in home-reared children with Down's Syndrome (mongolism). *American Journal of Mental Deficiency*, 74, 341–350.

Cullen, S., Cronk, C., Pueschel, S., Schnell, R., & Reed, R. (1981). Social development and feeding milestones of young Down Syndrome children. *American Journal of Mental Deficiency*, 85, 410–415.

DeMyer, M.K., Hintgen, J.N., & Jackson, R.K. (1981). Infantile autism reviewed: A decade of research. *Schizophrenia Bulletin*, 7, 388–451.

Detterman, D. (1979). Memory in the mentally retarded. In N.R. Ellis (Ed.), *Handbook of mental deficiency: Psychological theory and research* (2nd ed.). Hillsdale, NJ: Erlbaum.

Detterman, D. (1987). Theoretical notions of intelligence and mental retardation. *American Journal of Mental Deficiency*, 92, 2–11.

Dingman, H.F. (1959). Some uses of descriptive statistics in population analysis. *American Journal of Mental Deficiency*, 64, 291–295.

Dingman, H.F., & Tarjan, G. (1960). Mental retardation and the normal distribution curve. *American Journal of Mental Deficiency*, 64, 991–994.

Down, J.L. (1887). *Mental affections of children and youth*. London: J. & A. Churchill.

Dykens, E.M., Hodapp, R.M., & Leckman, J.F. (1987). Strengths and weaknesses in the intellectual functioning of males with fragile X syndrome. *American Journal of Mental Deficiency*, 92, 234–236.

Ellis, N.R. (1963). The stimulus trace and behavioral inadequacy. In N.R. Ellis (Ed.), *Handbook of mental deficiency*. New York: McGraw-Hill.

Ellis, N.R. (1969). A behavioral research strategy in mental retardation: Defense and critique. *American Journal of Mental Deficiency*, 73, 557–566.

Ellis, N.R., & Cavalier, A.R. (1982). Research perspectives in mental retardation. In E. Zigler & D. Balla (Eds.), *Mental retardation: The developmental – difference controversy*. Hillsdale, NJ: Erlbaum.

Fisher, M.A., & Zeaman, D. (1970). Growth and decline of retardate intelligence. *International Review of Research in Mental Retardation*, 4, 151–191.

Fisher, M.A., & Zeaman, D. (1973). An attention–retention theory of retardate discrimination learning. In N.R. Ellis (Ed.), *International review of research in mental retardation* (Vol. 6). New York: Academic Press.

Fraser Roberts, J.A., Norman, R.M., & Griffiths, R. (1938). Studies on a child population. IV. The form of the lower end of the frequency distribution of Stanford–Binet intelligence quotients and the fall of low intelligence quotients with advancing age. *Annals of Eugenics*, 8, 319–337.

Gibson, D. (1978). *Down's Syndrome: The psychology of mongolism*. Cambridge, MA: Cambridge University Press.

Goddard, H. (1912). The Kallikak family: A study in the heredity of feeble-mindedness. New York: Macmillan.

Goodman, J. (1977). Medical diagnosis and intelligence levels in young mentally retarded children. *Journal of Mental Deficiency Research*, 21, 205–212.

Gottesman, I.I. (1963). Genetic aspects of intelligent behavior. In N.R. Ellis (Ed.), *Handbook of mental deficiency*. New York: McGraw-Hill.

Grossman, H. (Ed.). (1983). *Classification in mental retardation* (3rd ed.). Washington, DC: American Association on Mental Deficiency.

Guilford, J.P. (1954). *Psychometric methods* (2nd ed.). New York: McGraw-Hill.

Heal, L.W., & Johnson, J.T., Jr. (1970). Inhibition deficits in retardate learning. In N.R. Ellis (Ed.), *International review of research in mental retardation* (Vol. 4). New York: Academic.

Ireland, W.W. (1877). *On idiocy and imbecility.* London: J. & A. Churchill.

Jacobs, P., Baikie, A., Court-Brown, W., & Strong, J. (1959). The somatic chromosomes in mongolism. *Lancet, 1*, 710.

Joseph, M.C., & Parrott, D. (1958). Severe infantile hypercalcaemia with special reference to the facies. *Archives of Disease in Childhood, 33*, 385–395.

Junkala, J. (1977). Teacher assessments and team decisions. *Exceptional Children, 44*, 32–38.

Kahn, J.V. (1985). Evidence of the similar-structure hypothesis controlling for organicity. *American Journal of Mental Deficiency, 89*, 372–378.

Kaufman, A., & Kaufman, N. (1983). *K-ABC Kaufman Assessment Battery for Children.* Circle Pines, MN: American Guidance Services.

Kephart, N.C., & Strauss, A.A. (1940). A clinical factor influencing variations in IQ. *American Journal of Orthopsychiatry, 10*, 343–350.

Kopp, C. (1983). Risk factors in development. In P. Mussen (Ed.), *Handbook of child psychology.* Vol. 2, *Infancy and developmental psychobiology.* New York: Wiley.

Kounin, J. (1941). Experimental studies of rigidity: II. The explanatory power of the concept of rigidity as applied to feeble-mindedness. *Character and Personality, 9*, 273–282.

Krakow, J., & Kopp, C. (1982). Sustained attention in young Down syndrome children. *Topics in Early Childhood Special Education, 2*, 32–42.

Leifer, J., & Lewis, M. (1984). Acquisition of conversational response skills by young Down Syndrome and nonretarded young children. *American Journal of Mental Deficiency, 88*, 610–618.

Leland, H. (1969). The relationship between intelligence and mental retardation. *American Journal of Mental Deficiency, 73*, 533–535.

Lewin, K. (1936). *A dynamic theory of personality.* New York: McGraw-Hill.

Lewis, E.O. (1933). Types of mental deficiency and their social significance. *Journal of Mental Science, 79*, 298–304.

Lewis, V. (1987). *Development and handicap.* New York: Blackwell.

Lubbs, H.A. (1969). A marker-X chromosome. *American Journal of Human Genetics, 21*, 231–244.

Lubs, M.L.E., & Maes, J. (1977). Recurrence risk in mental retardation. In P. Mittler (Ed.), *Research to practice in mental retardation* (Vol. 3). Baltimore: University Park.

Luria, A. (1963). *The mentally retarded child.* New York: Pergamon.

MacMillan, D.L. (1977). *Mental retardation in school and society.* Boston: Little, Brown.

MacMillan, D.L. (1982). *Mental retardation in school and society* (2nd ed.). Boston: Little, Brown.

Martin, N.A., Snodgrass, G., & Cohen, R. (1984). Idiopathic infantile hypercalcaemia – A continuing enigma. *Archives of Disease in Childhood, 59*, 605–613.

Milgram, N.A. (1969). The rationale and irrationale of Zigler's motivational approach to mental retardation. *American Journal of Mental Deficiency, 73*, 527–532.

Mosley, J.L. (1980). Selective attention of mildly mentally retarded and nonretarded individuals. *American Journal of Mental Deficiency, 84*, 568–576.

O'Connor, N., & Hermelin, B. (1959). Discrimination and reversal learning in imbeciles. *Journal of Abnormal and Social Psychology, 59*, 409–413.

Pearson, K. (1931). On the inheritance of mental disease. *Annals of Eugenics, 4*, 362.

Pearson, K., & Jaederholm, G.A. (1914). *On the continuity of mental defect.* London: Delau & Co.

48   J.A. BURACK

Penrose, L. (1949). *The biology of mental defect.* New York: Grune & Stratton.
Penrose, L. (1954). *The biology of mental defect.* London: Sidgwick & Jackson.
Penrose, L. (1963). *The biology of mental defect.* London: Sidgwick & Jackson.
Pueschel, S. (1983). The child with Down Syndrome. In M. Levine, W. Carey, A. Crocker, & R. Gross (Eds.), *Developmental pediatrics.* Philadelphia: Saunders.
Pueschel, S., Gallagher, P., Zartler, A., & Pezullo, J. (1987). Cognitive and learning processes in children with Down syndrome. *Research in Developmental Disabilities, 8,* 21–37.
Scheerenberger, R.C. (1983). *A history of mental retardation.* Baltimore: Brookes.
Spitz, H. (1963). Field theory and mental deficiency. In N. Ellis (Ed.), *Handbook of mental deficiency.* New York: McGraw-Hill.
Stephen, E., & Hawks, G. (1974). Cerebral palsy and mental subnormality. In A.M. Clarke & A.D.B. Clarke (Eds.), *Mental deficiency: The changing outlook.* New York: Free Press.
Strauss, A.A., & Lehtinen, L.E. (1947). *Psychopathology and education of the brain-injured child.* New York: Grune & Stratton.
Tarjan, G. (1959). Prevention, a program goal in mental deficiency. *American Journal of Mental Deficiency, 64,* 4–11.
Tarjan, G. (1960). Research in mental retardation with emphasis on etiology. *Bulletin of the Menninger Clinic, 24,* 57–69.
Tarjan, G. (1970). Some thoughts on socio-cultural retardation. In H.C. Haywood (Ed.), *Social-cultural aspects of mental retardation: Proceedings of the Peabody–NIMH Conference.* New York: Appleton-Century-Crofts.
Thomson, G.H. (1953). *Social implications of the 1947 Scottish method survey.* London: University of London Press.
Tredgold, A.F., (1908). *A textbook of mental deficiency.* London: Bailliere, Tindall, & Cox.
Udwin, O., Yule, W., & Martin, M. (1987). Cognitive abilities and behavioural characteristics of children with idiopathic infantile hypercalcaemia. *Journal of Child Psychology and Psychiatry, 28,* 297–309.
Wechsler, D. (1944). *The measurement of adult intelligence.* Baltimore: Williams & Wilkins.
Weisz, J.R., & Yeates, K.O. (1981). Cognitive development in retarded and nonretarded persons: Piagetian tests of the similar structure hypothesis. *Psychological Bulletin, 90,* 153–178.
Zeaman, D., & House, B.J. (1963). The role of attention in retardate discrimination learning. In N.R. Ellis (Ed.), *Handbook of mental deficiency.* New York: McGraw-Hill.
Zeaman, D., & House, B.J. (1979). A review of attention theory. In N.R. Ellis (Ed.), *Handbook of mental deficiency, psychological theory and research.* Hillsdale, NJ: Erlbaum.
Zigler, E. (1967). Familial mental retardation: A continuing dilemma. *Science, 155,* 292–298.
Zigler, E. (1969). Developmental versus difference theories of mental retardation and the problem of motivation. *American Journal of Mental Deficiency, 73,* 536–556.
Zigler, E., Balla, D., & Hodapp, R.M. (1984). On the definition and classification of mental retardation. *American Journal of Mental Deficiency, 89,* 215–230.
Zigler, E., & Cascione, R. (1984). Mental retardation: An overview. In E.S. Gollin (Ed.), *Malformations of development.* New York: Academic Press.
Zigler, E., & Hodapp, R. (1986). *Understanding mental retardation.* New York: Cambridge University Press.

3   One road or many? Issues in the similar-sequence hypothesis

Robert M. Hodapp

Workers interested in children's behavior have long disagreed about the idea that there is one, fixed, and invariant sequence of development in any particular domain. On the one hand, workers such as Piaget (1954), Kohlberg (1969), and Slobin (1970) and Lenneberg (1967) have argued that there are invariant sequences in cognition, morality, and language, respectively. From observations of children from one culture or a small set of cultures, these workers have asserted that their particular sequences of development constitute the single orderings of achievements that lead to more adaptive and higher-level functioning. Some have even argued that the search for so-called universals in development is the true mission of the developmental psychologist.

On the other hand, the quest for universals has been derided as simplistic by certain workers interested in cross-cultural (Shweder, 1984) and atypical (Switzsky, Rotatori, Miller, & Freagon, 1979) development. These workers have asserted that there are many roads to the same end point, that development is variable and individualized across children. For example, behaviorists argue that environmental conditions should be able to guide change in a number of directions – that is, in the appropriate rearing environment, any particular child could be made into "a doctor, lawyer, artist, merchant-chief and yes, even into a beggar-man and thief" (Watson, 1926, p. 10). Other workers have emphasized that the speed of development is strongly influenced by the environment (Hunt, 1980), and even that developmental sequences and end points differ from one culture to another (Miller, 1986). Dewey (1920) and his modern adherents (e.g., Kessen, 1984) have gone so far as to question whether universal development exists, whether all "development" solely involves the processes by which children come to be imbued with the values and behaviors of the local adult culture.

The issue of universal development versus more contextual or individual development is in part a difference in personal orientation among workers

49

interested in children. Like many scientific disciplines, the field of child development can be divided into "lumpers" and "splitters" (Breslow, 1986) – those searching for more general scientific laws and those examining smaller, more specific, and context-dependent manifestations of a particular phenomenon. Thus, lumpers emphasize that all children from all cultures undergo similar changes from infancy to adulthood, that children everywhere get bigger, stronger, more verbal, and more intelligent. They are "struck by ... the orderliness, sequentiality, and apparent lawfulness of the transition taking place from the birth or conception of the organism to the attainment of maturity" (Zigler, 1963, p. 344). The splitters, meanwhile, emphasize the diversity among different children, different cultures, and among definitions of "the highest level of development" from one culture to another. These workers tend to deemphasize structural, or more abstract, commonalities across cultures, noting that "the more we attend to surface content, the less common is the culture of man" (Shweder, 1984, p. 48). Their mission is to explain the within-system workings of specific cultural "frames," and the ways in which these culture-specific world views get passed on to children within each particular culture.

The issue of universal development versus individual development also has important implications when examining the functioning of retarded individuals. In particular, the possibility of universal sequences of development has provided both researchers (Weisz, Yeates, & Zigler, 1981; Woodward, 1979; Zigler & Hodapp, 1986) and interventionists (e.g., Dunst, 1980; McLean & Snyder-McLean, 1978) with an important vantage point onto the functioning of retarded persons. At the same time, a focus on those aspects of development that are not universal – that differ from individual to individual or from culture to culture – permits a view of retarded development that uses the theories, knowledge, and research strategies of normal development, but that recognizes the individuality of each retarded (and nonretarded) child.

This chapter will therefore attempt to balance these two perspectives – universal and individual development – even as its goal is to evaluate universal developmental sequences. It will begin with a discussion of whether universal sequences of development exist, whether retarded (or any) children proceed from step A to B to C in a single, universal, and invariant order. The reasons why such sequences might be expected, why they might not be, and a preliminary guess as to which ages and domains show universal sequences will all be considered. A brief review of studies on the similar-sequence hypothesis with mentally retarded children will then be presented. The chapter will conclude with a general discussion of the advantages and limitations of applying the similar-sequence approach to studying and intervening with retarded children.

Theoretical rationale for and against universal sequences

Arguments in favor of universal sequences

There are at least four reasons to expect that there might be universal sequences of development in any of several domains. The first concerns biological development, and the relationship between certain sorts of psychological functioning and the child's biological development. This relationship can be shown either as an analogy between different types of development or as an actual dependence of one type of development on another. In the original developmental metaphor, the idea of differentiation and hierarchic integration (e.g., Werner, 1948) was considered to be analogous to processes of development found in embryology and other fields, such as neurophysiology, physiological psychology, and neurobiology (see Cicchetti, 1986). The argument is simply that psychological development becomes more complex in a way that is analogous to the developmental progressions seen in biological development; all development, according to this view, "proceeds from a state of relative globality and lack of differentiation to a state of increasing differentiation, articulation, and hierarchic integration" (Werner, 1957, p. 126). The communicative progression from single words signifying complete sentences ("holophrases") to individual words organized within sentences (Werner & Kaplan, 1963) is an example of this movement from global and undifferentiated to differentiated and hierarchically organized, but there are other examples. This progression (called the "orthogenetic principle" by Werner) is thought to characterize all instances of development, in all living systems.

The relationship between biological development and psychological development can also be seen directly, as much psychological development seems directed or channeled by biological constraints. Piaget (1954) has documented how the earliest reflexes of the infant come to be differentiated one from another, coordinated, and, eventually, come under conscious control. At slightly older ages (i.e., at about 10 months), the child is able to coordinate attention to another person, a desired object, and a gesture (pointing, showing, vocalization), thereby allowing for intentional communication (Bates, Camaioni, & Volterra, 1975). In reviewing the literature on infant intelligence, Scarr-Salapatek (1975) has proposed that many developments within the infancy period are highly canalized – that is, they are set to occur in a biologically predisposed manner that is very difficult to deflect (see also McCall, 1981). At least for some periods of time and for some areas of development, then, psychological development is thought to be dependent upon biological constraints.

A second reason for universal sequences involves logic. As Flavell (1972) notes, one of the relationships between two subsequent behaviors is inclusion, such that the earlier behavior (behavior A) is embedded in a later behavior (behavior B). An infant will be unable to perform sensorimotor stage IV object permanence (i.e., uncovering an object hidden under a screen) without first being able to perform visual tracking of objects (sensorimotor stage II) (Uzgiris & Hunt, 1975). Similarly, Flavell notes that later behaviors are often modifications of earlier ones – for example, the infant's uncoordinated swiping at objects eventually changes to an ability to smoothly reach out and grasp the desired object (Uzgiris, 1987). Other relationships, such as the addition and coordination of one behavior to an already existing behavior (addition) also occur, with the logical prediction that the behavior composed of fewer components will develop before the behavior with a greater number of components. In each of these cases, some behaviors are logically easier than others, and children in every culture and with varying developmental disabilities might be expected to perform the easier before the harder task.

A third argument for universal sequences involves human information-processing capacities and the nature of the world. Humans in every culture share a certain (albeit difficult to define) humanity, and the world has certain laws and relationships that transcend culture, geography, or language. Consistent with the orienting response of newborns, young children are more likely to notice (Graham & Jackson, 1970) and talk about (Snyder, 1978) novel objects and events than old ones. Thus, the finding that one- and two-word utterances encode novel information (Greenfield & Smith, 1976) should hold true for all children, in all cultures. Similarly, all children should speak of the "here and now" in their first sentences, with language describing past, future, abstract, and hypothetical events developing only at later ages. Given the need of all human beings to discuss the manner in which the world works, all languages contain sentences involving actors, actions, and objects (Fillmore, 1968; Hockett, 1960); simple sentences involving these case relations appear to characterize the first sentences in every language (Brown, 1973; Slobin, 1972). Common ways of processing information and of experiencing the world should lead to universal sequences of development.

A fourth reason for universal sequences involves possible environmental similarities across different cultures. At the most basic level, all environments are similar in that societies everywhere must take care of young children enough so that they survive. Beyond this obvious cross-cultural similarity, various workers have postulated more interesting similarities across environments. Kenneth Kaye (1982) proposes that the "burst-pause" rhythm of early breastfeeding (mothers quietly holding the baby during the sucking portion of breastfeeding, but jiggling and talking to the infant during pauses) might be universal; this interactive behavioral pattern might also, according to Kaye, constitute the original "conversation" between mothers and their children. Within Western cultures, mothers do seem to demonstrate behaviors appropriate to the child's level of ability. They utter shorter and simpler sentences to children just beginning to produce language, and provide more advanced language only when children's skills develop (e.g., Phillips, 1973; Snow, 1972; see Rondal, 1985, for a review). Thus, in addition to possible biological and logical constraints forcing development in one and only one direction, there may be certain environmental similarities across cultures that foster development along universal stages.

Arguments against universal sequences

There are also several reasons to doubt the existence of universal sequences of development. The first – a counterargument to the first argument for universal sequences – is that there are many domains of development that can best be characterized as nonbiological. In discussing the concept of epigenesis in developmental psychology, for example, Kitchener (1978) notes that there are many domains in which there will probably be no genetically based program guiding development. "It seems implausible to claim ... that moral development has a developmental program resident in the genes, for it is precisely in areas such as moral development that social and cultural factors play an essential role – you cannot have ego and moral development without interpersonal relations ..." (p. 157). This effect of the environment on moral development goes beyond its influence as a material condition (as air is for life) or as a factor affecting the speed of developmental change, a role that even the most maturationist of thinkers (e.g., Gesell, 1934) allows for the environment. There may be some domains for which biologically based developmental models are not appropriate.

A second counterargument to universal sequences involves the possibility that many areas of development do not possess necessary sequences based on logic, human processing constraints, or on real-world considerations. The best candidates for such nonbiological, or cultural, domains involve those areas of "nonrationality" (Shweder, 1984) that are separate from pure cognition or language per se. For instance, it has been difficult to smoothly apply Kohlberg's (1969) stages of moral development to non-Western cultures (Simpson, 1974), as these groups appear to hold sets of values, beliefs, and explanations for human action that differ from those held in Western countries. Buck-Morss (1975) has criticized even the idea that Piagetian cognitive development is universal, arguing that Piaget's distinction between the formal structure and the content of one's thought is valued predominantly in industrialized societies. At the very least, it would seem that there are certain domains that are strongly influenced by contextual factors, and that the wide differences across cultures should make universal sequences problematic in these areas.

This interest in cultural factors signifies a changing emphasis from universal development to a focus on development in context. Although the best known of this work examines children's development within families (Bronfenbrenner, 1979; Kaye & Furstenberg, 1985) and other environments, there has also been a movement to examine the value systems of the developmentalists themselves. In this regard, Wertsch and Youniss (1987) argue that researchers studying the development of children are very much affected by the sociohistorical context and cultural surroundings in which they live. They note by way of example the divergent histories of developmental psychology in the United States and the Soviet Union, and how the larger issue of building a nation in both countries has had profound implications for each society's views of development. Other developmentalists are similarly interested in one or another type of context (Bronfenbrenner, Kessel, Kessen & White, 1986). Although universal development continues to be an important area of study, workers are noting that contextual factors influence both how the child develops and how the child is conceptualized as developing.

Finally, the degree of cross-cultural similarity across child-rearing environments has recently been called into question. Ochs and Schiefflin (1984) have argued that even such a basic "universal" as adult input language to children may not in fact occur in all cultures (although see Ferguson, 1978, for an overview of findings that "in every speech community people modify their speech when talking to young children," p. 203). Furthermore, John-Steiner and Souberman (1978), in reviewing Vygotsky (1962, 1978), note that "different patterns of interaction may lead to radically different outcomes in development" (p. 126). To the extent that this is true, and assuming that there is little or no consistency in the environment of different cultural groups, one would expect few environmentally induced instances of universal development.

Integrating universal and nonuniversal development

One way to reconcile the data showing both universal and nonuniversal domains in development is to follow Vygotsky (1962; 1978) in differentiating between "natural" (biologically based) lines of development, and "cultural" (higher-level) developmental lines. At the earliest ages (and in reference to less culturally based achievements), developments would predominantly be of the first kind – under the control of biological processes. These natural functions, although receiving less weight (or attention) by Vygotsky, consist of those early developments that occur in all cultures, along an invariant universal sequence. In his review of Vygotsky, Wertsch (1985) nominates Piagetian sensorimotor development as one area of natural development. Later achievements, such as the development of internalized language, social cognition, and morality, occur along the cultural line of development; as such, they require for their appearance interpersonal contact with adult members of the culture, and are more variable in occurrence and in sequence across different societies. At all times, the two lines are separate but interacting, but one or the other line might take precedence at different periods in the child's life.

With the additional idea that there may be some domains (e.g., social–moral) that are *more* dominated by cultural influences and others (e.g., cognition) that are *less* so, this formulation of biology into culture seems to account for the relevant findings. It does appear that the earliest cognitive (Dasen, 1972) and linguistic (Slobin, 1972) achievements follow a universal sequence of stages; later achievements in either area may not so closely follow universal sequences. Even in some areas that are heavily dependent on culture, young children's less-sophisticated cognitive abilities may make early – but not later – developments universal. Miller (1986) has shown, for example, that when judging the reasons given to explain another's social or antisocial behavior, 8-year-old Indian and American children give identical types of concrete, instance-oriented explanations. At later ages, responses in the two cultures diverge, with Indians providing more contextual explanations for human actions, whereas Americans give more traitlike attributional responses. Thus, we see an interplay between the degree to which a domain is biological and the age of the child; earlier behavior in more biologically dependent domains will show more universal sequences, whereas later behavior in more culturally dependent domains are likely to be culturally distinct.

It should be noted that the movement from biology to culture does not imply that cultural factors are lacking from early development or, conversely, that biological factors are missing from later development. Concerning the first issue, anthropologist Theodore Schwartz (1981) has criticized much of developmental work as examining a "pristine" child who only comes into contact with environmental forces at later ages. Yet, recent work on mother–infant interaction (Bruner, 1978; Hodapp, Gold-field & Boyatzis, 1984; Kaye, 1982) highlights the idea that there is an adult "scaffold" supporting and encouraging infant development, at least for Western children. From the opposite perspective, Bronfenbrenner (1986) notes that in most developmental work, "once we get beyond early childhood, genetics and biology are forgotten; indeed, the notion of a complex, integrated organism is forgotten" (p. 1219) in most studies of older children. It seems clear that both biology and culture act on the organism in numerous ways throughout early and later development.

Still, at least for heuristic purposes, it is possible to distinguish between early and later development and between domains that are more and less biological. Granted, such an approach muddles domains such as language, in which ample numbers of biological and cultural forces are operating. These distinctions do, however, serve to acknowledge the role of cultural factors and of "context-specific" changes in childhood; at the same time, universal sequences in development and the accumulated data over the past quarter century are retained in developmental work.

The similar-sequence hypothesis in relation to mentally retarded children

In the preceding discussion of universal sequences, most findings were taken from the cross-cultural literature. The assumption was that if development proceeds in the same sequence across widely divergent cultures, then (literal) evidence for universals has been demonstrated. Weisz (1978) has called this the problem of transcontextual validity, noting that this form of validity is demonstrated when "a developmental principle can be shown to hold good across physical and cultural setting, time, or cohort" (p. 2). In the next section, the issue of universal sequences of development is further expanded to include retarded children.

As discussed in earlier chapters, the rationale for conceptualizing retarded children within a developmental framework has long been debated within the field of mental retardation. A first set of workers has assumed that all retardation involves one or another set of particular defects. These defects – in verbal mediation (Luria, 1963), attention (Zeaman & House, 1979), or some other circumscribed area – have been thought to characterize functioning in all retarded individuals. As a result, it is hypothesized that retarded children differ in their development from nonretarded individuals. Another set of workers emphasizes the importance of normal development as a vantage point from which to view functioning in retarded persons (e.g., Zigler, 1967; 1969). They hypothesize that mentally retarded children develop in the same way as nonretarded children, albeit at a slower rate. From this debate, two questions arise: (1) Do retarded children traverse the same sequences of developments as those traversed by nonretarded children (the similar-sequence hypothesis)?, and (2) Do retarded children, when matched with nonretarded children on overall mental age, demonstrate identical performance on Piagetian, information processing, or other cognitive tasks (the similar-structure hypothesis)? Both questions involve empirically testable hypotheses about the similarity or difference of retarded children compared with their nonretarded peers.

Even within the developmental camp itself, workers have disagreed about the applicability of the developmental perspective to all types of retarded individuals. In Zigler's (1967; 1969) original formulation, only those persons showing no organic etiology (the so-called familial or cultural–familial retarded person) were considered to show similar sequences and structures to those of nonretarded individuals; those children showing clear organic etiologies for their retardation were excluded from the original developmental formulation. Although later workers (e.g., Beeghly & Cicchetti, 1987; Cicchetti & Beeghly, in press; Cicchetti & Pogge-Hesse, 1982; Hodapp & Zigler, in press) have attempted to apply the developmental perspective to both organically and nonorganically retarded individuals, its original application was more delimited.

With this abbreviated background as a starting point, the review that follows focuses on the similar-sequence hypothesis as it affects all retarded individuals. Following a brief overview of the Weisz and Zigler (1979) findings, recent studies will be described more fully. In line with the focus of this chapter, studies of development in retarded children will be reviewed both to see if they show a similar sequence of developments to those shown by nonretarded children, and to contrast earlier and more biologically based developments with sequences shown in later and more culturally based areas. In this way, we can use evidence from studies of retarded children to judge the degree of transcontextual validity for different types of supposedly universal sequences in various domains.

The Weisz and Zigler review (1979)

In evaluating data on the similar-sequence hypothesis for retarded children, Weisz and Zigler (1979) summarized a host of studies from the 1940s until the late 1970s. Even though they restricted their review to examinations of the performance of mentally retarded children on Piagetian-based tasks, a wide variety of tasks was examined. Studies included tests of sensorimotor spatial concepts, object permanence, causality, imitation, affective responding, identity and equivalence conservation (of many properties), seriation, transitivity, moral reasoning, comparison processes, time, space, relative thinking, role-taking, mental imagery, geometric concepts, and classification and inclusion. All together, 28 cross-sectional and three longitudinal studies were reviewed.

Across both the cross-sectional and longitudinal studies, evidence was amassed demonstrating that retarded children traverse the same sequences of development as shown by nonretarded children. In cross-sectional studies, children with higher mental ages passed items at a higher level than did lower-MA children, and rank orderings of items (i.e., percentages of the sample passing each item) were identical to the rankings predicted from Piagetian theory. More importantly, Guttman (1950; Green, 1956) scalogram analyses indicated that for individual children, the passing of higher-level items generally implied the passing of all lower-level items. Similarly for the three longitudinal studies, development seemed to follow universal sequences, such that children performed higher-level behaviors only when they were older; as younger children, they could perform only lower-level behaviors. Although more will be mentioned about scaling and longitudinal studies versus cross-sectional studies, suffice it to say that Weisz and Zigler (1979) concluded that the similar-sequence hypothesis – the idea that retarded children traverse the same sequences of development as shown by nonretarded children – held up across all types of Piagetian tasks.

Weisz and Zigler (1979) also contrasted the extent to which familial and organically retarded persons showed similar sequences in development. In general, both organically and familial retarded children traverse the same universal, invariant sequences as do nonretarded children. The single possible exception to this finding involved children with seizure disorders in addition to their retardation. For these children, evidence of the sequential nature of development was unclear, occurring in some studies, but being absent in others. All other etiological groups showed similar sequences to those found in nonretarded children. The finding of similar sequences of development across all types of organically (and familial) retarded individuals allows for a more "liberal" developmental approach' (Cicchetti & Pogge-Hesse, 1982) than Zigler's (1969) original formulation, at least in terms of the similar-sequence hypothesis.

Contrasting earlier, biologically based and later, culturally based developments in retarded children

In entertaining the hypothesis that early and biologically based developments are more likely to be sequential in their courses of development compared with later, more cultural achievements, it is easiest to examine the two extremes. Concerning psychological functioning, these extremes consist of cognitive sensorimotor development, as described by Piaget (1954), and moral development, as described by Kohlberg (1969), Piaget (1962), and others. Although arguments have been made both for the influence of environmental forces on infant development (Hunt, 1971) and for the underlying structural universality of moral development (Kohlberg, 1971), these two concepts seem most dissimilar in terms of domains that occur earlier and are more biologically based compared with those occurring later, with greater influence coming from environmental factors. The degree of sequentiality of the development of retarded children in these two areas should therefore vary enormously.

Sensorimotor cognitive development during the infancy period has been described by Piaget (1954) as progressing along six substages in each of six domains. The six substages are thought to occur in an invariant order; they proceed from reflexive movements soon after birth, through symbolic and insightful behaviors at about 2 years of age. More importantly, behaviors at each substage are thought to reflect the child's underlying concepts or understanding of the world.

The six domains involve the most basic of all human skills. *Object permanence*, probably the best-known sensorimotor domain, involves the increasing ability to understand that objects continue to exist when outside one's visual field. Vocal and gestural imitation (*imitation*), understanding of basic *spatial relations*, human causality (*causality*), *means–ends relationships* (i.e., the ability to use one object as a means to obtain another object), and appropriate uses of common objects (*symbolic uses*) constitute the remainder of the six Piagetian sensorimotor domains. Tests of these domains have been devised by Uzgiris and Hunt (1975), Casati and Lezine (1968), and Corman and Escalona (1968).

Restricting the analysis only to cross-sectional studies, it is not immediately so clear that retarded children show lower-level items if they show later items, the basic test for scalability. Reviewing a series of studies by himself and others, Kahn (1987) notes that only the domain of object permanence has been shown to be ordinal when examined according to Guttman procedures. The problem, however, may be methodological. It may be the case that the most widely used Piagetian infant test – the Ordinal Scales of Infant Development (Uzgiris & Hunt, 1975) – is ordinal in that infants (and, presumably, mentally retarded children) progress in an invariant sequence, but that the presence of one item does not necessarily imply the presence of all lower-level items. Some items build on prior items, such that the child who can uncover an object completely hidden under one screen can also uncover a partially hidden object. But other items are superseded by higher-level items. Thus, the ability to give a wind-up toy to an adult to rewind replaces the lower-level causality behavior of simply banging or waving the object to keep it functioning. In statistical terms, the Ordinal Scales combine items that are additive (i.e., Guttman-like) with those that are disjunctive (item A drops out once item B is achieved), making cross-sectional analyses difficult (Uzgiris, 1987). Not surprisingly, the evidence is contradictory about whether retarded children show scalable attainments of Piagetian sensorimotor developments using purely cross-sectional data.

Examining the few studies that longitudinally test sensorimotor developments in retarded children, the evidence is less murky. Cicchetti and Sroufe (1976) and Cicchetti and Mans-Wagener (1987) found that many sensorimotor developments are scalable across time. When Down syndrome children in their studies were tested six times throughout the first 2 years of life, average scale scores increased on each of the six domains at each successive test (see Cicchetti & Mans-Wagener, 1987, Table 8.1). Combining this with Cicchetti and Sroufe's (1976) earlier results showing sequentiality in early affective developments, there seems to be evidence that early development proceeds along invariant sequences.

Other studies, while not totally consistent in their findings, also point to a high degree of sequentiality in early cognitive development. Wohlhueter and Sindberg (1975) examined 1- to 6-year-old moderately to profoundly retarded children at monthly intervals over a 1-year period. They found that while there were some instances of skipping of stages and some children (generally those with EEG abnormalities) who showed variable performance from month to month, most children traversed the predicted sequence of object permanence. Items characteristic of earlier stages were passed at younger ages than those of later stages, and at least general support for the Piagetian sequence of object permanence was found with this population. Similarly, in a longitudinal study of sensorimotor development in younger retarded and at-risk children, Mundy, Seibert, and Hogan (1980) found that mean stage-scores increased with repeated testings. Comparing performance at two different times, 3 to 6 months apart, Mundy et al. (1980) found that the mean stage-level score for the Uzgiris–Hunt Scales increased for 16 children, showed no change for 5, and regressed for 3 (from Kahn, 1987). Although these scores consisted of mean scores derived from pooling across the different sensorimotor domains, there again seems fairly strong evidence of sequential development when heterogeneous samples of retarded children are examined longitudinally.

Reviewing each of these studies and adding his own data from 85 children with Down syndrome, Dunst (in press) has recently concluded that there is indeed strong evidence of ordinal acquisition of sensorimotor developments for both mixed-etiology and Down syndrome children. His evidence is drawn from four types of data:

1. Age-related changes, such that retarded children (like their nonretarded peers) acquire more difficult items in each of the six sensorimotor domains at later ages than they acquire easier items.
2. A strong relationship between the level of acquisition of sensorimotor behaviors and increasing mental ages and, for children, chronological ages.
3. Guttman scalability for most domains.
4. Most importantly, longitudinal evidence for sequential development when the same retarded children were tested from five to nine times over a span of several years.

Although Dunst notes that groups of retarded children may show more variability across domains, as well as regressions and spurts or lags at different levels of development, his overview provides support for the sequential acquisition of achievements in the six sensorimotor domains of infant development.

In contrast, studies of moral development do not show sequential development as clearly. Following Piaget (1962), Mahaney and Stephens (1974) examined whether retarded children advance along three stages of moral development – from being controlled by adult expectations to eventually having their own autonomous moral systems. Mildly retarded and non-retarded children at three age levels were examined on two occasions, 2 years apart.

Although generally supportive of sequential development, Mahaney and Stephens's results were dependent on the type of moral question asked. On questions dealing with whether an entire group should be punished for the actions of a single individual (i.e., collective responsibility), retarded children at all three age levels advanced over the 2-year span. In contrast, on questions involving the difference between the consequences of an action and the actor's intent, retarded children made either no progress or, in some cases, even regressed. They continued to interpret lying, stealing, and clumsiness in terms of their consequences, not the intent of the actor. Mahaney and Stephens (1974) suggest that the "immaturity in the judgment of intent vs. consequences in the type of situations presented in the stories tends to maintain or perhaps increase over time in retarded persons" (p. 139). Thus, although some instances of sequential development were observed in moral reasoning, there were many instances in which retarded children either stayed the same or decreased vis-a-vis Piagetian moral stages. At the very least, there was variability in terms of sequential acquisition of moral stages in this population.

In criticizing this study, Kohlberg (1974) noted that Piaget's "stages" of moral development are not true stages in that one stage is not logically higher than another. He concluded that "by way of contrast, my own moral judgment measures do define true stages and meet the criteria the Piaget measures fail to meet" (p. 142). Even concerning nonretarded development, however, this claim of sequential development for moral reasoning is open to debate (see Gilligan, 1982; Kurtines & Grief, 1974). But with no longitudinal studies directly employing Kohlberg's stages, it remains unclear whether the development of moral reasoning in retarded children is as sequential in its appearance as is early cognitive development.

It therefore seems a safe conclusion that there are some areas of development that are more sequential in nature, whereas other achievements are more variable. Earlier developments, especially in more biologically based areas, seem to show invariant sequences across cultures and with retarded children; later and more culturally determined achievements are more variable.

Applying the data and theories of nonretarded development to the retarded population

In reviewing the evidence from studies examining development both across cultures and with retarded children, there is a tendency to consider the similar-sequence issue as being of concern only to those interested in developmental theory. This view could not be further from the truth. Similar sequences are important for all sorts of interventions with retarded individuals; if one follows the dictum that normal development informs retardation work (and vice versa), the similar-sequence hypothesis is of particular interest.

Similar sequences are of immediate value in that they help designate areas that are important in development. The fact that children in all cultures and with varying impairments traverse identical sequences in early cognitive or linguistic development at least suggests the importance of these areas for human functioning. For example, the cognitive ability to use a person or object to reach a particular goal (means–ends) and to understand that people cause events to occur (causality) leads to concepts that are crucial in meeting, and getting others to meet, one's personal needs. Similarly, imitation skills (both gestural and vocal) have been implicated in both human and animal learning (Kaye, 1982; Piaget, 1954). Even the attainment of object permanence seems an important accomplishment, with Flavell (1977) commenting, "If any concept could be regarded as indispensable to a coherent and rational mental life, this one [object permanence] would be. Imagine what your life would be like if you did not believe that objects continued to exist when they left your visual field" (p. 42).

In addition to their intrinsic importance, achievements showing similar sequences in one particular area often serve as prerequisite skills to later developments in other domains. Curcio (1978) has found that for autistic children, certain levels of means–ends and causality skills, along with minimal levels of imitation, are important as prerequisite skills for the earliest intentional communication. Children who were able to use a rake as a means to reach a desired object (a sensorimotor stage V behavior) were able to make eye contact when offering objects to the teacher for help; children unable to perform sensorimotor stage V means–ends and causality behaviors either took the teacher's hand to work the object or banged the object on the table. Skill levels in other areas (e.g., object permanence) were not as closely related to the child's levels of early communication. Mundy, Seibert, and Hogan (1984) have shown that means–ends skills and the ability to use objects appropriately (e.g., to drink from a cup or hug a doll) are important prerequisites for particular communicative behaviors of developmentally delayed infants and toddlers operating at mental age levels from 8 to 13 months. Although much more work needs to be done on the issue of prerequisites, skills taught in developmental programs might be important in themselves and as prerequisites to later developments.

It may also be that the relationship between two areas of functioning is predictive of successful intervention. In comparing early cognitive and communicative development, Miller, Chapman, and Bedrosian (1977) and Mahoney and Snow (1983) propose that some children can be expected to advance more quickly in language once their cognitive level is taken into account. "That is, if a child's communication skills are lower than would be expected from his or her cognitive level, that child would be expected to learn to communicate at a relatively rapid rate. However, if a child's communication skills are in line with his or her cognitive level, the child would be expected to learn communication at a relatively slower rate" (Kahn, 1987, p. 269). Such findings, which are now only preliminary, point again to the importance of certain (usually universal) cognitive skills for the attainment of other (also usually universal) linguistic behaviors.

The evaluation of retarded individuals is also enhanced when domains that show universal sequences of development are included. For the most part, psychologists and educators currently employ psychometric instruments such as the Stanford–Binet and WISC-R to assess functioning in retarded children. These measures are useful in comparing the retarded child with others of his or her age, for determining a mental age equivalent, and for estimating an understanding of the child's cognitive functioning. Yet for severely and profoundly retarded children, psychometric measures are of only limited value. Too often, children are described as "untestable" using these instruments, and even when tested, global IQ scores or mental ages are difficult to translate into strategies of intervention. More Piagetian-based tests of early abilities are therefore useful because they provide theoretically interesting areas to be evaluated, and provide profiles of abilities across diverse sensorimotor domains. Several scales based on Piagetian sensorimotor development have been devised (e.g., Uzgiris & Hunt, 1975), and these scales have been adapted to allow the testing of retarded and otherwise handicapped children (Dunst, 1980). Results based on these scales provide interventionists with detailed descriptions of what the child can do in several areas of importance to future development.

Armed with such information, interventionists have at their disposal ready-made curricula on how to proceed in an intervention program. But because of Piaget's stage-structural model of infant development, interventionists are provided with more than simply "cookbook" approaches in their work with young retarded children. The teaching of specific behaviors per se is subordinated to attempts to foster the child's ability to understand and make use of basic concepts in the various domains. For example, whereas Piaget's idea of object permanence has generally been tested by hiding a desired object under one or more screens, there are numerous other manifestations of the object concept. Children who cry when their mothers leave the room or who laughingly uncover the mother in peek-a-boo are also thought to demonstrate object permanence. Such use of different behaviors to examine and intervene around an underlying concept illustrates Seibert's (1987) notion of "expanding one's categories" of intervention through the application of Piagetian-based sequences of development.

By analogy, optimal environments for development are implied within Piagetian-based programs. By providing problems just at or slightly above the child's current levels of ability, children themselves can presumably be prompted to structure their environments in new and higher level ways. Interventions can make use of various games (Hodapp & Goldfield, 1983) or tasklike procedures (Robinson & Rosenberg, 1987) closely tied to the child's level of functioning in any number of domains. Parents and interventionists can be taught the types of activities, styles of presentation, and levels of language best able to foster development (Bromwich, 1980; Hansen, 1984). Thus, evidence of universal sequences is indispensable for both intervention and assessment purposes.

This idea of a ready-made curriculum does, however, involve a major and somewhat controversial assumption. Even if all children (retarded and nonretarded in all cultures) show identical sequences in their developments, curricula based on developmental sequences will not necessarily be easier to teach than those based on other criteria. Consider the following statement describing the sequences of language intervention within a behaviorist program:

> Generally, the subject is first taught noun labels and then other forms of grammar. There are, however, no data to aid in deciding the proper temporal sequence for introducing various grammatic forms. The only guidelines thus far are convenience and developmental norms. (Harris, 1975, p. 571)

Clearly, a reliance on "developmental norms" (i.e., on the age at which certain behaviors generally occur) or on universal sequences of development is deemphasized in behaviorist intervention programs.

The use of developmentally based sequences, then, assumes that orderings of achievements that have been found across cultures and with retarded children are easier to implement. Intervention efforts are thought to proceed best if they go "with the grain" of the child's natural developmental processes (as shown in similar sequence studies). To date, however, there are few studies that have examined the efficacy of developmental intervention compared with other types of intervention programs for the development of young retarded children.

Finally, the idea that not all areas of development show universal sequences should not deter interventionists from employing "locally applicable" sequences to intervention work. Moral or social development may not occur uniformly across cultures, but this need not signal the exclusion of these areas by the sensitive interventionist. One could even argue that the lack of attention to culturally specific areas has hampered work with retarded children. We know very little, for example, about the degree to which retarded children adopt roles and behaviors considered to be chronologically age-appropriate in our culture. This inattention to such an obvious culturally dependent area of children's behavior needs to be addressed, and a focus on culture can highlight these issues.

Making use of the culturally specific sequences would seem, then, to be an important adjunct to work emphasizing universal sequences of development. It is also in line with those workers (e.g., Kessen, 1984; 1986) who view development as local adaptation to adult culture. Thus, although this chapter has focused predominantly on the issue of universal sequences, local and more contextual sequences can also be profitably employed. Furthermore, the use of local sequences to bring retarded children into the adult culture is an important implication of the idea of developmental psychology as a "moral science," currently proposed by Kessen and others.

In a similar vein, the lack of development sequences in some areas of development implies an acceptable, albeit more humble, vision of the developmental enterprise. Whereas developmental sequences or principles may not apply to all changes, they do apply to some important domains at certain times during childhood. Such a restricted vision of the utility of universal developmental principles – while unique in developmental work – is not new in the field of mental retardation. Historically, developmentally oriented workers have been very influential in designing interventions addressing skills in domains such as early cognition (e.g., Dunst, 1980) and language (Bricker & Bricker, 1974; MacDonald & Blott, 1974; McLean & Snyder-McLean, 1978; Miller & Yoder, 1974). At the same time, they have had little influence on the development of adaptive behaviors; in this area, adherents of behavior modification (Baker, 1984) have designed effective programs to teach toileting, grooming, and feeding behaviors to severely and profoundly retarded children. Thus, although the developmental formulation may not be all-inclusive, it continues to maintain an important role in intervention work. I would argue further that universal sequences play an important, if not all-inclusive, role in examinations of development in nonretarded children as well.

References

Baker, B. (1984). Intervention with families with young, severely handicapped children. In J. Blacher (Ed.), *Severely handicapped children and their families: Research in review*. New York: Academic Press.

Bates, E., Camaioni, L., & Volterra, V. (1975). The acquisition of performatives prior to speech. *Merrill-Palmer Quarterly, 21*, 205–226.

Beeghly, M., & Cicchetti, D. (1987). An organizational approach to symbolic development in children with Down syndrome. In D. Cicchetti & M. Beeghly (Eds.), *Symbolic development in atypical children*. San Francisco: Jossey-Bass.

Breslow, L. (1986). Lumping and splitting in developmental theory: Comments on Fischer and Elmendorf. In M. Perlmutter (Ed.), *Cognitive perspectives on children's social and behavioral development. The Minnesota Symposium on Child Psychology, 18*. Hillsdale, NJ: Erlbaum.

Bricker, W., & Bricker, D. (1974). An early language training strategy. In R. Schiefelbusch & L. Lloyd (Eds.), *Language perspectives: Acquisition, retardation, and intervention*. Baltimore: University Park Press.

Bromwich, R. (1980). *Working with parents of infants*. Baltimore: University Park Press.

Bronfenbrenner, U. (1979). *The ecology of human development*. Cambridge, MA: Harvard University Press.

Bronfenbrenner, U. (1986). Discussion. In U. Bronfenbrenner, F. Kessel, W. Kessen, & S. White (1986). Toward a critical social history of developmental psychology: A propaedeutic discussion. *American Psychologist, 41*, 1218–1230.

Bronfenbrenner, U., Kessel, F., Kessen, W., & White, S. (1986). Toward a critical social history of developmental psychology: A propaedeutic discussion. *American Psychologist, 41*, 1218–1230.

Brown, R. (1973). *A first language.* Cambridge, MA: Harvard University Press.

Bruner, J. (1978). Learning how to do things with words. In J. Bruner & A. Garton (Eds.), *Human growth and development.* Oxford, England: Oxford University Press.

Buck-Morss, S. (1975). Socio-economic bias in Piaget's theory and its implications for cross-culture studies. *Human Development, 18*, 35–49.

Casati, I., & Lezine, I. (1968). *Les etapes de l'intelligence sensori-motrice.* Paris: Les Editions du Centre de Psychologie Appliquée.

Cicchetti, D. (1986). Foreword. In E. Zigler & M. Glick, *A developmental approach to adult psychopathology.* New York: Wiley.

Cicchetti, D., & Beeghly, M. (Eds.) (in press). *Children with Down Syndrome: A developmental perspective.* New York: Cambridge University Press.

Cicchetti, D., & Mans-Wagener, L. (1987). Sequences, stages, and structures in the organization of cognitive development in infants with Down Syndrome. In I. Uzgiris & J.McV. Hunt (Eds.), *Infant performance and experience: New findings with the Ordinal Scales.* Urbana, IL: University of Illinois Press.

Cicchetti, D., & Pogge-Hesse, P. (1982). Possible contributions of the study of organically retarded persons to developmental theory. In E. Zigler & D. Balla (Eds.), *Mental retardation: The developmental-difference controversy.* Hillsdale, NJ: Erlbaum.

Cicchetti, D., & Sroufe, L.A. (1976). The relationship between affective and cognitive development in Down syndrome infants. *Child Development, 47*, 920–929.

Corman, H., & Escalona, S. (1969). Stages of sensorimotor development: A replication study. *Merrill-Palmer Quarterly, 15*, 351–361.

Curcio, F. (1978). Sensorimotor functioning and communication in mute autistic children. *Journal of Autism and Childhood Schizophrenia, 8*, 281–292.

Dasen, P. (1972). Cross-cultural Piagetian research: A summary. *Journal of Cross-Cultural Psychology, 3*, 23–29.

Dewey, J. (1920). *Reconstruction in philosophy.* New York: Holt.

Dunst, C. (1980). *A clinical and educational manual for use with the Uzgiris–Hunt Scales for infant development.* Baltimore: University Park Press.

Dunst, C. (in press). Sensorimotor development of infants with Down syndrome. In D. Cicchetti & M. Beeghly (Eds.), *Children with Down Syndrome: A developmental perspective.* New York: Cambridge University Press.

Ferguson, C. (1978). Talking to children: A search for universals. In J. Greenberg (Ed.), *Universals of human language* (Vol. 1). *Method and theory.* Stanford, CA: Stanford University Press.

Fillmore, C. (1968). The case for case. In E. Bach & T. Harms (Eds.), *Universals in linguistic theory.* New York: Holt.

Flavell, J. (1972). An analysis of cognitive-developmental sequences. *Genetic Psychology Monographs, 86*, 279–350.

Flavell, J. (1977). *Cognitive development.* Englewood Cliffs, NJ: Prentice-Hall.

Gesell, A. (1934). *Infant behavior: Its genesis and growth.* New York: McGraw-Hill.

Gilligan, C. (1982). *In a different voice.* Cambridge, MA: Harvard University Press.

Graham, F., & Jackson, J. (1970). Arousal systems and infant heart rate responses. In L. Lipsett & H.W. Reese (Eds.), *Advances in child development and behavior* (Vol. 5). New York: Academic Press.

Green, B. (1956). A method of scalogram analysis using summary statistics. *Psychometrika, 21*, 79–88.

Greenfield, P., & Smith, J. (1976). *The structure of communication in early language development.* New York: Academic Press.

Guttman, L. (1950). The basis of scalogram analysis. In S.A. Stouffer et al. (Eds.), *Measurement and prediction* (Vol. 4). Princeton, NJ: Princeton University Press.

Hansen, M. (Ed.) (1984). *Atypical infant development*. Baltimore: University Park Press.

Harris, S. (1975). Teaching language to nonverbal children, with emphasis on problems of generalization. *Psychological Bulletin, 82*, 565–580.

Hockett, C. (1960). The origin of speech. *Scientific American, 203*, 87–97.

Hodapp, R.M., & Goldfield, E. (1983). The use of mother–infant games as therapy with delayed children. *Early Child Development and Care, 13*, 27–32.

Hodapp, R.M., Goldfield, E.C., & Boyatzis, C. (1984). The use and effectiveness of maternal scaffolding in mother–infant games. *Child Development, 55*, 772–781.

Hodapp, R.M., & Zigler, E. (in press). Applying the developmental perspective to individuals with Down Syndrome. In D. Cicchetti & M. Beeghly (Eds.), *Children with Down Syndrome: A developmental perspective*. New York: Cambridge University Press.

Hunt, J.McV. (1971). Parent and child centers: Their basis in the behavioral and educational sciences. *American Journal of Orthopsychiatry, 41*, 13–38.

Hunt, J.McV. (1980). *Early psychological development and experience* (Vol. X, Heinz Werner Lecture Series). Worcester, MA: Clark University Press.

John-Steiner, V., & Souberman, E. (1978). Afterword. In L.S. Vygotsky, *Mind in Society*. Cambridge, MA: Harvard University Press.

Kahn, J. (1987). Uses of the Scales with mentally retarded populations. In I. Uzgiris & J. McV. Hunt (Eds.), *Infant performance and experience: New findings with the Ordinal Scales*. Urbana, IL: University of Illinois Press.

Kaye, K. (1982). *The mental and social life of babies*. Chicago: University of Chicago Press.

Kaye, K., & Furstenberg, F. (1985). Family development and the child [Special issue]. *Child Development, 56*(2).

Kessen, W. (1984). Introduction: The end of the age of development. In R. Sternberg (Ed.), *Mechanisms of cognitive development*. New York: Freeman.

Kessen, W. (1986). Discussion. In U. Bronfenbrenner, F. Kessel, W. Kessen, & S. White (1986). Toward a critical social history of developmental psychology: A propaedeutic discussion. *American Psychologist, 41*, 1218–1230.

Kitchener, R. (1978). Epigenesis: The role of biological models in developmental psychology. *Human Development, 21*, 141–160.

Kohlberg, L. (1969). Stage and sequence: The cognitive-developmental approach to socialization. In D. Goslin (Ed.), *Handbook of socialization theory and research*. Chicago: Rand McNally.

Kohlberg, L. (1974). Discussion: Developmental gains in moral judgment. *American Journal of Mental Deficiency, 79*, 142–146.

Kurtines, W., & Greif, E. (1974). The development of moral thought: Review and evaluation of Kohlberg's approach. *Psychological Bulletin, 81*, 453–470.

Lenneberg, E. (1967). *Biological foundations of language*. New York: Wiley.

Luria, A. (1963). Psychological studies of mental deficiency in the Soviet Union. In N. Ellis (Ed.), *Handbook of mental deficiency*. New York: McGraw-Hill.

MacDonald, J., & Blott, J. (1974). Environmental language intervention: A rationale for diagnostic and training strategy through rules, context, and generalization. *Journal of Speech and Hearing Disorders, 39*, 395–415.

Mahaney, E., & Stephens, B. (1974). Two-year gains in moral judgment by retarded and nonretarded persons. *American Journal of Mental Deficiency, 79*, 134–141.

Mahoney, G., & Snow, K. (1983). The relationship of sensorimotor functioning to children's responses to early language training. *Mental Retardation, 6*, 248–254.

McCall, R. (1981). Nature–nurture and the two realms of development: A proposed integration with respect to mental development. *Child Development, 52*, 1–12.

McLean, J., & Snyder-McLean, L. (1978). *A transactional approach to early language training.* Columbus, OH: Bobbs-Merrill.

Miller, J.F., Chapman, R., & Bedrosian, J. (1977). *Defining developmentally disabled subjects for research: The relationships between etiology, cognitive development, language, and communicative performance.* Paper presented at the Boston University Conference on Language Development.

Miller, J.F., & Yoder, D. (1974). An ontogenetic language teaching strategy for retarded children. In R. Schiefelbusch & L. Lloyd (Eds.), *Language perspectives: Acquisition, retardation and intervention.* Baltimore: University Park Press.

Miller, J.G. (1986). Early cross-cultural commonalities in social explanation. *Developmental Psychology, 22,* 514–520.

Mundy, P., Seibert, J., & Hogan, A. (1980). Reliability and validity of the ordinal scales and the Early Social-Communication Scales. In J. Seibert, P, Mundy, & A. Hogan (Eds.), *Communication research project: Year II progress report.* Report to the Bureau of Education for the Handicapped. Mailman Center for Child Development, University of Miami, FL.

Mundy, P., Seibert, J., & Hogan, A. (1984). Relationship between sensorimotor and early communication abilities in developmentally delayed children. *Merrill-Palmer Quarterly, 30,* 33–48.

Ochs, E., & Schiefflin, B. (1984). Language acquisition and socialization: Three developmental stories and their implications. In R. Shweder & R. LeVine (Eds.), *Culture theory: Essays on mind, self, and emotion.* Cambridge: Cambridge University Press.

Phillips, J. (1973). Syntax and vocabulary of mothers' speech to young children: Age and sex comparisons. *Child Development, 44,* 182–185.

Piaget, J. (1954). *The construction of reality in the child.* New York: Ballantine.

Piaget, J. (1962). *The moral judgment of the child.* New York: Collier Books.

Robinson, C., & Rosenberg, S. (1987). A strategy for assessing infants with motor impairments. In I. Uzgiris & J. McV. Hunt (Eds.), *Infant performance and experience: New findings with the Ordinal Scales.* Urbana, IL: University of Illinois Press.

Rondal, J. (1985). *Adult–child interaction and the processes of language acquisition.* New York: Praeger.

Scarr-Salapatek, S. (1975). An evolutionary perspective on infant intelligence: Species patterns and individual variations. In M. Lewis (Ed.), *Origins of intelligence.* New York: Plenum.

Schwartz, T. (1981). The acquisition of culture. *Ethos, 9,* 4–17.

Seibert, J. (1987). Uses of the Scales in early intervention. In I. Uzgiris & J. McV. Hunt (Eds.), *Infant performance and experience: New findings with the Ordinal Scales.* Urbana, IL: University of Illinois Press.

Shweder, R. (1984). Anthropology's romantic rebellion against enlightenment, or there's more to thinking than reason and evidence. In R. Shweder & R. LeVine (Eds.), *Culture theory: Essays on mind, self, and emotions.* Cambridge: Cambridge University Press.

Simpson, E. (1974). Moral development research: A case study of scientific culture bias. *Human Development, 17,* 81–106.

Slobin, D. (1970). Universals of grammatical development in children. In G.B. Flores d'Arcais & W.J.M. Levelt (Eds.), *Advances in psycholinguistics.* New York: American Elsevier.

Slobin, D. (1972). Language change in childhood and history. In J. Macnamara (Ed.), *Language learning and thought.* New York: Academic Press.

Snow, C. (1972). Mothers' speech to children learning language. *Child Development, 43,* 549–565.

Snyder, L. (1978). Communicative and cognitive abilities and disabilities in the sensorimotor period. *Merrill-Palmer Quarterly, 24*, 161–180.

Switsky, H., Rotatori, A., Miller, T., & Freagon, S. (1979). The developmental model and its implications for assessment and instruction for the severely/profoundly handicapped. *Mental Retardation, 17*, 167–170.

Uzgiris, I. (1987). The study of sequential order in cognitive development. In I. Uzgiris & J. McV. Hunt (Eds.), *Infant performance and experience: New findings with the Ordinal Scales.* Urbana, IL: University of Illinois Press.

Uzgiris, I. & Hunt, J. McV. (1975). *Assessment in infancy: Ordinal Scales of psychological development.* Urbana, IL: University of Illinois Press.

Uzgiris, I. & Hunt, J. McV. (Eds.) (1987). *Infant performance and experience: New findings with the Ordinal Scales.* Urbana, IL: University of Illinois Press.

Vygotsky, L.S. (1962). *Thought and language.* Cambridge, MA: MIT Press.

Vygotsky, L.S. (1978). *Mind in society.* Cambridge, MA: MIT Press.

Watson, J. (1926). What the nursery has to say about instincts. In C. Murcheson (Ed.), *Psychologies of 1925.* Worcester, MA: Clark University Press.

Weisz, J. (1978). Transcontextual validity in developmental research. *Child Development, 49*, 1–12.

Weisz, J., Yeates, K., & Zigler, E. (1982). Piagetian evidence and the developmental–difference controversy. In E. Zigler & D. Balla (Eds.), *Mental retardation: The developmental–difference controversy.* Hillsdale, NJ: Erlbaum.

Weisz, J., & Zigler, E. (1979). Cognitive development in retarded and nonretarded persons: Piagetian tests of the similar-sequence hypothesis. *Psychological Bulletin, 86*, 831–851.

Werner, H. (1948). *Comparative psychology of mental development* (rev. ed.). New York: Follett.

Werner, H. (1957). The concept of development from a comparative and organismic point of view. In D. Harris (Ed.), *The concept of development.* Minneapolis, MN: University of Minnesota Press.

Werner, H., & Kaplan, B. (1963). *Symbol formation.* New York: Wiley.

Wertsch, J. (1985). *Vygotsky and the social formation of mind.* Cambridge, MA: Harvard University Press.

Wertsch, J., & Youniss, J. (1987). Contextualizing the investigator: The case of developmental psychology. *Human Development, 30*, 18–31.

Wohlhueter, M.J., & Sindberg, R. (1975). Longitudinal development of object permanence in mentally retarded children: An exploratory study. *American Journal of Mental Deficiency, 79*, 513–518.

Woodward, W. (1979). Piaget's theory and the study of mental retardation. In N. Ellis (Ed.), *Handbook of mental deficiency research* (2nd ed.). Hillsdale, NJ: Erlbaum.

Zeaman, D., & House, B. (1979). A review of attention theory. In N.R. Ellis (Ed.), *Handbook of mental deficiency* (2nd ed.). Hillsdale, NJ: Lawrence Erlbaum.

Zigler, E. (1963). Metatheoretical issues in developmental psychology. In M. Marx (Ed.), *Theories in contemporary psychology.* New York: Macmillan.

Zigler, E. (1967). Familial mental retardation: A continuing dilemma. *Science, 155*, 292–298.

Zigler, E. (1969). Developmental versus difference theories of mental retardation and the problem of motivation. *American Journal of Mental Deficiency, 73*, 536–566.

Zigler, E., & Hodapp, R.M. (1986). *Understanding mental retardation.* New York: Cambridge University Press.

4 The similar-structure hypothesis and differential rate of development in mental retardation

Peter Mundy and Connie Kasari

The formulation or recognition of contrasting models is an essential process in any scientific enterprise. Just as the juxtaposition of color and line may intensify the perception of elements in a painting, so the contrast of models in science brings the fundamental principles and questions of a field of inquiry into clearer focus. Within the field of mental retardation the debate over the developmental and difference models has exemplified this process (Baumeister, 1987).

Two fundamental questions are commonly associated with this debate. The first concerns the etiology of mental retardation. Advocates of difference theories of mental retardation often maintain that mental retardation is the result of a distinct organic disturbance that leads to deficits in intellectual development. For example, Ellis and Cavalier (1982) have argued that mental retardation is presumptive evidence of organic pathology.

Alternatively, the developmental model suggests that there are two groups of mentally retarded individuals – one resulting from a distinct disturbance of physiology (e.g., Down syndrome or hydrocephaly), the other with an unknown etiology. It is assumed that for a significant number of individuals in this latter group, mental retardation results not from a distinct disturbance of organic process, but rather from natural, genetic variation in processes associated with intellectual development (Zigler, 1967; Zigler, 1982; Zigler & Hodapp, 1986).

The second question concerns the cognitive characteristics of mentally retarded individuals. The difference model assumes that all mentally retarded individuals display specific cognitive deficits that distinguish them

This chapter was prepared while Peter Mundy was on the staff of Olive View Medical Center, Sylmar, California. Preparation of the chapter was also supported by NICHD grant #31629 and NINCDS grant #30526. Appreciation is extended to Jim McKraken, Marian Sigman, and the editors of this volume for their constructive comments on the initial drafts of the chapter.

71

from the normal population (e.g. Spitz, 1982; Weir, 1967). In contrast, adherents of the developmental model agree that organically impaired individuals may display pathognomonic cognitive deficits, but suggest that those mentally retarded individuals whose abilities reflect the low end of natural variation in intellectual development should display a slowed but essentially normal course of cognitive development (Zigler, 1982). Therefore, the cognitive performance of these mentally retarded individuals is expected to be exactly the same as the cognitive performance of non-retarded individuals when equated on some measure of general cognitive developmental level (e.g., psychometric MA). This principle of the model has been called the similar-structure hypothesis (Weisz, Yeates, & Zigler, 1982).

Recently, the debate between the developmental and difference models of mental retardation has reached a significant juncture. The results of studies comparing mentally retarded and nonretarded individuals on Piagetian tasks of logical problem solving have supported the similar-structure hypothesis (Weisz & Yeates, 1981; Weisz et al., 1982). In contrast, the results of studies comparing mentally retarded and nonretarded individuals on measures of information-processing skills have not been consistent with the similar-structure hypothesis (Weiss, Weisz, & Bromfield, 1986).

These results present an obvious challenge to the validity of the developmental model (Weiss et al., 1986). The central question of this chapter is whether the developmental model provides a framework that allows for the integration of these contradictory findings. In answer to this question we propose that the model can accommodate these divergent findings if a fundamental but neglected component of the model – the differential rate hypothesis – is taken into consideration.

The similar-structure hypothesis emphasizes the similarity between the content and pattern of cognitive achievements of mildly mentally retarded and nonretarded persons (Weiss et al., 1982; Zigler & Hodapp, 1986). Nevertheless, the developmental model formally recognizes that mentally retarded persons also experience a slower rate of cognitive achievement than nonretarded persons (Zigler, 1982). This differential-rate hypothesis is a very important feature of the model, but an articulation of the nature of processes related to differential rate have heretofore received little attention.

To understand the processes that may be related to differences in rate of cognitive achievement, it is useful to return to one of the foundations of the developmental model – Piaget's stage theory of development. Piaget (1952) distinguished between cognitive functions associated with different levels of cognitive achievement and cognitive functions that play a role in mediating the rate of cognitive achievement.[1] In this chapter we suggest that incorporating this distinction into the developmental model of mental retardation enhances the model's utility. It provides a framework both for understanding the relation between the similar-structure and differential rate hypotheses, and enables the model to parsimoniously account for the disparity in recent research on the similar-structure hypothesis. We will also argue that this distinction suggests new hypotheses on the relations between Piagetian and information-processing measures of cognition and psychometric IQ.

To provide a context for this discussion, the chapter begins with a review of the basic tenets of the developmental model. Following comments on the theoretical and methodological contributions associated with this model, the importance of the differential-rate hypothesis for the prospective utility of the model is examined.

Mental retardation and the natural-variation hypothesis

Based on a polygenic model of variation in human intelligence (Gottesman, 1963), a normal distribution of human intelligence is expected with 2.3% of the population manifesting IQs within the 50–70 range. This range of intelligence coincides with the classification of "mild mental retardation" in our society (APA, 1980; Grossman, 1983). Therefore, a significant number of individuals should function in the mild range of mental retardation as the result of natural variation within the species.

However, the epidemiology of mental retardation shows that the prevalence of individuals with very low IQs (less than 50) is higher than predicted by a polygenic, normally distributed model of intelligence. This phenomenon has been explained in terms of a second distribution of intelligence comprised of individuals whose intellectual capacities have been compromised by a distinct disturbance of normal organic processes (Penrose, 1963; Zigler, 1967). The distribution of this organic group of mentally retarded individuals presumably overlaps with the low end of the normal distribution of intelligence. Thus, according to the developmental model, two groups of individuals fall within the mild range of mental retardation – those whose mental retardation is associated with organic morbidity, and

---

[1] Examples of the former include sensorimotor schemes and concrete logical operations. Examples of the latter include the reciprocal processes of accommodation and assimilation.

those whose mental retardation presumably reflects natural variation in intellectual development (see Zigler & Hodapp, 1986).

Epidemiological data currently present mixed results on the validity of the natural-variation hypothesis. Prevalence estimates of mentally retarded individuals with identifiable organic pathology have increased over the last 20 years. Zigler and Hodapp (1986) suggest that the accepted estimates of a 3 : 1 ratio favoring individuals with unknown etiology should be revised to a 1 : 1 estimate. This ratio is obtained even among mildly mentally retarded people (Blomquist, Gustavson, & Holmgren, 1981[2]; Hagberg, Hagberg, Lewerth, & Lindberg, 1981).

Advocates of the difference model may argue that the higher estimates of organic causes in mental retardation reflect the process of slowly uncovering the true nature of retardation, and that, ultimately, organic pathology will be recognized in all cases of retardation. For example, the recognition of fetal alcohol syndrome is a relatively recent event, and this unfortunate organic syndrome makes a significant contribution to the incidence of mild mental retardation (Cooper, 1987). Nevertheless, research continues to indicate that a substantial number of mildly retarded individuals fall within unknown etiology or nonorganic subgroups. For example, of the 50 children with mild mental retardation with unknown etiology identified in one recent epidemiological study, 26 had at least one parent or sibling who was of borderline or lower intelligence according to school records (Hagberg et al., 1981). That is, a significant portion of individuals with mild mental retardation displayed a familial or polygenic inheritance pattern.

In summary, the developmental model suggests that there are two distinct groups of mentally retarded individuals, and presents a methodological contribution by providing one rationale for subgrouping mildly mentally retarded individuals (Kopp & Krakow, 1982; Zigler, 1982). This rationale has been sufficiently persuasive to encourage some advocates of the difference model to include a similar two-group approach in recent research (e.g., Meador & Ellis, 1987).

The natural-variation hypothesis of the developmental model also makes a more general contribution to the study of human development. It suggests that the study of mental retardation and normal development is a reciprocal or complementary enterprise, because some forms of mental retardation may be part of normal individual variation in intellectual and cognitive development. That is, it promotes the view that information gained in the

---

[2] These studies involved Swedish samples. Estimates of the prevalence of mild mental retardation in Sweden fall well below similar estimates of prevalence in the U.S. Because this difference may reflect an assessment bias (Gallagher, 1985), the possibility exists that these studies underestimate the prevalence of mild mental retardation with unknown etiology.

attempt to understand nonorganic[3] forms of mental retardation is relevant to work in normal cognitive development and vice versa. For example, Detterman (1987) notes that the implicit position of many cognitive psychologists is that their theories should be exempt from explaining the behavior of mentally retarded people. The developmental model makes this position less tenable.

The similar-structure hypothesis

If many individuals with mild mental retardation are part of the normal distribution of intellectual development, they are likely to display a delayed but essentially normal process of cognitive development (Zigler, 1967). This logical assumption was formalized as the similar-structure hypothesis. Within a context provided by Piaget's stage theory of cognitive development, this hypothesis proposed that once a mentally retarded individual had achieved a certain cognitive stage or level, regardless of the time required for this achievement, his or her performance on cognitive tasks should be comparable with that of nonretarded individuals at the same cognitive level (Zigler, 1982).

The similar-structure hypothesis has been stated in both strong and weak terms. In the strong form of the hypothesis, mildly mentally retarded individuals should behave exactly the same as cognitive-level matched normals on *all* types of cognitive tasks including problem-solving tasks and information-processing tasks (Zigler, 1982; Weiss et al., 1986). In a weaker form of the hypothesis, the cognitive tasks on which equal performance is expected are limited to tasks measuring processes associated with reasoning and problem-solving (Zigler & Hodapp, 1986; Weisz & Yeates, 1981).

To operationalize the similar-structure hypothesis, Zigler (1967, 1969) suggested the use of psychometric mental age (MA) to estimate and match individuals on cognitive level. This use of MA for matching is another fundamental methodological contribution of the developmental model. Differences in developmental level are associated with differences in cognitive performance on a variety of tasks (Flavell, 1977). Thus, the necessity to control for developmental level often exists in comparative studies of mental retardation and other types of developmental disorders (e.g., Sigman, Ungerer, Mundy, & Sherman, 1987).

---

[3] We have focused our efforts on a discussion of nonorganic, mild mental retardation in this chapter. However, as illustrated in several chapters within this volume as well as in some of our own work (Mundy, Sigman, Ungerer, & Sherman, 1987), the reciprocal nature of the study of normal development and mental retardation is not necessarily restricted to the nonorganic subgroup, but may also involve organic subgroups of developmental disabilities.

This method of matching has been criticized as imperfect because equivalent MAs may be derived from different performance patterns on psychometric assessments (Baumeister, 1967). However, MA-matched groups of mildly retarded and nonretarded individuals exhibit few differences on the items passed or failed on the Stanford–Binet (Achenbach, 1970) and few differences on the factor scores obtained on the WISC-R (Groff and Linden, 1982).

The similar-structure hypothesis has been criticized on another methodological issue. The initial formulation of the hypothesis stated that no difference is expected between MA-matched groups of mildly retarded and nonretarded individuals (Zigler, 1982). Therefore, it seems to require for support the methodologically difficult task of proving the null hypothesis (Spitz, 1983). The pros and cons of this issue have been debated at length (Weiss et al., 1986; Zigler, 1982; also see Dar, 1987). However, an elaboration of the similar-structure hypothesis suggests a solution to this problem based on the use of two groups of retarded individuals. In this strategy, MA-matched groups of mildly retarded subjects – those who are organically impaired and those who are not – would be compared with non-retarded controls. The nonorganic mildly retarded and nonretarded individuals would not be expected to differ from each other on cognitive tasks. However, these groups would be expected to differ from MA-matched organic, mildly retarded individuals. This prediction of a nonlinear order may be tested directly, alleviating the problems associated with testing the null hypothesis. As we shall see, this type of design has recently been employed in at least one test of the similar-structure hypothesis (Kahn, 1985).

Piagetian research

Differences in research methods and the great variety of cognitive tasks used in the comparison of mentally retarded and nonretarded groups have made it difficult to isolate a few critical studies on the similar-structure hypothesis. Therefore, it has fallen to the task of research review to attempt to determine the validity of the similar-structure hypothesis. Weisz and his colleagues (Weisz & Yeates, 1981; Weisz et al., 1982) began this process with a review of studies using Piagetian tests of reasoning and problem-solving skills. Thus, this review examined the validity of the weak form of the similar-structure hypothesis noted earlier.

Weisz and Yeates (1981) used two of the basic methodological contributions of the developmental model to guide their review. First, they only selected studies that attempted to control for between-group developmental effects by matching on psychometric MA. Second, they separately examined studies involving samples that were screened for organicity and studies that included individuals with known organic impairments. This sampling method yielded 30 studies involving 104 group comparisons. These studies focused on a variety of preoperational and concrete operational cognitive processes, and most often examined the performance of children.

Weisz and Yeates pooled the data from the 104 group comparisons to determine if the number of significant differences obtained exceeded the number expected by chance. When the data from the group comparisons that did not control for organic etiology were analyzed ($N = 71$), a significantly greater number of comparisons than expected by chance favored the performance of the nonretarded children. In contrast, when the group comparisons that did attempt to control for organicity were analyzed ($N = 33$), the nonretarded children did not display a significant performance advantage.

These results support the similar-structure and two-group assumptions of the developmental model. On the two-group assumption, however, it is important to note that the mean IQs in the samples with organically impaired children were lower than in the samples excluding children with known organic impairment. Thus, IQ and organicity were confounded across these studies (Weisz & Yeates, 1981; Spitz, 1983).

Kahn's (1985) study addressed these results. He compared four groups, primarily composed of children, on tasks of moral reasoning and conservation. The four groups were matched on MA, and included a nonretarded group, a moderately retarded group, and two mildly retarded groups matched for IQ as well as MA. One of the latter was comprised of children with known organic etiology. The other group included children with no evidence of organic etiology. The results indicated that the moderate MR group and the organic, mild MR group performed worse on both the moral reasoning and conservation measures than the nonretarded group. However, the performance of the unknown etiology, mild MR group did not differ from the nonretarded group, and was significantly superior to the other MR groups on the conservation measure. Thus, this study provides additional support for the similar-structure hypothesis and the organic versus nonorganic group dichotomy of the developmental model.

Although Kahn's (1985) study supports the similar-structure hypothesis, it is important to bear in mind the limits of this literature. As we noted, it only applies to the weak form of the similar-structure hypothesis. Moreover, given a developmental perspective, it should be recognized that the studies described predominantly involved children with mental ages of between 5 and 12 years, and only apply to the preoperational and concrete operational periods as defined by Piaget (1952). They do not address the question of whether similar structure is observed when the developmental level of the groups is within the sensorimotor or formal operational stage.

Research on sensorimotor skills suggests that similar structure may be typical even among samples including children with organic disturbances (Cicchetti & Mans-Wagner, 1987; Mundy, Seibert, & Hogan, 1984; Seibert, Hogan, & Mundy, 1984). However, research also suggests that young mentally retarded children exhibit more variability across tasks within a sensorimotor stage than do nonretarded children (Dunst & Rheingrover, 1983; Morss, 1983). We are not aware of any study that clearly demonstrates similar structure in a comparison of nonretarded and nonorganic, mildly retarded children on measures of Piagetian sensorimotor skill. This is most likely because of the difficulty of identifying the latter group at a sufficiently early age. Thus, the status of the similar-structure hypothesis with respect to Piagetian sensorimotor skills remains unclear at present.

Similarly, few data are available on the formal operational capacities of mentally retarded people. The extent to which formal operational skills are expressed varies by task experience, and formal operations are not necessarily displayed even by individuals who do well on standardized tasks of intelligence (Wagner & Sternberg, 1984). These findings complicate efforts to compare the formal operational capacity of mentally retarded and nonretarded individuals. Nevertheless, this comparison appears to be an important arena for investigation. Formal operations represent the highest stage of cognitive development in Piaget's theory. Because the developmental model predicts that mildly retarded individuals will display a constrained upper limit of cognitive achievement (Zigler, 1982), this upper limit may well be apparent on tests of formal operations.

In spite of these limits of the literature, current research supports the similar-structure hypothesis when retarded and nonretarded groups are compared on Piagetian measures of cognitive skills. Piagetian measures, however, provide a measure of only one important domain of cognitive development. Information-processing measures provide an index of an alternative, but equally important domain of cognitive development (Case, 1985; Wagner & Sternberg, 1984). Therefore, to appraise the validity of the strong version of the similar-structure hypothesis, it is also necessary to examine the literature on information-processing skills among mentally retarded individuals (Weisz & Yeates, 1981). A recent survey of the literature in this area is Weiss et al., 1986.

Information-processing research

Weiss et al. (1986) identified 24 studies of mentally retarded children that employed MA-matching designs, excluded individuals with known organic impairments, and involved noninstitutionalized samples. The latter selection criterion was used to control for reduced task motivation that may be associated with institutionalization (Zigler & Balla, 1977). As was the case in Weisz and Yeates (1981), the MA of the majority of subjects in these studies ranged between 5 and 12 years. The 24 studies reviewed covered a variety of information-processing and learning tasks, including tests of memory, paired-associate learning, selective attention, discriminative learning, and incidental learning.

In contrast to the survey of Piagetian tests of the similar-structure hypothesis, Weiss et al. (1986) found that significantly more studies than expected by chance demonstrated that the mentally retarded children performed worse than MA-matched groups of nonretarded children on the information-processing tasks. Similarly, meta-analysis of the data from these studies indicated that the performance of the mentally retarded children, averaged across tasks and samples, was significantly worse than the performance of the nonretarded children. On specific skill deficits, the literature reviewed by Weiss et al. suggests that nonorganic, mentally retarded children consistently displayed deficits on discrimination tasks, distractibility/attention tasks, and especially memory tasks.

These findings appear to be inconsistent with the strong version of the similar-structure hypothesis, and therefore, present problems for the developmental position. Alternatively, they appear to be consistent with difference theories that suggest that deficits in components of information processing such as attentional or memory processes are characteristic of all mentally retarded individuals (e.g., Ellis & Cavalier, 1982). Therefore, in assessing the implication of these findings, Weiss et al. thoroughly explored alternative explanations of the apparent deficit in information-processing skills among mentally retarded children. They suggested that it would be premature to reject the similar-structure hypothesis or accept the difference position until these alternative explanations are addressed.

One alternative explanation stands out. Weiss et al. (1986) argue that extracognitive variables such as task motivation or expectancy for success may influence cognitive performance on some types of tasks (e.g., information-processing measures) more than others (e.g., Piagetian). Zigler (Zigler, 1982; Zigler & Balla, 1982) has long argued that it is necessary, from a methodological point of view, to acknowledge that mentally retarded individuals frequently differ from nonretarded individuals in task-related motivation. Lowered task motivation may occur after mentally retarded individuals experience failure experiences sufficiently often to develop a lowered expectancy for success on tasks. Thus, the process of learned helplessness may attenuate task performance even in situations where the individual has the necessary cognitive skills (Weisz,

1982). Lower task motivation among mentally retarded individuals may also be associated with the presence of psychopathology. Studies suggest that the incidence of emotional and behavioral disorder is higher within groups of mentally retarded people than in control groups (Russell, 1985). Therefore, if proper control is not exercised, interpretation of mentally retarded performance deficits on cognitive tasks may be obfuscated by the potentially confounding influence of group difference in motivation and associated phenomena.

To accept the motivational explanation espoused by Weiss et al., it would be necessary to demonstrate that variance in motivation is more closely associated with performance on information-processing tasks than on Piagetian tasks. We are not aware of any data that address this issue. However, one approach would be to compare the degree that Piagetian and information-processing task performance covaries with measures associated with the construct of motivation. In this type of study, measures of task persistence (e.g., Sigman, Cohen, Beckwith & Topinka, 1986), self-esteem (Silon & Harter, 1985), or behavioral expectations (Gibbons & Kassin, 1982) may be useful. Measures of emotional disturbance such as the depression inventories (e.g., Kovacs, 1981) or behavioral problem checklists (e.g., Achenbach & Edelbrock, 1983) may also be useful to examine the degree of covariance between task performance and indexes of psychopathology.

Although some may disagree with these findings (Anderson, 1986; Spitz, 1983), we believe that recognition of the possible effects of motivation on the task performance of mentally retarded individuals is another methodological contribution of the developmental model.[4] However, while the motivational explanation is open to empirical inquiry, recourse to motivational factors to explain the findings of Weiss et al. (1986) appears to be problematic in the light of the literature on infant information processing skills.

The effects of motivation have been tied to experience. Thus, with experience and age, the impact of lower motivation on task performance may be expected to increase among mentally retarded people compared with the nonretarded (Weiss et al., 1986; Weisz, 1982). However, group differences on measures of visual attention and information processing have been obtained even in studies of infants. In one study of children under 30 months of age, samples both of mildly retarded children with unknown etiology and of Down syndrome children displayed less well-organized

---

[4] See Mundy, Seibert, and Hogan (1985) for a related discussion of motivational and sociolinguistic factors in the development of communication skills among retarded individuals.

attentional control than an MA-matched sample of nonretarded infants (Krakow & Kopp, 1983). Other studies have demonstrated that infants at risk for developmental delays (i.e., preterm, low birth weight infants) perform more poorly than matched samples of full-term infants on measures of visual attention and discrimination in the first 6 months of life (e.g., Rose, 1983; Sigman & Parmelee, 1974). The early age at which these differences are observed presents a challenge to the motivation–experience explanation of group differences on information-processing tasks.

Motivational factors may not provide the most parsimonious explanation of the poor performance of mentally retarded individuals on measures of attention and information-processing tasks. Instead, the differences between the performance of mildly retarded individuals on Piagetian and information-processing tasks may be understood within the context of the relationship between the similar-structure hypothesis and the differential rate hypothesis of the developmental model.

The differential rate hypothesis

The developmental model predicts that MA-matched groups of nonorganic, mildly retarded and nonretarded individuals will be similar in terms of cognitive achievement or structure. However, the model also recognizes that some aspect of cognition distinguishes all individuals with mild mental retardation from individuals with higher IQs. Zigler (1967, 1982) proposed that mildly retarded individuals proceeded through the same sequence of cognitive stages as nonretarded individuals, but at a *slower rate* and with a lower final level of achievement. As Zigler (1982) stated:

> "... my developmental theory can itself be called a cognitive difference theory ... individuals of differing IQ ... differ in rate of cognitive development and upper level of achievement." (p. 167)

The importance of motivational and experiential factors as mediators of cognitive change were noted. However, in keeping with a polygenic model of determination, it was assumed that differences in rate of cognitive development reflect individual differences in genotype to a greater extent than individual differences in environment or experience (Zigler, 1982). We call this aspect of the developmental model the differential rate hypothesis.

The nature of the processes associated with differences in rate of cognitive development was not explicitly addressed in previous formulations of the developmental model. Nevertheless, an implicit but critical assumption appears to have been made in this regard. The developmental model assumed that rate of development was a maturational phenomenon, but not one that was mediated to any significant degree by cognitive functions. Hence, when level of cognitive achievement was controlled by matching individuals on MA, the variance associated with rate of development in psychometric IQ performance was not expected to affect cognitive performance (Zigler, 1982). However, as noted at the beginning of this chapter, this assumption of the developmental model is not completely consistent with its foundation in Piagetian theory.

Piaget (1952) described cognitive development in terms of stage transitions, and acknowledged the importance of maturational factors in mediating these transitions. However, he also suggested that the cognitive process of equilibration plays a fundamental role in mediating stage transitions within the individual. Equilibration involves the complementary functions of assimilation and accommodation. The former refers to the process of changing or interpreting external information in order to incorporate the information within the internal cognitive system. The latter refers to the process of changing the internal cognitive system in order to incorporate external information. Through the processes of assimilation and accommodation, Piaget envisioned individuals as active participants in their own development.

In addition to those cognitive functions that were involved in the mediation of developmental transitions, Piaget also described cognitive functions that marked the milestones of developmental achievement. These were referred to as structural elements, and reflected stage-dependent logical operations such as conservation in the concrete operational stage.

We suggest that the utility of the developmental model may be enhanced if it accommodates Piaget's notion that different cognitive functions are associated with cognitive structure and the mechanisms of developmental change. In such a modification of the model, it may be assumed that the differential rate hypothesis and the similar-structure hypothesis apply to different aspects of cognition. Moreover, it may be assumed that the cognitive factors associated with developmental rate are to some degree independent factors associated with cognitive structure. That is, individuals may vary on rate-related cognitive phenomena while not varying on the performance of stage-dependent logical operations or problem-solving skills.

The accommodation of Piagetian theory with regard to the differential rate hypothesis has a number of implications for the developmental model. On the distinction between the strong and weak forms of the similar-structure hypothesis, this interpretation of the model suggests that the weak form of the hypothesis is likely to be the more valid. That is, the similar-structure hypothesis may not apply to all aspects of cognition, but rather may apply only to some forms of cognition such as the logical operations used in problem solving.

A second implication of this modified developmental model is that it suggests that comparative research on MA-matched groups of nonorganic, mildly mentally retarded and nonretarded groups may make a valuable contribution to research on the nature of intelligence. In particular, comparisons of MA-matched mildly retarded and nonretarded individuals provide one method for isolating cognitive skills that are related to rate phenomena as opposed to structural phenomena in intellectual development.

In this context, current literature on the similar-structure hypothesis (Weiss et al., 1986; Weisz & Yeates, 1981) suggests a specific proposition about the nature of psychometric measures of intelligence. Psychometric IQ may reflect two important but partially independent components of cognitive development.[5] One component reflects level of cognitive achievement. This component is commonly indexed by estimates of mental age, and is closely associated with structural features of cognition such as the development of qualitatively different types of problem-solving skills as measured by Piagetian tasks. The second component is less closely associated with *level* of achievement and MA. Instead, this component is associated with cognitive functions that play a role in determining the rate of cognitive achievement. Moreover, these cognitive functions are apparently associated with processes indexed by performance on some types of information-processing tasks (see Weir, 1967).

These arguments may appear to some to be a rather post hoc attempt to achieve congruence between the findings of Weiss et al. (1986) and the developmental model. However, as previously noted, this modification of the model follows from Piagetian theory. In addition, this modification follows from current research on the nature of intelligence and neo-Piagetian formulations of the processes that determine cognitive development. In the next sections we turn our attention to a brief survey of this literature.

The correlates of IQ

In the preceding section it was suggested that research on the developmental model of mild mental retardation may be interpreted as indicating

---

[5] It is important to remember that in Weisz and Yeates (1981) and Weiss et al. (1986), the preponderance of the data reviewed was on the performance of children with chronological ages between 5 and 16 years. Accordingly, the suggestion made here and throughout this chapter – that a component of IQ may be related to rate of development – refers to the psychometric intelligence performance of children rather than adults.

that both Piagetian and information-processing measures of cognitive skills index important components of psychometric IQ. The current literature is consistent with this assumption.

Humphreys and Parsons (1979) have provided data on the relationship between Piagetian task performance and psychometric IQ. Using factor analysis, this re-analysis examined the relationship between performance on 27 reasoning assessments and performance on the Wechsler intelligence scale by children with a wide range of abilities. This study yielded a remarkably high estimate of the correlation between Piagetian and Wechsler composite scores (.80), suggesting that these were virtually overlapping measures of a single common factor. More recently, though, data from Carrol, Kohlberg, and Devries (1984) suggest that Piagetian measures and measures of psychometric IQ assess both common and linearly independent factors. Moreover, different types of Piagetian tasks appear to vary with respect to whether they load on a factor in common with psychometric IQ or a factor independent of IQ.

The literature also suggests that performance on information-processing tasks shares a common source of variance with psychometric IQ performance. Measures of IQ are correlated with performance on reaction-time measures of speed of execution of information-processing skills (Vernon, 1983). These findings may be attributed to the fact that IQ measures themselves often include timed task-performance measures (Sternberg, 1986). However, two studies indicate that reaction time and speed of information-processing measures correlate with both timed and untimed IQ measures (Vernon & Kantor, 1986; Vernon, Nador, & Kantor, 1985).

Studies have examined both the size of the association and the nature of the processes leading to the correlation between IQ and reaction-time measures. Nettlebeck and Kirby (1983) examined the correlations between reaction time and IQ in samples of 41 retarded and 141 nonretarded adults. The former were mildly retarded and had neither significant physical disabilities nor specific brain damage associated with retardation. Multiple correlation estimates of the variance shared between reaction-time task and IQ scale performance ranged from 20% for the retarded group to 25% for the nonretarded group. Thus, speed of information-processing measures shared a component of variance with IQ, but did not index a source of variance that is completely redundant with IQ.

About the nature of the processes that underlie these correlations, one study reports that measures of speed of processing are associated with measures of attentional control as well as with IQ (Carlson, Jensen, & Widman, 1983). Thus, attentional control may be a mediator of the relationship between reaction time or speed of information-processing measures and IQ.

The foregoing literature suggests that performance on both information-processing tasks and Piagetian problem-solving tasks are significant correlates of psychometric IQ performance. However, what is the relationship between all three types of measures? The modified developmental model, advocated here, suggests that Piagetian tasks are associated with cognitive achievement variance that is also associated with IQ scores (i.e., MA). Alternatively, information-processing tasks index a source of variance associated with rate of achievement rather than level of achievement.

This dichotomy is not necessarily absolute. Piagetian and information-processing task performance may share a significant source of variance with psychometric IQ performance. However, the current model also predicts that information-processing task performance and Piagetian task performance will display significant, independent paths of association with IQ. Moreover, information-processing task performance and Piagetian task performance may be expected to differ in their association with MA. Although performance on both types of tasks may be correlated with MA, the latter may be expected to correlate more strongly with MA than the former.

These predictions, for the most part, are currently untested. For example, the former prediction – that Piagetian and information-processing tasks display significant, independent paths of association with IQ – may be tested by examining the concurrent multiple correlations of Piagetian and information processing tasks with IQ. However, our survey of the literature failed to reveal studies that addressed this issue. Concerning the latter prediction – that Piagetian tasks correlate more strongly with MA than do information-processing tasks – one study has indicated that a measure of Piagetian sensorimotor skills was more highly correlated with MA ($r = .90$) than was a visual attention/information-processing measure ($r = .58$) in a sample of young mentally retarded children (Mundy, Seibert, Hogan, & Fagan, 1983). These data are consistent with the expectations we have noted. However, they were derived from a group of mentally retarded children that was heterogeneous with respect to organicity, thereby limiting the applicability of these data to the developmental model. Although the foregoing predictions are largely untested, they represent an important area of inquiry for the developmental model.

Mechanisms of cognitive development

The finding that concurrent measures of information-processing skills and IQ correlate is consistent with, but hardly proof of, the assumption that information-processing skills are associated with processes that mediate differences in rate of cognitive development. However, theory on the mechanisms of cognitive development and data that indicate that infant information-processing measures predict rate of cognitive development also support this assumption.

As indicated earlier, paradigms for assessing individual differences in infant attention capacity and information-processing capacity have been developed. Studies using these paradigms have shown that performance on measures administered in the first 6 months of life is a significant predictor of psychometric IQ between 2 and 8 years of age (Bornstein & Sigman, 1986; Fagan & Singer, 1983).

The predictive validity of infant information-processing measures has been demonstrated for infants at risk for developmental delays (Rose & Wallace, 1985; Sigman, Cohen, Beckwith, & Parmelee, 1986) as well as for samples of normal infants (Fagan & McGrath, 1981; Lewis & Brooks-Gunn, 1981). Of course, the predictive validity of these measures is not perfect. Most of the correlations obtained in research to date suggest that infant information-processing tasks predict between 10% and 40% of the variance in childhood IQ (Bornstein & Sigman, 1986). Moreover, as with the relationship between reaction-time measures and IQ (Carlson et al., 1983), it is not clear whether this predictive association occurs because the infant measures index efficiency of information processing or attentional control (Bornstein & Sigman, 1986). Nevertheless, these correlations suggest that processes associated with ontogenetically primary attentional or information-processing skills provide an important foundation for individual differences in the rate of development of the verbal and conceptual tasks indexed by performance on psychometric IQ.

Although it is clear that information-processing skills are associated with individual differences in rate of cognitive development, understanding the mechanisms for this association is a complex endeavor. Recently, several theorists have made progress on this issue. Especially noteworthy for the discussion here are the theorists who have developed neo-Piagetian stage theories of developmental process (Case, 1984; Fischer & Pipp, 1984). Of these, the model developed by Robbie Case is most explicit on the mechanisms of development.

Like Piaget and the developmental model of mental retardation, Case (1984, 1985) suggests that intellectual development in childhood is best conceived as a sequence of qualitative shifts in increasingly sophisticated mental structures. However, Case (1985) suggests that Piaget's constructs of accommodation and assimilation are not adequate to explain these qualitative shifts (i.e., stage transitions). Case argues that information-processing theory provides a more powerful explanatory tool. He suggests that the cognitive resources of an individual are limited, and must be divided between two functions: executing current cognitive operations, and storing or retrieving the products of operations. Using the processing space metaphor of the computer, he refers to the former as operating space and the latter as short-term storage space (STSS).

The critical proposal of Case's theory is that growth of STSS plays an important role in the regulation of stage transitions, and hence, rate of cognitive development. This growth in STSS may result from a developmental change in the size or capacity of total operating space. Alternatively, developmental decreases in the proportion of total processing space that must be devoted to executing operations (i.e., increased operational efficiency) may result in increased STSS. Case (1984, 1985) suggests that current research supports the latter explanation. Case (1985) also proposes that increased efficiency of information processing is associated with maturational changes in the central nervous system (CNS) (e.g., degree of neuronal myelination). Similarly, others have argued that cognitive stage transitions are associated with physical, maturational changes in the CNS (see Goldman-Rakic, 1987; Fischer, 1987).

Case suggests that rate of development or stage transition is determined by components of the individual's information-processing system. However, this is not to say that developments in the information-processing system occur *only* in conjunction with major stage transitions in logical operations. Instead, quantitative changes in information-processing efficiency may also occur within a stage (Case, 1985). Hypothetically, the accumulation of these within-stage changes in information-processing efficiency potentiates major stage transitions in logical operations. Thus, within major cognitive stages, individuals may differ on measures of information-processing efficiency.[6]

Case's theory may have important implications for a developmental model of retardation. His theory of change in efficiency of information processing may be heuristic with regard to attempts to explore the mechanisms of slowed rate of cognitive development among the mildly mentally retarded (see Anderson, 1986). Moreover, if Case is correct about the relationship between cognitive development, efficiency of information processing, and maturation of the CNS, an integration of Case's (1985) theory into the developmental model would suggest that mild mental re-

---

[6] Given the results of Weiss et al. (1986), attempts to integrate information-processing and stage models of cognitive development have obvious relevance for the continued growth of the developmental model of mental retardation. Extrapolating from Case's model, one possibility here is to view the development of information-processing functions as a relatively continuous process throughout childhood. Discontinuous changes or stage transitions in logical operations may be a related, but not isomorphic path of development that is superimposed upon the continuous path of change in information-processing skills.

tardation may result from natural variation in CNS processes rather than a pathological disruption of CNS processes, as suggested by some difference theorists.

Conclusion

All models and theories in science have a growth cycle in which, in response to accumulated data, they are modified. We have suggested that in order to parsimoniously account for the findings of Weisz and Yeates (1981) and Weiss et al. (1986), the developmental model may be modified. Following Piaget's (1952) theory of cognitive development, the similar-structure hypothesis may apply to a domain of cognitive development that is specific to the achievement of problem-solving skills. Alternatively, the differential rate hypothesis may apply to separate cognitive functions that mediate cognitive change. About the latter, we have noted that differences in information-processing skills may be related to individual differences across the normal distribution of psychometric IQ performance. Moreover, we have suggested that among children, some types of information-processing measures and IQ measures may share a source of variance associated with individual differences in rate of cognitive development.

This is not to say that organismic, cognitive functions are the only mechanisms of cognitive development or the only source of differences between mentally retarded individuals and nonretarded individuals. In later chapters in this volume, the important role of environmental and extracognitive factors in development and mental retardation are also discussed. Nevertheless, the assumption that cognitive functions play an important role in the complex, multivariate mechanisms of cognitive development is consistent with theory (e.g., Case, 1985; Piaget, 1952) and data on cognitive development (e.g., Bornstein & Sigman, 1986). Therefore, it is important to attempt to integrate this assumption into the framework of the developmental model of mental retardation.

If some types of information-processing skills are associated with the cognitive functions that mediate individual differences in rate of cognitive achievement, the recognition and identification of these functions is an important goal in the process of developing the most effective intervention programs for mentally retarded children. The notion of developing interventions to target information-processing skills may appear to be a daunting prospect. However, the educational implications of individual differences in information-processing skills is an arena of expanding inquiry and understanding (Case, 1985; Wagner & Sternberg, 1984).

The significant changes in fundamental assumptions of the developmental model proposed in this chapter may lead to a rapprochement with difference theorists. These changes are consistent with other efforts leading to rapprochement (Detterman, 1987) but do not simply duplicate them. Nevertheless, the modified developmental model is not indistinguishable from the difference model. In contrast to the difference position, this modification of the model continues to acknowledge the importance of the two-group approach and individual differences in motivation in research on mental retardation. It also provides a framework that emphasizes the importance of understanding the similarities as well as the differences manifested by retarded and nonretarded groups.

In this regard, the difference model suggests that MA is a relatively unimportant feature of psychometric IQ (Baumeister, 1987). However, this developmental position continues to assume that level of achievement is an important descriptor of individual cognitive functioning. It is to be expected that there will be numerous similarities between the cognitive functioning of MA-matched mildly retarded and nonretarded individuals. Therefore, a complete understanding of the differences of mildly retarded individuals will only be possible in concert with a detailed understanding of the similarities in function between mentally retarded and nonretarded children and adults.

References

Achenbach, T. (1970). Comparisons of Stanford–Binet performance of nonretarded and retarded persons matched for MA and sex. *American Journal of Mental Deficiency, 74,* 488–499.

Achenbach, T., & Edelbrock, C. (1983). *Manual for the child behavior checklist and revised child behavior profile.* Burlington, VT: University Associates in Psychiatry.

Anderson, M. (1986). Understanding the cognitive deficit in mental retardation. *Journal of Child Psychology and Psychiatry, 27,* 297–306.

APA (1980). *American Psychiatric Association Diagnostic and Statistical Manual of Mental Disorders – III.* Washington. DC.

Baumeister, A. (1967). Problems in comparative studies of mental retardates and normals. *American Journal of Mental Deficiency, 71,* 869–875.

Baumeister, A. (1987). Mental retardation: Some conceptions and dilemmas. *American Psychologist, 42,* 796–800.

Blomquist H., Gustavson, K., & Holmgren, G. (1981). Mild mental retardation in children in a northern Swedish county. *Journal of Mental Deficiency Research, 25,* 169–186.

Bornstein, M. & Sigman, M. (1986). Continuity in mental development from infancy. *Child Development, 57,* 251–274.

Carlson, J., Jensen, M. & Widman, K. (1983). Reaction time, intelligence, and attention. *Intelligence, 7,* 329–344.

Carrol, J., Kohlberg, L., & Devries, R. (1984). Psychometric and Piagetian intelligences: Toward a resolution of the controversy. *Intelligence, 8,* 67–91.

Case, R. (1984). The process of stage transition: A neo-Piagetian view. In R. Sternberg (Ed.), *Mechanisms of cognitive development* (pp. 19–44). New York: Freeman.

Case, R. (1985). *Intellectual development: Birth to adulthood.* New York: Academic Press.

Cicchetti, D., & Mans-Wagner, L. (1987). Sequences, stages, and structures in the organization of cognitive development in infants with Down syndrome. In I. Uzgiris & J. Hunt (Eds.), *Infant performance and experience* (pp. 281–310). Urbana: University of Illinois Press.

Cooper, S. (1987). The fetal alcohol syndrome. *Journal of Child Psychology and Psychiatry, 28,* 223–227.

Dar, R. (1987). Another look at Meehl, Lakatos, and the scientific practice of psychologists. *American Psychologist, 42,* 145–151.

Detterman, D. (1987). Theoretical notions of intelligence and mental retardation. *American Journal of Mental Deficiency, 92,* 2–11.

Dunst, C. & Rheingrover, R. (1983). Structural characteristics of sensorimotor development among Down's syndrome infants. *Journal of Mental Deficiency Research, 27,* 11–22.

Ellis, N., & Cavalier, A. (1982). Research perspective in mental retardation. In E. Zigler & D. Balla (Eds.), *Mental retardation: The developmental–difference controversy* (pp. 121–154). Hillsdale, NJ: Erlbaum.

Fagan, J., & McGrath, S. (1981). Infant recognition memory and later intelligence. *Intelligence, 5,* 121–130.

Fagan, J., & Singer, L. (1983). Infant recognition memory as a measure of intelligence. In L. Lipsett (Ed.), *Advances in Infancy Research* (vol. 2, pp. 31–78). Norwood, NJ: ABLEX.

Fischer, K. (1987). Relations between brain and cognitive development. *Child Development, 58,* 623–632.

Fischer, K., & Pipp, S. (1984). Processes in cognitive development: Optimal level and skill acquisition. In R Sternberg (Ed.), *Mechanisms of cognitive development* (pp. 45–80). New York: Freeman.

Flavell, J. (1977). *Cognitive development.* Englewood Cliffs, NJ: Prentice-Hall.

Gallagher, J. (1985). The prevalence of mental retardation: Cross-cultural considerations from Sweden and the United States. *Intelligence, 9,* 97–108.

Gibbons, F., & Kassin, S. (1982). Behavioral expectations of retarded and nonretarded children. *Journal of Applied Developmental Psychology, 3,* 85–104.

Goldman–Rakic, P.S. (1987). Development of cortical circuitry and cognitive function. *Child Development, 58,* 601–622.

Gottesman, I. (1963). Genetic aspects of intelligent behavior. In N. Ellis (Ed.), *Handbook of Mental Deficiency.* New York: McGraw-Hill.

Groff, M., & Linden, K. (1982). The WISC-R factor score profiles of cultural–familial mentally retarded and nonretarded youth. *American Journal of Mental Deficiency, 87,* 147–152.

Grossman, H. (Ed.) (1983). *Manual on terminology and classification in mental retardation.* (3rd rev.). Washington, DC: American Association on Mental Deficiency.

Hagberg, B., Hagberg, G., Lewerth A., & Lindberg, U. (1981). Mild mental retardation in Swedish school children. *Acta Paediatrica Scandinavia, 70,* 445–452.

Humphreys, L., & Parsons, C. (1979). Piagetian tasks measure intelligence and intelligence tests assess cognitive development: A re-analysis. *Intelligence, 3,* 369–382.

Kahn, J. (1985). Evidence of the similar-structure hypothesis controlling for organicity. *American Journal of Mental Deficiency, 89,* 372–378.

Kopp, C., & Krakow, J. (1982). The issue of sample characteristics: Biologically at risk or developmentally delayed infants. *Journal of Pediatric Psychology, 7,* 361–374.

Kovacs, M. (1981). Rating scales to assess depression in school aged children. *Acta Paedopsychiatrica, 46,* 305–315.

Krakow, J., & Kopp, C. (1983). The effects of developmental delay on sustained attention in young children. *Child Development, 54,* 1143–1155.

Lewis, M., & Brooks-Gunn, J. (1981). Visual attention at three months as a predictor of cognitive functioning at two years of age. *Intelligence*, 5, 131–140.

Meador, D., & Ellis, N. (1987). Automatic and effortful processing by mentally retarded and nonretarded persons. *American Journal of Mental Deficiency*, 91, 613–619.

Morss, J. (1983). Cognitive development in the Down's syndrome infant: Slow or different. *British Journal of Educational Psychology*, 53, 40–47.

Mundy, P., Seibert, J., & Hogan, A. (1985). Communication skills in mentally retarded children. In M. Sigman (Ed.), *Children with emotional disorders and developmental disabilities* (pp. 45–70). New York: Grune and Stratton.

Mundy, P., Seibert, J., & Hogan, A. (1984). Relationships between sensorimotor and early communication abilities in developmentally delayed children. *Merrill-Palmer Quarterly*, 30, 33–48.

Mundy, P., Seibert, J., Hogan, A., & Fagan, J. (1983). Novelty responding and behavioral development in young, developmentally delayed children. *Intelligence*, 7, 163–174.

Mundy, P., Sigman, M., Ungerer, J., & Sherman, T. (1987). Nonverbal communication and play correlates of language development in autistic children. *Journal of Autism and Developmental Disabilities*, 17, 349–364.

Nettlebeck, T., & Kirby, N. (1983). Measures of timed performance and intelligence. *Intelligence*, 7, 39–52.

Penrose, L. (1963). *The biology of mental defect*. London: Sidgwick & Jackson.

Piaget, J. (1952). *The origins of intelligence in children*. New York: International Universities Press.

Rose, S. (1983). Differential rates of visual information processing in full-term and pre-term infants. *Child Development*, 54, 1189–1198.

Rose, S., & Wallace, I. (1985). Visual recognition memory: A predictor of later cognitive functioning in preterms. *Child Development*, 56, 843–852.

Russell, A. (1985). The mentally retarded and emotionally disturbed child and adolescent. In M. Sigman (Ed.), *Children with emotional disorders and developmental disabilities* (pp. 111–136). New York: Grune & Stratton.

Seibert, J., Hogan, A., & Mundy, P. (1984). Mental age and cognitive stage in young handicapped and at-risk children. *Intelligence*, 8, 11–29.

Sigman, M., Cohen, S., Beckwith, L., & Topinka, C. (1986). Task persistence in two-year-olds in relation to subsequent attentiveness and intelligence. Paper presented at the International Conference on Infant Studies, Los Angeles.

Sigman, M., Cohen, S., Beckwith, L., & Parmelee, A. (1986). Infant attention in relation to intellectual abilities in childhood. *Developmental Psychology*, 22, 788–792.

Sigman, M., & Parmelee, A.H. (1974). Visual preferences of four-month-old premature and full-term infants. *Child Development*, 45, 959–965.

Sigman, M., Ungerer, J., Mundy, P., & Sherman, T. (1987). Cognition in autistic children. In D. Cohen, A. Donnellan, & R. Paul (Eds.), *Handbook of autism and pervasive developmental disorders* (pp. 103–120). New York: Wiley.

Silon, E., & Harter, S. (1985). Assessment of perceived competence, motivational orientation, and anxiety in segregated and mainstreamed educable mentally retarded children. *Journal of Educational Psychology*, 77, 217–230.

Spitz, H. (1982). Intellectual extremes, mental age, and the nature of human intelligence. *Merrill-Palmer Quarterly*, 28, 167–192.

Spitz, H. (1983). Critique of the developmental position in mental retardation research. *Journal of Special Education*, 17, 261–294.

Sternberg, R. (1986). Haste makes waste versus a stitch in time: A reply to Vernon, Nador, and Kantor. *Intelligence*, 10, 265–270.

Vernon, P. (1983). Speed of information processing and general intelligence. *Intelligence, 7,* 53–70.

Vernon, P., & Kantor, L. (1986). Reaction time correlations with intelligence test scores obtained under either timed or untimed conditions. *Intelligence, 10,* 315–330.

Vernon, P., Nador, S., & Kantor, L. (1985). Reaction times and speed-of-information processing: Their relationship to timed and untimed measures of intelligence. *Intelligence, 9,* 357–374.

Wagner, R., & Sternberg, R. (1984). Alternative conceptions of intelligence and their implications for education. *Review of Educational Research, 54,* 179–223.

Weir, M. (1967). Mental retardation. *Science, 157,* 576–578.

Weiss, B., Weisz, J., & Bromfield, R. (1986). Performance of retarded and nonretarded persons on information processing tasks: Further tests of the similar-structure hypothesis. *Psychological Bulletin, 100,* 157–175.

Weisz, J. (1982). Learned helplessness and the retarded child. In E. Zigler & D. Balla (Eds.), *Mental retardation: The developmental–difference controversy* (pp. 27–40). Hillsdale, NJ: Erlbaum.

Weisz, J., & Yeates, K. (1981). Cognitive development in retarded and nonretarded persons: Piagetian tests of the similar-structure hypothesis. *Psychological Bulletin, 90,* 153–178.

Weisz, J., Yeates, K., & Zigler, E. (1982). Piagetian evidence and the developmental difference controversy. In E. Zigler & D. Balla (Eds.), *Mental retardation: The developmental–difference controversy* (pp. 213–276). Hillsdale, NJ: Erlbaum.

Zigler, E. (1967). Familial mental retardation: A continuing dilemma. *Science, 155,* 292–298.

Zigler, E. (1982). Developmental versus difference theories of mental retardation and the problem of motivation. In E. Zigler and D. Balla (Eds.), *Mental retardation: The developmental–difference controversy* (pp. 163–188). Hillsdale, NJ: Erlbaum.

Zigler, E., & Balla, D. (1977). Impact of institutional experience on the behavior and development of retarded persons. *American Journal of Mental Deficiency, 82,* 1–11.

Zigler, E., & Balla, D. (1982). Motivational and personality factors in the performance of the retarded. In E. Zigler & D. Balla (Eds.), *Mental retardation: The developmental–difference controversy* (pp. 9–26). Hillsdale, NJ: Erlbaum.

Zigler, E., & Hodapp, R. (1986). *Understanding mental retardation.* New York: Cambridge University Press.

5   Neo-environmental perspectives on developmental theory

Arnold J. Sameroff

The role of the environment in human development can never be discussed without a complementary discussion of the role of the individual's constitution. What is outside an individual can only be defined with reference to what is inside. Historically, this dialectical relationship between the organism and its environment has been discussed in mechanistic terms that perpetuate a nature–nurture debate. The mechanistic orientation was based on the view that there are entities such as nature and nurture that can be defined independently of each other, as in the Newtonian concept of objects in space. The contrasting modern view that will be promoted here is that objects are only defined in relation to each other, as in the Einsteinian concept of the relativity of space and time. From this transactional perspective, organism and environment are always in intimate connection, not only in the ontogenetic development of each human, but in the phylogenetic evolution that produced both the human species – a commonly accepted idea – and the human environment – a less commonly accepted or understood idea.

Evolution and development

The theory of evolution led to major changes in the understanding of human behavior across all the disciplines that dealt with the life sciences. The history of changes in biological organization was seen to result from the success or failure of a species' behavior. The existence of every organism is regulated by both internal and external influences. The internal factors are the result of evolution in the way living beings are organized from molecules to single-celled organisms to multicelled and then multiorganed individuals. The external influences are the result of the same processes because the context of each individual evolved as well. Environments differentiated from primordial soup to sea and land, to forest and savannah, to farm and city. Included in the external context of each individual were other lives – of the same and different species – that supported and were supported by each other as care givers or as food. Throughout evolution, each living individual existed on the interface of these two worlds – the inner and the outer – and no development could take place in the absence of either.

In development and in evolution, individuals have never existed outside an environment. The classic egg-and-chicken paradox is a dialectical truism. Even the fertilized single-celled zygote contains both the genotype – the egg – and an organized biochemical environment provided by the mother – the chicken – that was not produced by that genome. Each species evolved in intimate relationship to some environment. Moreover, those environments were *organized*. There was an organization of existing forms into which each new species had to fit. On the one hand, the organization may have been a biological one in terms of the food sources or predators available, a physical one related to the geographic context, or a temporal one related to the seasons of the year. On the other hand, species played an active role in selecting among niches within that environment to reduce the variance in life attributable to the environment – in summer, an animal can search for relatively cool locales; in winter, it can seek out relatively warm ones.

For humans, as well, there is no development without an organized environment. Someone has to feed, protect, and provide warmth to infants. There are environmental codes in each society that provide an agenda of experiences for the developing child aimed at producing an adult suitable to fill a role in that society (Sameroff, 1983). Behavioral development is regulated by the interplay between the individual and the social system. Neither can be said to dominate the other. A lot of attention has been paid to the organization of internal control systems – the biological ones – but relatively little to the organization of external control systems – the social ones. It is the purpose of this chapter to elaborate on what we know about the environment and how it influences individual development.

One of the main questions in the study of development is why certain individuals in our society do not achieve an average level of intellectual and social–emotional competence. To answer this question, I will begin with a discussion of causal models in behavioral development to examine the idea that an individual's present condition, whether normal or deviant, is rooted in the past. A review of research exploring constitutional and environmental determinants will be presented indicating that neither perspective can ever provide a complete explanation of development, a conclusion that will surprise few readers. However, what is less obvious is that although different in kind, nature and nurture fit into a single developmental model where the processes by which biological and social factors affect individual development are analogous. A dynamic view of developmental influences will be presented within a "neo-environmental" perspective that incorporates the various sources of regulation that shape human growth – both inside and outside the individual.

Developmental deviancy

Linear causal models of child development have been used to explain the origins of a variety of abnormal mental conditions, as well as to offer rationales for the design of intervention programs to prevent or ameliorate such conditions. Although such efforts have frequently been categorized as applied rather than basic science, they have been very informative about gaps in our understanding of normative developmental processes. Two such areas of research provide examples of how our understanding of the determinants of child growth have changed. Studies of the relationship between birth complications and later developmental disabilities, and studies of the effectiveness of early child intervention programs in preventing such mental problems, were instrumental in these reconceptualizations.

Epidemiological studies (Pasamanick & Knobloch, 1961) suggested that children with a variety of disorders from mental retardation to schizophrenia had significantly greater rates of birth complications than children who did not have these disorders. To test this hypothesis based on retrospective data, a large number of prospective studies were conducted in which infants with birth complications were followed longitudinally to observe their outcomes (Sameroff & Chandler, 1975). Surprisingly, the vast majority of these children grew up to show no evidence of their poor biological origins (Sameroff, 1986). What was even more surprising was that social conditions were much better predictors of outcome for these children than either their early biological status, as measured by birth and pregnancy complications (Wilson, 1985), or their psychological status, as measured by developmental scales (Broman, Nichols, & Kennedy, 1975).

The theory that poor early social conditions produced developmental problems was reinforced by a series of epidemiological studies of mild mental retardation. Surveys in Sweden found a prevalence of *severe* mental retardation in childhood of about 3 in 1,000, compatible with rates of severe mental retardation in the United States. On the other hand, the prevalence of *mild* mental retardation in Sweden is about 4 in 1,000, 8 or 10 times lower than rates recorded in the United States. Susser. Hauser, et al. (1985) point out that these rates are related to the reduction in Sweden of retardation from family and cultural influences, and provide evidence for the powerful impact of social environment on mental performance.

Another indication of the role of environment in mild mental retardation is the percentage these of children with detectable clinical abnormalities. In Sweden, 40% of mildly retarded children had identifiable conditions (Hagberg et al., 1981), whereas the comparable percentage in the United States is only 10%. Comparisons between countries that may have different criteria for a diagnosis of mental retardation may be suspect (Zigler & Hodapp, 1986), so greater credence should be given to comparisons within the same society. In the Collaborative Perinatal Project of the National Institute of Neurological Diseases and Stroke, the percentage of cases in the United States with mild mental retardation and detectable abnormalities was 14% for white children and 6% for black children (Broman, 1979). Similarly, an English study found that the percentage of mildly retarded children with organic conditions was twice as high in schools with low social standing, but the percentage of mildly retarded children without clinical abnormalities was 15 times as high (Stein & Susser, 1963).

The belief that social disadvantage produced mental deficiency and school failures led to a large number of intervention programs that proposed to modify the early environment of children of lower socioeconomic status (SES), with a major goal of increasing their intellectual performance. Early intervention programs were based on traditional models of child development in which children who were identified as doing poorly early in life were expected to continue to do poorly. The early childhood education movement as exemplified in the Head Start program was designed to improve the learning and social competence of children during the preschool years, with the expectation that these improvements would be maintained into later life. Unfortunately, follow-up research of these children has shown that the major changes in their behavior that resulted from their preschool experience began to disappear as soon as they entered their regular elementary school system, and only moderate gains were maintained into adolescence (Zigler & Trickett, 1978). Some later effects were found in reduced rates of school failure and the need for special education by children with preschool experience (Lazar, Darlington, Murray, Royce, & Snipper, 1982; Schweinhart & Weikart, 1980).

In both research areas, early characteristics of the child have been overpowered by factors in the later environmental context of development. Where family and cultural variables have fostered development, children with severe perinatal complications have been indistinguishable from children without complications. Where these variables have hindered development, children from the best preschool intervention programs have developed severe social and cognitive deficits. When predictions on how children will turn out are based on their early behavior, the predictions are generally wrong. When such predictions are based on their life circumstances, the predictions are generally right (Sameroff, Seifer, Barocas, Zax, & Greenspan, 1987). In this domain, an understanding of the context may have greater developmental importance than an understanding of the child.

When the birth condition of a variety of infants is examined, a common expectation is one of continuity – that is, those children who appeared normal as infants should continue to be normal; those who were handicapped should end up retarded; and those who suffered from a variety of perinatal insults should perform somewhere in between. Indeed, that is the case for a number of such infants. However, it is also the case that most handicapped children will end up either normal or only moderately impaired, and a number of normal infants will end up as retarded children.

How do we explain these surprises? The explanations center around transitions. The judgment of normality or abnormality during the newborn period is based on biological functioning. The judgment of normality or abnormality in later childhood is based on psychological functioning. Most biologically handicapped newborns will continue to be biologically handicapped. They will continue to be blind, deaf, or motor impaired. But what is the relevance of these biological handicaps to these children's psychological functioning? Will such handicaps also produce intellectual and social–emotional handicaps? For most infants, the answer is no. There is a transition in functioning from a biological level to a behavioral level, where the status during one phase does not have a necessary connection to the status during the next. There are further transitions within behavioral development – for example, from sensorimotor to linguistic or logical functioning, where similar discontinuities also are evident. The basic question to be answered here is not whether there are continuities or discontinuities in development, but rather "under what conditions is development continuous or discontinuous?"

Environmental risk

In defining the developmental risk associated with any specific child, the characteristics of the child must be related to the ability of the environment to regulate the development of that child toward social norms. In some cases of massive biological abnormality, such regulations may be ineffectual. At the other extreme, disordered social environments might convert biologically normal infants into caretaking casualties.

The Kauai study of Werner and her colleagues (Werner, Bierman, & French, 1971; Werner & Smith, 1977; Werner & Smith, 1982) provides a good description of the interplay between risk factors in the child and those in the environment. A sample of children was followed from birth through adolescence. Assessments were made of the birth condition of the children and their developmental progress at 2, 10, and 18 years of age. Of the predominantly lower SES sample, more than half had learning or emotional problems by 18 years of age. The first reports of this study (Werner et al., 1971; Werner & Smith, 1977) helped to dispel the notion that birth complications had a determining effect on behavioral outcomes. Children with severe early trauma frequently showed no later deficits unless the problems were combined with persistently poor environmental circumstances such as chronic poverty, family instability, or maternal mental health problems.

In the third report of the Kauai study, Werner and Smith (1982) divided all the children who had been at high clinical risk at 2 years of age into three groups: those who developed problems by 10 years of age, those who did not develop problems until 18 years of age, and those who did not develop problems at all. This latter "resilient" group was the target of analyses to determine what factors in development protected them from the disorders that characterized the children who did have problems. Most of the protective factors that were identified were not surprising: good temperament, favorable parental attitudes, low levels of family conflict, counseling and remedial assistance, small family size, and a smaller load of stressful life experiences. What was surprising was the variety of interactions among the factors and the complexity of analysis needed to match the complexity of variables that affected the course of a child's development. For example, Werner and Smith attempted to separate those factors that led to healthier outcomes both in the presence or absence of risk conditions from those factors that only had an interactional effect – that is, a positive impact in the presence of risk factors, but no impact when risk factors were absent. These latter protective factors were not found to discriminate between positive and negative outcomes for middle-class children whose lives were relatively free of stress, but they were very important in the lives of children who were growing up in poverty and subject to a large number of negative life events.

The Kauai study is in tune with others (Sameroff & Chandler, 1975) in targeting family mental health and especially social class as important moderators of child development (Broman, Nichols, & Kennedy, 1975; Golden & Birns, 1976). In the Rochester Longitudinal Study (RLS), my colleagues and I also found social class and parental mental health to be associated with developmental risk (Sameroff, Seifer, & Zax, 1982). The RLS is a study of the development of several hundred children from birth through early adolescence assessing environmental factors as well as the cognitive and social competence of the children. We decided to subdivide the global variable of social class to see if we could identify factors more directly connected to the child that acted as environmental risks. These factors ranged from proximal variables such as the mother's interaction with the child, to such intermediate variables as the mother's mental health, to distal variables such as the financial resources of the family.

Although causal models have been sought in which singular variables uniquely determine aspects of child behavior, a series of studies in a variety of domains have found that except at the extremes of biological dysfunction, it is the *number* rather than the *nature* of risk factors that are the best determinants of outcome. Parmelee and Haber (1973) found this to be true for neurological factors in samples of infants with many perinatal problems, Rutter (1979) for family factors in samples of children with many psychosocial problems, and Greenspan (1981) for both biological and family factors in multirisk families.

When the sample of children in the RLS were 4 years old, we assessed a set of 10 environmental variables that are correlates of SES but not equivalents (Sameroff et al., 1987). We then tested whether poor cognitive development in our preschool children was a function of low SES or the compounding of environmental risk factors found in low-SES groups. The 10 environmental risk variables were (1) a history of maternal mental illness, (2) high maternal anxiety, (3) a parental perspectives score derived from a combination of measures that reflected rigidity in the attitudes, beliefs, and values that mothers had in regard to their child's development, (4) few positive maternal interactions with the child observed during infancy, (5) head of household in an unskilled occupation, (6) minimal maternal education, (7) disadvantaged minority status, (8) reduced family support, (9) stressful life events, and (10) large family size.

When these risk factors were related to social–emotional and cognitive competence scores, major differences were found between those children with few risks and those with many. In terms of intelligence, children with no environmental risks scored more than 30 points higher than children with eight or nine risk factors (Figure 5.1).

These data support the view that IQ scores for 4-year-old children are multidetermined by variables in the social context, but the possibility exists that poverty may still be an overriding variable. To test for this possibility, two additional analyses were completed. The first analysis was to deter-

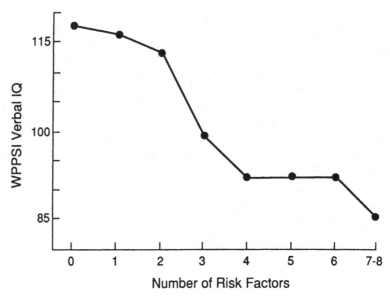

Figure 5.1. Effects of multiple-risk scores on intelligence of 4-year-old children (Sameroff, Seifer, Barocas, Zax, and Greenspan, 1987).

mine if there were consistencies in the distribution of risk factors – i.e., were there always the same factors present? The second analysis was to determine if the relationship between high risk and lower intelligence was to be found in high-SES families as well as in low-SES families.

For the first type of analysis, the data from the families that had a moderate score of three, four, or five risk factors were cluster-analyzed. The families fell into five clusters with different sets of high-risk conditions, listed in Table 5.1. Different combinations of factors appear in each cluster. Cluster 2 has no overlapping variables with clusters 3, 4 or 5. Minority status is a risk variable in clusters 3, 4, and 5, but does not appear in clusters 1 or 2. Despite these differences in the specific risks among families, the mean IQs were not different for children in the five clusters, ranging from 92.8 to 97.7. Thus, it seems that it was not any single variable but the combination of multiple variables that reduced the child's intellectual performance. If this is the case, it is unlikely that a universal single factor will be found that explains either good or bad developmental outcomes for children. In every family situation, a unique set of risk or protective factors will be related to how the children turn out.

For the second analysis, the sample was split into high and low SES groups, and the effect of an increased number of risks was examined within each social-class group. The effects of the multiple-risk scores were as clear within SES groups as for the population at large. The more risk factors, the worse the child outcomes for both high and low SES families.

These analyses of the RLS data were attempts to elaborate on environmental risk factors by reducing global measures – for example, SES – to component social and behavioral variables. We were able to identify a set of risk factors that were found predominantly in lower SES groups, but affected child outcomes in all social classes. Moreover, no single variable was determinant of outcome. Only in families with multiple-risk factors was the child's competence placed in jeopardy. In the analyses of intellectual outcomes, none of the children in the low multiple-risk group had an IQ below 85, whereas 24% of the children in the high multiple-risk group did.

The multiple pressures of (1) the amount of stress from the environment, (2) the family's resources for coping with that stress, (3) the number of children that must share those resources, and (4) the parents' flexibility in understanding and dealing with their children all play a role in the fostering or hindrance of child intellectual and social competencies.

Environmental continuity

Within the RLS, our attention has been devoted to the source of continuities and discontinuities in child performance. We have recently completed

Table 5.1. *Cluster analysis of families with moderate multiple-risk scores*

Cluster 1	Mental health
	Family support
	Mother education
	Anxiety
Cluster 2	Mother–infant interaction
	Mental health
	Anxiety
Cluster 3	Family support
	Minority status
Cluster 4	Mother education
	Minority status
	Occupation
Cluster 5	Parental perspectives
	Minority status
	Mother education

Source: Sameroff, Seifer, Barocas, Zax, & Greenspan, 1987.

a new assessment of the sample in which the children were 13 years of age (Baldwin, Baldwin, Sameroff, & Seifer, 1988). We were especially interested in those children from multiple-risk families who had managed to overcome early difficulties and reach normal or above-average levels of intellectual or social–emotional competence. We were very disappointed to find little evidence of these resilient or invulnerable children. When we recreated our multiple-risk score at age 13, we found the same powerful relationship between environmental adversity and child behavior – children with the most environmental risk factors had the lowest competence ratings.

The typical statistic reported in longitudinal research is the correlation between early and later performance of the children. We too found such correlations. Intelligence at 4 years correlated .72 with intelligence at 13 years, and the social competence scores at the two ages correlated .43. The usual interpretation of such numbers is that there is a continuity of competence or incompetence in the child. Such a conclusion cannot be challenged if the only assessments in the study were of the children. In the RLS, both environmental and child factors were examined. We were able to correlate environmental characteristics across time as well as child ones. We found that the correlation between environmental risk scores at the two ages was .76, as great or greater than any continuity within the child. Children who had poor family and social environments at 4 years still had them when they were 13 years, and probably would continue to have them for the foreseeable future. Whatever the child's ability for achieving high levels of competence, it was severely undermined by the continuing paucity of environmental support. Whatever the capabilities provided to the child by individual factors, it is the environment that limits the opportunities for development.

The importance of the regulatory function of parents became clear when we examined discontinuities in our data. We expected that children from demographically high-risk families would be below average in cognitive achievement. This was true for the majority of such children, but we were able to identify a small group (20%) that was doing better than average on their cognitive outcome scores (Baldwin, Baldwin, & Cole, in press). When we searched among our measures to find the factors that permitted these children to do better than their peers, we found differences in the attitudes and practices of their parents. A pattern of restrictiveness with little democracy, clarity of rules, and emotional warmth characterized the parents in these families. The parents had constructed a safe family environment in which their children could develop in the midst of the social chaos that typified their neighbors. The environment was modified to foster development rather than hinder it.

Regulatory systems in development

What kind of theory would be necessary to integrate our understanding of internal and external influences on development? It must explain how the individual and the context work together to produce patterns of adaptive or maladaptive functioning, and relate how such past or present functioning influences the future.

The first principle to emerge in such a general theory of development is that individuals can never be removed from their contexts. Whether the goal is understanding causal connections, predicting outcomes, or intervention, it will not be achieved by removing the individual from the conditions that regulate development. A great deal of attention has been given to the biological influences on development. It has now become necessary to give equal attention to the environmental influences.

The development of each individual is constrained by interactions with regulatory systems acting at different levels of organization. The two most prominent of these systems are the biological and social regulatory systems. From conception to birth, interactions with the biological system are most prominent. Changes in the contemporary state of the organism's embryonic phenotype trigger the genotype to provide a series of new biochemical experiences. These experiences are regulated by the turning on and off of various gene activities directed toward the production of a viable human child. These processes continue less dramatically after birth with some exceptions – for example, the initiation of adolescence and possibly senility.

The period from birth to adulthood is dominated by interactions with the social system. Again, the state of the child triggers regulatory processes, but now in the social environment. Examples of such coded changes are the reactions of parents to their child's ability to walk or talk, and the changes in setting provided when the child reaches preschool or school age. These regulations change the experience of the child in synchrony with changes in the child's physical and behavioral development.

The result of these regulatory exchanges is the expansion of each individual's ability for biological self-regulation and the development of behavioral self-regulation. Advances in motor development permit children to control their temperature and nutrition that initially could only be regulated by care givers. The children soon are able to dress themselves and reach into the refrigerator. Despite this burgeoning independence, each individual is never freed from a relationship to an internal and external context. Should we forget this connection, it only takes a bout of illness or a social transgression to remind us of our constraints.

The environtype

Just as there is a biological organization – the genotype – that regulates the physical outcome of each individual, there is a social organization that regulates the way human beings fit into their society. This organization operates through family and cultural socialization patterns and has been postulated to constitute an "environtype" analogous to the biological genotype (Sameroff, 1985; Sameroff & Fiese, in press).

The environtype is composed of subsystems that not only transact with the child but also with each other. Bronfenbrenner (1977) has provided the most detailed descriptions of environmental organizations that have an impact on developmental processes within categories of microsystems, mesosystems, exosystems, and macrosystems. The *microsystem* is the immediate setting of a child in an environment with particular features, activities, and roles – for example, the home or the school. The *mesosystem* comprises the relationships between the major settings at a particular point in an individual's development – for example, between home and school. The *exosystem* is an extension of the mesosystem that includes settings that the child may not be a part of, but that affect the settings in which the child does participate – for example, the world of work and neighborhoods. Finally, the *macrosystem* includes the overarching institutional patterns of the culture, including the economic, social, and political systems of which the microsystems, mesosystems, and exosystems are concrete expressions. Bronfenbrenner's ecological model has been fruitfully applied in the analysis of a number of developmental issues (Belsky, 1980; Kurdek, 1981).

Despite the promising consequences for understanding behavior by using the ecological models (Bronfenbrenner, 1986), most behavioral research on the effects of the environment have focused narrowly on analyses of interaction patterns of pairs of individuals. Parke and Tinsley (1987), in an extensive review of family interaction research, have pointed to an important new trend of adding not only father–child interaction to the study of mother–child interaction, but the combination of these into studies of triadic interactions and entire family behavioral patterns. Behavioral research is slowly overcoming the technological difficulties embodied in analyses of multiple interacting individuals. Another growing empirical base comes from the direction of beliefs rather than behavior

(Sigel, 1985; Goodnow, 1988). Investigators have become increasingly articulate at defining the dimensions of parental belief systems, with the goal of describing the effects of these belief systems on parental behavior, and ultimately on the behavior of the child.

For our purpose now, the discussion will be directed to the organization of environmental factors in codes contained within the culture, the family, and the individual parent. These codes are hierarchically related in their evolution and in their current influence on the child. The experience of the developing child is partially determined by the beliefs, values, and personality of the parents; partially by the family's interaction patterns and transgenerational history; and partially by the socialization beliefs, controls, and supports of the culture. Developmental regulations at each of these levels are carried within codes that direct cognitive and social–emotional development so that the child will ultimately be able to fill a role defined within society.

Although at any point in time the environtype can be conceptualized independently of the child, changes in the abilities of the developing child are major triggers for regulatory changes, and most likely were major contributors to the evolution of each culture's timetable of reactions to behavioral milestones – that is, the society's *developmental agenda*.

Cultural code

The ingredients of the cultural code are the complex of characteristics that organize a society's child-rearing system, incorporating elements of socialization and education. These processes are embedded in sets of social controls and social supports based on beliefs that differ in the amount of community consensus, ranging from mores and norms to fads and fashions. It is beyond the scope of this chapter to elucidate the full range of cultural regulatory processes. As a consequence, only a few points will be highlighted to flesh out the description of the cultural code.

Although the common biological characteristics of the human species have produced similar developmental agendas in most cultures, there are differences in many major characteristics that often ignore the biological status of the individual. In most cultures, on the one hand, formal education begins between the ages of 6 and 8 years (Rogoff, 1981) when most children have developed the cognitive ability to learn from structured experiences. On the other hand, informal education can begin at many different ages depending on the culture's attributions to the child. The Digo and Kikuyu are two East African cultures that have different beliefs about infant capacities (Sameroff & Chandler, 1975). The Digo believe that infants can learn within a few months after birth and begin socialization at that time. The Kikuyu wait until the second year of life before they believe serious education is possible. Closer to home, some middle-class parents have been convinced that prenatal experiences will enhance the cognitive development of their children. Such examples demonstrate the variability of human developmental contexts.

Family code

Just as cultural codes regulate the fit between individuals and the social system, family codes organize individuals within the family system. Family codes provide a source of regulation that allows a group of individuals to form a collective unit in relation to society. As the cultural code regulates development so that an individual may fill a role in society, family codes regulate development to produce members who fulfill a role within the family and ultimately are able to introduce new members into the shared system. Traditionally, new members are incorporated through birth and marriage. In recent years, remarriage has more frequently provided new family members.

The family regulates the child's development through a variety of forms that vary in their degree of explicit representation. Families have rituals that prescribe roles, stories that transmit orientations to each family member as well as to whomever will listen, shared myths that influence individual interactions, and behavioral paradigms that change individual behavior in the presence of other family members (Reiss, in press). The regulations that family members are most aware of are family rituals, and they are least aware of family paradigms. At intermediate levels are stories and myths. Research efforts are only beginning to explore the exact nature of how these forms are transmitted behaviorally among family members and how they are represented in cognition.

Individual parent code

There is good evidence that individual behavior is influenced by the family context. When individuals operate as part of a family, the behavior of each member is altered (Parke & Tinsley, 1987), frequently without awareness of the behavioral change (Reiss, 1981). There is also no doubt that all individuals bring their own distinct contribution to family interactions. The contribution of parents is much more complexly determined than that of young children, given the multiple levels of parents' behavior. Although the socializing regulations embodied in the cultural and family codes have been discussed, the individualized interpretations that each parenting figure imposes on these codes has not. To a large extent, these interpretations are conditioned by the parents' past participation in their own family's coded interactions, but they are captured uniquely by each member of the family. These individual influences further influence parents' responses to their own children. The richness of both health and pathology embodied in these responses are well described in the clinical literature (Fraiberg, 1980).

Parental problems have long been recognized as contributors to the poor developmental status of children. Although we acknowledge that influence, we must also be careful to note the effects of the contexts in which parental behavior is rooted – family and cultural codes. It is important to recognize the parent as a major regulating agency of child development, but it is equally important to recognize that parental behavior is itself embedded in regulatory contexts.

Understanding development

To understand the course of the human species since the evolution of civilization, one must consider social factors, not biological factors, as the major motivating force. The evolution of the "environtype" – the familial and social external regulators of development – has progressed at a much greater rate than the evolution of the genotype – the internal biological developmental regulator. Even E.O. Wilson (1975), a leading sociobiologist, described human society as autocatalytic. He saw civilization as fueled by positive feedback from its own social products. The evolution of the human species now operates independently of the typical environmental constraints that influenced all other evolutionary progressions.

The key to understanding development is understanding how each individual integrates inner biological and outer social factors. The inner organization produces capability, the outer organization produces opportunity. For example, the development of the child's digestive system provides the capability for using nutrients, but the context provides the set of nutrients that will be eaten; the development of the visual and auditory system provides the capability for using perceptual information, but the context provides the set of sights and sounds that will be perceived; the development of the brain will provide the capability to conceptualize the universe, but the context provides the collected wisdom that will be the content of advanced thought.

Research on the causal matrix of individual human behavior reveals that neither internal nor external determinants can operate independently.

Bidirectional or transactional processes dominate every level of life. In molecular biology, clear evidence of the effects of gene activity on the biochemical composition of the cell is matched by clear evidence of the effects of cellular composition on gene activity. At the behavioral level, these same transactions have been identified between parent and child. Changes in child behavior are related to antecedent parental activity, and there is clear evidence that changes in parental activity are related to antecedent child behavior.

When one expands the time line and studies causal relations in development between the individual and internal and external factors across generations, there is clear evidence that these factors have been organized through their evolution into coherent regulatory systems. We have long been accustomed to recognize the genotype's regulation of individual growth. In the short run, the genes respond to their local biochemical context. But in the long run, the regulated organization of these local interactions produces normative species-specific characteristics of the whole individual through feedback systems that have evolved over eons. We have been less accustomed to recognize the environtype's regulation of psychosocial growth that in the long run produces culture-specific characteristics of the individual through analogous family and cultural buffering systems. As the genotype regulates the development of the individual's capabilities, so the environtype regulates the individual's opportunities. To study individuals who are incapacitated, the search must include both biological and psychosocial factors. To study individuals who have no opportunities, the focus is more restricted to the social conditions of life.

The environment plays an active role in regulating development. Most individuals can only grow up to fill existing roles in a culture. If one does not blind oneself to history, there were vast periods of human existence when the number of roles were highly limited, either in absolute number or in the number available to certain parts of society. Feudal society was not a meritocracy. Serfs, no matter what their talents, could not fill intellectual, political, or intellectual roles in their societies.

To the extent that roles are open to individuals in our own day and age, there are usually selection systems to determine who would be most appropriate for available positions in the existing social organization. Academic tests allow or prevent certain children from entering certain tracks, but so may discrimination. The same may be true for athletic or artistic efforts. In these situations, the contributions of the genotype to the selection process may be large, but it is the environment that decides which developmental tracks are permissible for a given individual. In a society where artistic achievement is proscribed, that aspect of the genotype will have little positive effect on developmental outcomes. Within our own culture, the environment still places major restrictions on individual development based on characteristics other than talent. Race, social status, and sex are examples of such restrictive criteria.

We all would like to believe that decisions about admission to schools and employment are all *influenced* by our individual competencies, but we all realize that our competencies do not *determine* those decisions. To the extent that we can shape our behavior to fit in with the constraints of the educational and occupational environment, we can be said to be controlling our destiny, but that is a far cry from believing that we, as individuals, have major roles in shaping the nature of the environment we are trying to fit into.

An understanding of the developmental process requires an appreciation of the transactions between individuals, their biological inner workings, and their social outer workings. Continuities and discontinuities are a joint function of three systems – the genotype, the phenotype, and the environtype (see Figure 5.2). The *genotype* is an organized biological system that transacts with the phenotype to produce the biological organization that supports an individual's capacities for behavior. The *environtype* is the cultural code that provides the developmental opportunities for individuals growing up in any given society. The *phenotype* – in this case the individual person – transacts with both the genotype and environtype in order to develop. To the extent that the three systems are in a state of equilibrium, continuity of performance is to be expected. To the extent that one of the systems undergoes a reorganization, there is a corresponding reorganization of development itself. In normal development on the biological side, re-

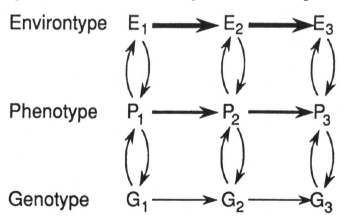

Figure 5.2. Regulation model of development with transactions between genotype, phenotype, and environtype (Sameroff, 1985).

organizations are required in changes such as walking or adolescence. From the environmental side, such normative transitions include beginning school and graduation. It is in the individual that the inner and the outer are brought into accord, either by seeking opportunities to use capacities or by fostering capacities to meet opportunities. In nonnormative development, either the capacities or the opportunities are missing. The plasticity of the environtype permits compensatory regulations such as providing wheelchairs for those who cannot walk or Braille books for those who cannot see. Equally, this same plasticity can deny education to those who are of the "wrong" race, or even of the "wrong" sex.

The appeal of models of development based on the individual stems from our purported lack of sophistication in defining meaningful environmental variables that explain significant amounts of variance. This lack of sophistication should be taken as a challenge for future research rather than as an excuse for eliminating the environment as an organized contributor to our destinies.

The future

Because of the more rapid evolution of the environtype than the genotype in human society, in studying the future of human development much greater attention must be paid to the social constraints than to the biological ones. Strong evidence for this position is found in a series of studies on increases in IQ scores during the last several generations in which Flynn (1984, 1987) found massive gains over the last 50 years. In one study of changes in test norms in the United States between 1932 and 1978, gains of 13.8 points were found. In another study of 14 nations over the last generation, gains of 5 to 25 points were found. What was even more surprising was that these large increases were not on IQ test subscales that would be influenced by schooling but on scales that were thought to reflect abstract problem solving ability. There is no biological model that can explain these increases in intelligence.

If we can understand the forces that increase the intelligence of whole societies, perhaps we can also understand the processes that will increase the intelligence of specific individuals within society. The research findings summarized here have identified the operation of major social factors that constrain human development. I have proposed that these environmental factors are part of an environtype that regulates human development by regulating developmental opportunities. Flynn (1987) concludes that potent unknown environmental factors must exist to produce these results. From the perspective of establishing a research agenda for the future, the key word here is "unknown." The task of research programs directed toward understanding human health and disorder is to make these potent factors "known."

References

Baldwin, A.L., Baldwin, C., & Cole, R.E. (in press). Stress-resistant families and stress-resistant children. In J. Rolf, D. Masten, D. Cicchetti, K. Neuchtherlin & S. Weintraub (Eds.), *Risk and protective factors in the development of psychopathology.* New York: Cambridge University Press.

Baldwin, A.L., Baldwin, C., Sameroff, A.J., & Seifer, R. (1988). Rochester Longitudinal Study progress report. Unpublished manuscript.

Belsky, J. (1980). Child maltreatment: An ecological integration. *American Psychologist, 35,* 430-435.

Broman, S.H. (1979). Perinatal anoxia and cognitive development in early childhood. In T.M. Field (Ed.), *Infants born at risk.* New York: Spectrum Publications.

Broman, S.H., Nichols, P.L., & Kennedy, W.A. (1975). *Preschool IQ: Prenatal and early development correlates.* Hillsdale, NJ: Erlbaum.

Bronfenbrenner, U. (1977). Toward an experimental ecology of human development. *American Psychologist, 32,* 513-531.

Bronfenbrenner, U. (1986). Ecology of the family as a context for human development: Research perspectives. *Developmental Psychology, 22,* 723-742.

Flynn, J.R. (1984). The mean IQ of Americans: Massive gains, 1932 to 1978. *Psychological Bulletin, 95,* 29-51.

Flynn, J.R. (1987). Massive IQ gains in 14 nations: What IQ tests really measure. *Psychological Bulletin, 101,* 171-191.

Fraiberg, S. (1980). *Clinical studies in infant mental health: The first year of life.* New York: Basic Books.

Golden, M., & Birns, B. (1976). Social class and infant intelligence. In M. Lewis (Ed.), *Origins of intelligence: Infancy and early childhood.* New York: Plenum.

Goodnow, J.J. (1988). Parents' ideas, actions, and feelings: Models and methods from developmental and social psychology. *Child Development, 59,* 286-320.

Greenspan, S.I. (1981). *Psychopathology and adaptation in infancy and early childhood: Clinical infant reports No. 1.* Hanover, NH: University Press of New England.

Hagberg, B. et al. (1981). Mild mental retardation in Swedish school children. I. Prevalence. *Acta Paediatrica Scandanavia, 70,* 445-452.

Kurdek, L.A. (1981). An integrative perspective on children's divorce adjustment. *American Psychologist, 36,* 856-866.

Lazar, I., Darlington, R., Murray, H., Royce, J., & Snipper, A. (1982). Lasting effects of early education: A report from the consortium for longitudinal studies. *Monographs of the Society for Research in Child Development, 47* (Serial No. 195).

Parke, R.D., & Tinsley, B.J. (1987). Family interaction in infancy. In J. Osofsky (Ed.), *Handbook of infant development* (2nd ed., pp. 579-641). New York: Wiley.

Parmelee, A.H., & Haber, A. (1973). Who is the at-risk infant? *Clinical Obstetrics and Gynecology, 16,* 376-387.

Pasamanick, B., & Knobloch, H. (1961). Epidemiologic studies on the complications of pregnancy and the birth process. In G. Caplan (Ed.), *Prevention of mental disorders in children.* New York: Basic Books.

Reiss, D. (in press). The represented and practicing family: Contrasting visions of family continuity. In A.J. Sameroff & R.N. Emde (Eds.), *Relationship disturbances in early childhood: A developmental approach.* New York: Basic Books.

Reiss, D. (1981). *The family's construction of reality.* Cambridge, MA: Harvard University Press.

Rogoff, B. (1981). Schooling and the development of cognitive skills. In H.C. Triandis and A. Heron (Eds.), *Handbook of cross-cultural psychology: Developmental psychology.* Vol. 4 (pp. 233–294). Boston: Allyn & Bacon.

Rutter, M.R. (1977). Protective factors in children's responses to stress and disadvantage. In M.W. Kent & J.E. Rolf (Eds.), *Primary prevention of psychopathology. Vol. 3: Social competence in children.* Hanover, NH: University of New England Press.

Sameroff, A.J. (1983). Developmental systems: Contexts and evolution. In W. Kessen (Ed.). *History, theories, and methods.* Volume 1 of P.H. Mussen (Ed.), *Handbook of child psychology* (pp. 237–294). New York: Wiley.

Sameroff, A.J. (1986). Environmental context of child development. *Journal of Pediatrics,* 109, 192–200.

Sameroff, A.J. (1985). *Can development be continuous?* Paper presented at Annual Meeting of American Psychological Association, Los Angeles.

Sameroff, A.J., & Chandler, M.J. (1975). Reproductive risk and the continuum of caretaking casualty. In F.D. Horowitz, M. Hetherington, S. Scarr-Salapatek, & G. Siegel (Eds.), *Review of child development research* (Vol. 4, pp. 187–244). Chicago: University of Chicago.

Sameroff, A.J., & Fiese, B.H. (in press). Transactional regulation and early intervention. In S.J. Meisels & J.P. Shonkoff (Eds.), *Early intervention: A handbook of theory, practice and analysis.* New York: Cambridge University Press.

Sameroff, A.J., Seifer, R., Barocas, R., Zax, M., & Greenspan, S. (1987). IQ scores of 4-year-old children: Social–environmental risk factors. *Pediatrics,* 79, 343–350.

Sameroff, A.J., Seifer, R., & Zax, M. (1982). Early development of children at risk for emotional disorders. *Monographs of the Society for Research in Child Development,* Vol. 47.

Sameroff, A.J., Seifer, R., Zax, M., & Barocas, R. (1987). Early indicators of development risk: Rochester longitudinal study. *Schizophrenia Bulletin, 13,* 383–394.

Schweinhart, L., & Weikart, D. (1980). Young children grow up: The effect of the Perry preschool program on youths through age 15. *Monographs of the High/Scope Educational Research Foundation,* No. 7, Ypsilanti, MI: High/Scope.

Sigel, E. (1985). *Parental belief systems: The psychological consequences for children.* Hillsdale, NJ: Erlbaum.

Stein, Z., & Susser, M. (1985). Effects of early nutrition on neurological and mental competence in human beings. *Psychological Medicine, 15,* 717–726.

Susser, M., Hauser, W.A., Kiely, J.L., Paneth, N., & Stein, Z. (1985). Quantitative estimates of prenatal and perinatal risk factors for perinatal mortality, cerebral palsy, mental retardation, and epilepsy. In J.M. Freeman (Ed.), *Prenatal and perinatal factors associated with brain disorders.* Washington DC: National Institutes of Health Publication No. 85–1149.

Werner, E.E., Bierman, J.M., & French, F.E. (1971). *The children of Kauai.* Honolulu: University of Hawaii Press.

Werner, E.E., & Smith, R.S. (1977). *Kauai's children come of age.* Honolulu: University of Hawaii Press.

Werner, E.E., & Smith, R.S. (1982). *Vulnerable but invincible: A longitudinal study of resilient children and youth.* New York: McGraw-Hill.

Wilson, E.O. (1975). *Sociobiology.* Cambridge, MA: Belknap Press.

Wilson, R.S. (1985). Risk and resilience in early mental development. *Developmental Psychology, 21*, 795–805.

Zigler, E., & Hodapp, R.M. (1986). *Understanding mental retardation.* New York: Cambridge University Press.

Zigler, E., & Trickett, P.K. (1978). IQ, social competence, and evaluation of early childhood intervention programs. *American Psychologist, 33*, 789–799.

6   The role of motivational factors in the functioning of mentally retarded individuals

Joseph Merighi, Mark Edison, and Edward Zigler

Investigators have long noted that personality factors are as important in the performance and adjustment of retarded individuals as cognitive factors (Penrose, 1963; Sarason, 1953; Tizard, 1953; Windle, 1962; Zigler, 1966b). Earlier workers, such as Potter (1922) and Fernald (1919), maintained that the difference between social adequacy and inadequacy in borderline retarded persons was a matter of personality rather than intelligence. Perhaps the first empirical study of this view was conducted by Weaver (1946), who examined the adjustment of 8,000 retarded persons inducted into the United States Army during World War II. Most of these recruits had IQs below 75, yet 54% of the males and 62% of the females made a satisfactory adjustment to military life. The median IQs of the successful and unsuccessful groups were 72 and 68, respectively. Weaver concluded that "personality factors far overshadowed the factor of intelligence" (p. 243) in the adjustment of retarded adults in the military.

At about the same time, a practical example of how intelligence is not the sole determinant of one's ability to function in society was provided by Harrell and Harrell (1945), who reported the IQ ranges for a variety of occupations. Persons involved in mining, trucking, farming, auto mechanics, bartending, sales, and tool making displayed a wide range of IQ scores. Although many of these persons had IQs in the average and above-average range, some individual miners, truckers, bartenders, and so on had IQs well below 70. For example, IQs ranged from 56 to 129 ($M = 93$) for miners and 43 to 131 ($M = 93$) for farmers. These jobs have certainly become more complex since that time, so workers in the lower reported IQ ranges might be unable to perform them in today's workplace. On the other hand, technological advances (particularly automation) have made many jobs easier and well within the ability of those with low IQs.

Despite existence of evidence such as Weaver's and the Harrells', there remained a tendency to overemphasize the importance of intellect in the adjustment of retarded persons. As late as 1962, Windle found that most

114

institutional personnel simply assumed that intellectual level was the critical factor in success after release. According to Windle, the relationship between IQ (range 40 to 80) and functioning in the community–nonschool environment is essentially zero. Once school has been completed, the level of cognitive functioning achieved by most retarded persons is adequate for at least a marginally self-sufficient existence in our society.

A more recent and definitive effort to explore the role of intelligence on overall adjustment was undertaken by Swedish researchers Granat and Granat (1973, 1978). They studied 19-year-old Swedish males with IQ scores below 84. Half of this population was found to be well adjusted and half displayed some adjustment problems. This study clearly demonstrates that the inability to assimilate in society is not totally dependent on below-average performance on psychometric measures of intelligence. In each of the studies described, personality factors such as dependency, wariness, and poor self-esteem were shown to influence the adjustment and functioning of retarded persons.

All of this does not mean that we can ignore the importance of lower intelligence per se, because personality traits and adaptive behavior patterns do not develop in a vacuum. In some instances, personality characteristics will reflect environmental factors that have little or nothing to do with intellectual endowment. In other instances, we must think in terms of an interaction; that is, given a lower intellectual ability, a person may well have certain experiences and develop certain behavior patterns differing from those of a person with higher intelligence. By exploring in more detail the factors that affect behavior, we hope to better understand the role of motivation in the life of retarded individuals.

This chapter has a two-part framework that explores issues relating to motivational aspects of retarded functioning. The first section outlines six major motivational factors thought to influence the behavior of retarded individuals, and presents empirical research showing how each factor operates. The second section presents new perspectives and future directions concerning motivational influences on the lives of those with below-average intelligence.

Studies of specific motivational factors

The focus of this section will be the discussion of motivational factors that have been shown to have a substantial impact on the lives of mentally retarded individuals. These factors include positive-reaction tendencies, negative-reaction tendencies, expectancy of success, reinforcer hierarchy, outerdirectedness, and self-concept. The section begins with a discussion of the environmental influence – social deprivation – that gives rise to these personality factors.

Social deprivation

Social deprivation is defined as a lack of continuity of care by parents or caretakers, an excessive desire by parents to separate from or institutionalize their child, impoverished economic circumstances, and/or a family history of marital discord, mental illness, abuse, or neglect. To incorporate these specific types of deprivation into a standardized measure, the Preinstitutional Social Deprivation Scale (PISD) was developed in 1966 and has been refined over the years (Butterfield & Zigler, 1970; Zigler, Butterfield, & Goff, 1966).

As shown by numerous empirical works (reviewed by Zigler & Hodapp, 1986), social deprivation has a noticeable effect on a variety of behaviors that retarded individuals display. Highly deprived retarded individuals have been found to be more verbally dependent and more wary than less-deprived children (Balla, Butterfield, & Zigler, 1974; Butterfield & MacIntyre, 1969). Although social deprivation can be experienced by any retarded child, most of the early work on this construct was performed in institutional settings. Retarded individuals enter institutions fully endowed with social and family histories that do not disappear as they pass through the institution gates. Indeed, preinstitutional social deprivation, where it exists, is clearly related to behavior once a person is institutionalized (Clarke & Clarke, 1954; Kaplun, 1935; Zigler, 1961; Zigler, Butterfield, & Capobianco, 1970; Zigler & Williams, 1963). Today, as institutions are replaced by home and homelike placements, the elements that comprise social deprivation may be shifting in prominence, or redefined altogether. Nonetheless, many retarded persons continue to be deprived in social realms, and their particular social experiences continue to affect their behavior.

Positive-reaction tendencies

An extensive line of research has shown that social deprivation results in a heightened motivation to interact with a supportive adult; this increased responsiveness to social reinforcement has been called the "positive-reaction tendency" (Balla & Zigler, 1975; Balla et al., 1974; Zigler, 1961; Zigler & Balla, 1972; Zigler, Balla, & Butterfield, 1968).

These studies have typically employed the use of adult–child interaction games in order to assess social responsiveness. The socially deprived child is thought to be more responsive than a less-deprived child and to be more persistent at a gamelike task if there is ample attention and support from the adult. For example, Zigler (1961) found that the greater the degree of social deprivation experienced by a retarded child, the more responsive this child will be to a supportive adult. Further, Harter and Zigler (1968) found that an adult examiner was a more effective social reinforcer than a peer examiner for institutionalized retarded children, but not for those who lived at home. Thus, the institutionalized retarded child's motivation to obtain social reinforcement appears to be based on a need for attention and praise dispensed by an adult, rather than on a more generalized desire for reinforcement dispensed by any social agent (e.g., a peer). In another study (Harter, 1967), institutionalized retarded individuals took significantly longer to solve a concept-formation problem in a social condition where they were face-to-face with a warm supportive examiner who praised their performance than in a standard condition where the examiner was silent and out of view. The retarded children in the social condition appeared highly motivated to interact with an approving adult, so much so that it seemed to compete with their attention to the learning task.

Some indication of the pervasiveness of the atypical dependency of institutionalized retarded persons may be found in a study by Zigler and Balla (1972). Retarded and nonretarded children of three MA levels (7, 9, and 12) were compared on their performance in an adult–child interaction game. In keeping with the general developmental progression from helplessness and dependence to autonomy and independence, both retarded and intellectually average children of higher MAs were found to be less motivated for social reinforcement than children of lower MAs. However, at each MA level, the retarded children were more dependent than the nonretarded children. This disparity in dependent behavior was just as marked at the highest MA level as at the lowest. Indeed, the oldest retarded group persisted at the adult–child interaction task almost twice as long as the youngest nonretarded group.

Institutions seem synonymous with social deprivation, but there is evidence that differences in the social–psychological climate of institutions can affect residents' behavior for better as well as for worse. For example, comparing two large residential schools in the same state with identical admission practices, Butterfield and Zigler (1965b) found that residents in an unenlightened and dehumanizing facility had a significantly higher motivation to receive attention from adults. The warmer, more homelike environment of the second institution helped make its residents less dependent on adult attention and approval.

To follow up this study, Zigler, Balla, and Kossan (1986) examined the behavioral effects of two large and five small institutions. The facilities were rated for demographic traits and for their social–psychological characteristics. The latter were assessed using King, Raynes, and Tizard's (1971) measure, which rates care practices on a scale from *institution-oriented* to *resident-oriented*. Outcome behaviors of interest were the individual's degree of wariness, imitation, and responsiveness to social reinforcement. As in prior research, MA was found to affect these motivational measures. Residents who had higher MAs were less dependent on adult social reinforcement; they were also less wary and less imitative of adults. Only one other personal variable related to the residents' behavior – the number of prior residential placements. The greater the number of previous residences, the more wary of adults the retarded residents became. For the most part, the demographic and social–psychological features of the institutions in this study did not affect the residents' behaviors that were measured.

We have addressed the socially deprived child's need for social reinforcement. This heightened motivation has also been viewed as an indicator of an important phenomenon discussed in the general child-development literature – namely, dependency. Thus, with a slight shift in terminology, we might conclude that a general consequence of social deprivation is overdependency. We cannot place enough emphasis on the role of such overdependency in the behavior of retarded persons. Given some minimal intellectual level, the shift from dependence to independence is perhaps the most important factor enabling retarded persons to become self-sustaining members of society (Zigler & Harter, 1969).

Negative-reaction tendencies

At variance with retarded individuals' increased desire for social reinforcement is their reluctance to interact with others (i.e., wariness). Wariness has been defined as an individual's watchful or cautious manner in social settings. This apparent inconsistency has raised questions about whether social deprivation leads to an increase in the desire for interaction or to apathy and withdrawal. Experimental work to date suggests that social deprivation results both in a heightened motivation to interact with supportive adults (positive-reaction tendency) and in a reluctance and wariness to do so (negative-reaction tendency).

The negative-reaction construct has been employed to explain some of the performance differences between retarded and nonretarded individuals originally reported by Kounin (1941a, 1941b). Kounin employed a simple two-part task in which both parts are highly similar and monotonous. A recurrent finding in studies utilizing such tasks (Kounin, 1941a, b; Zigler, 1958, 1961) is that retarded individuals show a much greater tendency than intellectually average individuals to spend more time on the second task than on the first. Zigler (1958) suggested that the institutionalized children learned during part one that the examiner was not like other strange adults, who initiated painful experiences (physical examinations, injections, etc.) while making supportive comments. This results in a reduction of the negative-reaction tendency. Part two is then met with a positive-reaction tendency; the child can now enjoy the social reinforcement, and so plays longer on part two than on part one. Evidence of this sort illustrates the effect positive social interaction has on the performance of retarded individuals.

A study by Zigler, Balla, and Butterfield (1968) illuminated some of the particular experiences that might make retarded children fear and mistrust adults. These investigators found that the parents' marital harmony factor in the PISD scale was most related to the manifestation of the negative-reaction tendency. The items in this factor include the nature of the parents' marital relationship, the father's and mother's mental health, and their general attitude toward the child. To further investigate the role of specific factors in the manifestation of wariness, Harter and Zigler (1968) employed both adult and peer examiners in the study described. Regardless of the examiner's age, institutionalized retarded children had a higher negative-reaction tendency than retarded children who lived at home. Thus, institutionalized retarded children exhibited a generalized wariness of strangers, and this could affect their ability to form friendships, which can lead to further social deprivation.

Another logical conclusion of the research on negative-reaction tendency is that wariness of adults and of the tasks they present leads to a general attenuation in the retarded child's social effectiveness. Retarded children's poor performance on tasks presented by adults is therefore not to be attributed entirely to intellectual factors, but must be interpreted in light of their atypically high negative-reaction tendency. This tendency motivates them toward behaviors (e.g., withdrawal) that reduce the quality of their performance to a level lower than that dictated by their intellectual capacity.

Expectancy of success

Another factor frequently noted as a determinant in the performance of retarded persons is their lowered expectancy of success. This characteristic is thought to be a consequence of regular encounters with tasks and situations that they are intellectually ill-equipped to handle. The pervasiveness of these feelings of failure can be seen in a series of studies by MacMillan and his colleagues (MacMillan, 1969; MacMillan & Keogh, 1971; MacMillan & Knopf, 1971). In these studies, children were prevented from finishing several tasks they had begun and were subsequently asked why the tasks were not completed. Retarded children consistently placed the blame on themselves, whereas nonretarded children attributed their failures to external causes.

In addition to work on attribution, other lines of research have focused on the effects of success and failure expectancies on problem-solving behavior. The task typically employed in these studies is called "probability learning," a three-choice discrimination problem in which one stimulus is reinforced about two-thirds of the time, while the remaining two stimuli are never reinforced. Children with low expectancies of success, as gauged by aspiration level or need-achievement measures, are more likely to use a maximizing strategy (persistent choice of the partially reinforced stimulus) on this task than children with high expectancies of success (Gruen, Ottinger, & Zigler, 1970; Kier, Styfco, & Zigler, 1977; Kreitler & Zigler, 1988; Luthar & Zigler, 1988; Ollendick & Gruen, 1971). Apparently, children with low aspirations settle for less than 100% success as an acceptable outcome, whereas those who expect 100% success, or a level of success greater than that allowed in the situation, try strategies other than maximizing in the hope of being right all the time.

Finally, Kreitler and Zigler (1988) tested two different age groups of nonretarded children to learn the effects of risk-taking and delay of gratification on performance. A high degree of risk-taking was associated with low maximizing, an effect possibly related to increased expectancy of success. Confident children who expected success on the task might trust their own choices a great deal and thus be willing to take risks on the choices, as opposed to children who expected failure, did not feel confident, and who would be willing to get any correct choices they could (thus increasing maximizing behaviors). In addition, children who were willing to delay gratification (e.g., wait for 6 days to receive five books rather than receive one book immediately) had a lower level of maximizing. Others who chose to receive a small, immediately available reward for participation increased maximizing because that strategy provided instant reinforcement. Further research in this area might also be used to understand the problem-solving approaches used by mentally retarded children to complete everyday tasks.

The reinforcer hierarchy

Because of experiential factors, the retarded individual's motivation for various incentives may differ from that of intellectually average individuals of the same MA. Moreover, the position of various reinforcers in the reinforcer hierarchy may differ in retarded and nonretarded children. For example, being correct may be more reinforcing for nonretarded children, whereas retarded youngsters may value the positive attention of the examiner much more than the satisfaction derived from performing the task correctly.

Such differences in reinforcer hierarchies can be seen in studies of tangible and intangible incentives. It has been argued that histories of failure and social deprivation cause retarded children to be less responsive to intangible reinforcement than are nonretarded children of equivalent mental age (Zigler, 1962; Zigler & deLabry, 1962; Zigler & Unell, 1962). This work is of special importance because intangible reinforcement (i.e., information that a response is correct) is the most immediate and frequently dispensed reinforcement in real-life tasks. When such a reinforcer is employed in experimental studies comparing retarded and nonretarded individuals, any group difference found might be attributable not to differences in intellectual capacity but rather to the different values that such reinforcement may have for the two types of individuals. The importance of the specific reinforcer dispensed in studies with retarded individuals was highlighted by both Plenderleith (1956) and Stevenson and Zigler (1957), who found that when tangible reinforcers were given, institutionalized retarded individuals were no more rigid than nonretarded persons on a discrimination reversal-learning task.

Support for the view that the retarded child is much less motivated to be correct for the sake of correctness can be found in a study by Zigler and deLabry (1962). MA-matched middle-SES, lower-SES, and retarded children were tested on a concept-switching task under two conditions of reinforcement: 1) the information that the child was correct, and 2) the reward of a toy if the child switched from one concept to another. In the "correct" condition, both the retarded and lower-SES groups were poorer in their concept-switching than the middle-SES children. However, no differences were found among the three groups that received tangible reinforcers. Furthermore, no differences in the ability to switch concepts were found among the three groups receiving what was assumed to be their optimal reinforcer (retarded, tangible; lower-SES, tangible; and middle-SES, intangible). Interestingly, both retarded and upper-SES children were found to switch concepts more readily in a tangible reinforcement condition than in an intangible condition (Zigler & Unell, 1962). One possible interpretation of this finding is that upper-SES children may value material rewards because they have learned that the receipt of such rewards is the true indicator of success. The familial retarded children, representing almost exclusively the lower SES, may value tangible rewards because they have been deprived of such rewards.

Another aspect of the value of different reinforcers concerns the intrinsic reinforcement that is inherent in being correct, regardless of whether an external agent dispenses a reinforcer for correctness. The work on this phenomenon owes much to White's (1959) formulation concerning the pervasive influence of the effectance or mastery motive. Effectance motivation is discerned in the pleasure people receive from having an effect on their environment. The effectance concept provides a rubric for a variety of behaviors that appear very central in an individual's behavioral repertoire (e.g., the desire for optimal levels of sensory stimulation, manipulation, exploration, and curiosity). A series of studies (Shultz & Zigler, 1970; Zigler, 1966a, 1966b; Zigler, Levine, & Gould, 1967) has given some support to this view that using one's own cognitive resources to their fullest is intrinsically gratifying, and thus motivating.

Further evidence on this point was provided by Harter and Zigler (1974). They presented MA-matched groups of nonretarded and retarded children who lived at home or in an institution with four tasks measuring various aspects of effectance motivation. Nonretarded children chose a nontangible reward (a "good player" certificate) over a tangible prize (candy) more often than did either retarded group. Furthermore, the nonretarded children showed the greatest desire to master a problem for the sake of mastery and to choose the most challenging task, and showed the greatest curiosity and exploratory behavior. The noninstitutionalized children showed less of these elements of effectance motivation, and the institutionalized children, in most cases, demonstrated the least. Thus, not only do retarded children differ from their nonretarded peers, but groups of retarded children, matched on intellectual functioning but differing in life experiences, also differ from one another in a general motive thought to influence a wide variety of behaviors.

Haywood and his colleagues extended work on the effectance motive by investigating "motivational orientation." This concept refers to a personality trait, probably learned and modifiable, by which persons may be characterized in terms of the sources of incentives that are effective in motivating their behavior, whether task-intrinsic or task-extrinsic. Persons who characteristically seek their satisfaction from task-intrinsic factors (e.g., responsibility, challenge, creativity) are referred to as intrinsically motivated. Those who tend instead to avoid dissatisfaction by concentrating on the ease, comfort, and practical aspects of the environment (i.e., task-extrinsic factors) are referred to as extrinsically motivated (Haywood & Switzky, 1985). Intrinsic motivational orientation is associated with greater task persistence (Haywood & Weaver, 1967); laboratory learning that is more effective and more resistant to extinction (Haywood & Wachs, 1966); higher school achievement (Dobbs, 1967; Haywood, 1968a, 1968b; Wooldridge, 1966); and preference for self-monitored rather than externally imposed control of performance and reinforcement (Haywood & Switzky, 1985; Switzky & Haywood, 1974).

Previous research on individual differences in motivational orientation has shown that retarded persons are, in general, less intrinsically motivated than are nonretarded persons. Haywood (1968a, 1968b) suggests that intrinsic motivational orientation is a function of both increasing chronological age and increasing MA. Given this complexity, the greater prevalence of "task-extrinsic" motivational orientation in retarded persons reflects yet another important motivational aspect in their day-to-day functioning.

Outerdirectedness

A history of an inordinate number of failure experiences borne by retarded individuals may lead to a style of problem solving characterized by outerdirectedness. That is, the child who frequently fails comes to distrust his or her own solutions to problems, and therefore seeks guides to action in the immediate environment. Three factors have been advanced as important in determining the child's degree of outerdirectedness: 1) the general level of cognitive development; 2) the incidence of success resulting from self-initiated solutions to problems; and 3) the extent of the child's attachment to adults (Balla, Kossan, & Zigler, 1980). Either too little or too much imitation of adults is viewed as a negative psychological indicator. Some intermediate level of imitation is seen as a positive developmental phenomenon reflecting the individual's healthy attachment to adults and responsivity to cues that adults emit, which can be utilized in the child's problem-solving efforts.

In general, the developmental aspect of the outerdirectedness formulation has received experimental support. Among nonretarded children, outerdirectedness has been found to decrease with increasing MA (MacMillan & Wright, 1974; Ruble & Nakamura, 1973; Yando & Zigler, 1971; Zigler & Yando, 1972). This developmental shift has also been found in institutionalized retarded persons (Turnure, 1970a, 1970b) and in noninstitutionalized mildly retarded children (Balla, Styfco, & Zigler, 1971; Gordan & MacLean, 1977). Apparently for younger children, outer-directedness is more conducive to problem-solving than is dependency upon poorly developed cognitive abilities. With growth and development, children should become more innerdirected, because their expanded abilities lessen their need for external cues. Furthermore, as children grow older and become more independent, adults gradually reduce their cues in both number and detail. This further decreases the effectiveness of an outerdirected style.

The success–failure aspect of the outer-directedness formulation has generated the prediction that retarded children, because of their histories of failure, are more outerdirected in their problem-solving behavior than are nonretarded children of the same MA, a prediction that has been confirmed in several studies (Achenbach & Zigler, 1968; Balla, Styfco, & Zigler, 1971; Sanders, Zigler, & Butterfield, 1968; Turnure & Zigler, 1964; Yando & Zigler, 1971). These studies have also indicated that both nonretarded and retarded children become more outerdirected following failure rather than success experiences.

An outerdirected style of problem solving might be modifiable based on the type of problem given. In a study by Bybee and Zigler (1988), mentally retarded children exhibited more outerdirectedness than nonretarded children, yet the groups did *not* differ in levels of outerdirectedness when easy tasks were presented before more difficult ones. Having an easy initial task may have raised retarded children's confidence level, expectations of success, and trust in their own cognitive abilities, those very traits and attributions thought to be lowered by their greater history of failure. It may be that the frequent failure experienced by retarded individuals makes them more sensitive to failure on tasks they are asked to perform, which leads to further failure, loss of confidence, and greater outerdirectedness. In addition, nonretarded children as opposed to retarded children were much more sensitive to characteristics such as task difficulty and external cues, and used outerdirected approaches in a strategic and benefical manner.

Whereas an outerdirected style of problem solving can apparently be reduced, sometimes it fails to materialize even when it is an age-appropriate behavior. There is some evidence that individuals who have not formed healthy attachments to adults will have atypically low levels of outer-directedness. Balla et al. (1980) found that institutionalized retarded individuals whose caretakers had negative attitudes concerning them were less outerdirected than those whose caretakers had positive attitudes. Thus, individuals who are responded to in a negative manner may learn to ignore cues provided by adults, and thus lose important models and guides to behavior.

The research on outerdirectedness teaches important lessons about the problem-solving approaches of mentally retarded individuals. First, having some level of outerdirectedness is useful in learning during early stages of development, whereas high levels foster dependency on adults. Second, outerdirectedness can to some extent be controlled by fostering a sense of success. The implications of outerdirectedness research in applied settings (e.g., classroom) are discussed in the last section of this chapter.

Self-concept

The self-concept construct has played a central role in general personality theory, but oddly enough has received relatively little attention in the mental retardation literature (Balla & Zigler, 1979). Traditionally, a person's self-concept has been viewed as heavily influenced by life experiences. Thus, one might expect that both perceived intellectual inadequacy and pervasive stigmatization of retarded persons would result in their having lower self-concepts than nonretarded individuals of the same mental age. This supposition, however, has been only partially confirmed.

One way to gauge the effect of experience on self-image is to compare retarded persons in different settings. For example, several investigators have compared institutionalized and noninstitutionalized retarded individuals on self-concept measures, but the results are mixed. For example, Gorlow, Butler, and Guthrie (1963) reported lower self-concepts in retarded persons living in institutions. The results of a similar study by Harrisón and Budoff (1972) indicated that when the issue was one of competence with a task, the institutionalized groups used their peers as a reference group, and felt superior. In issues concerning social status and affect, however, this group used the world at large for their frame of reference, and felt inferior.

An alternate view to the self-concept as a function of life experience is the developmental approach proposed by Zigler and his colleagues (Achenbach & Zigler, 1963; Glick & Zigler, 1985; Katz & Zigler, 1967). The central argument in this work is that the development of an individual must invariably be accompanied by a growing disparity between the assessment of the real self-image and the ideal self-image. Real self-image is defined as how one sees oneself. For example, a boy might consider himself a good person, or good at sports, academics, or socially popular. The ideal self-image is how one would ideally like to be. Thus, the boy would like to be popular, accomplished at sports, and excel in academics. According to developmental theory, the difference between the individual's real self-image and ideal self-image becomes greater with higher levels of development. In one study (Zigler, Balla, & Watson, 1972), retarded children reported less self-image disparity (difference between real and ideal self-image) and lower ideal self-image than nonretarded children. However, no differences emerged between the retarded and nonretarded groups on measures of real self-image.

Among subgroups, older retarded children had a more adverse self-concept than did their nonretarded peers matched on both CA and MA (see also Leahy, Balla, & Zigler, 1982). These findings seem to indicate that one consequence of being identified as retarded is a lowering of goals and aspirations, an interpretation certainly consistent with the expectancy-of-success literature cited earlier in this chapter. In addition, Phillips and Zigler (1980) examined differences among socioeconomic levels in four groups of low- and middle-SES black and white children. Consistent with earlier findings (Rosenberg & Simmons, 1971; Trowbridge, 1972), some evidence was found indicating lower ideal self-images in low-SES children than in middle-SES children. As with black children, the low-SES children did not exhibit depressed real self-images relative to middle-SES children of the same age. Apparently, the low-SES children also have developed a positive, self-protective orientation such that the rejection accorded their economic status by the society's majority is not directly internalized (see Rosenberg, 1979; Trowbridge, 1972).

New perspectives and future directions

Much of the past research on motivational variables affecting the performance of retarded persons has been limited because investigators have targeted specific groups (e.g., moderately or mildly retarded individuals) and dealt only with selected aspects of personality–motivational functioning. To expand our knowledge and understanding, we must begin to consider other motivational influences that affect behavior. In this section we will address four areas that may provide new insights: (1) motivational differences across levels of retardation, (2) assessment and intervention techniques, (3) the relationship between IQ and psychiatric disorders, and (4) the role of etiology.

Motivational differences across levels of retardation

A paramount issue in the study of motivational variables affecting performance has been the ability of persons with below-average intelligence to adapt successfully in their community. Studies conducted in Sweden by Granat and Granat (1973, 1978) produced important findings on how intellectual level relates to adaptation and functioning in society. The Swedish government maintains a well-organized system of compiling case record data on all Swedish citizens. From this registry, Granat and Granat reviewed the records of 2,000 nineteen-year-old males who were about to serve their mandatory military service. Although none of the men was officially identified as retarded, a fair percentage of them had IQ scores in the mentally retarded range. Their adjustment in the community was apparently such that their retardation had gone undetected. Thus, any straightforward link between intelligence and adaptability was called into question. Evidence of this kind casts a shadow on the validity of using psychometric measures to determine one's ability to adjust in society.

Additional analyses on a smaller sample of Swedish military recruits with IQs below 84 yielded four homogeneous clusters with respect to social and personal adjustment. These four clusters included a well-adjusted cluster (51.6%), a personal-problem cluster (25.0%), a crime cluster (11.7%), and a work-problem cluster (11.7%). Thus, individuals of any IQ can develop either adaptive or maladaptive social adjustment.

Although these findings do not indicate that intellectual level influences successful adaptation in society, Ross, Begab, Dondis, Giampiccolo, and Meyers (1985) concluded that IQ can be considered to be at least one important measure in determining degrees of "self-sufficiency." Ross et al. (1985) found no degree of self-sufficiency for persons with IQs 39 or lower. As one goes up the IQ spectrum, the percentage of persons with self-sufficiency increased. For example, at IQ 40 to 49, 20% of persons were self-sufficient; there were 42% at IQ 50 to 59; 71% at IQ 60 to 69; and at IQ 70 to 79, 84% were self-sufficient. In view of these results, one can conclude that a threshold exists at which IQ is a critical factor in predicting an individual's ability to be self-sufficient. Moreover, a person would seem to need an IQ somewhere at or near the moderate level of mental retardation in order to have the potential to care for himself or herself.

Supporters of motivational and personality factors that affect adjustment in society (e.g., Granat & Granat, 1978; Zigler, 1971) have not discounted the role that IQ plays in retarded functioning, but advocate that these nonintellectual factors are crucial to the understanding of retarded behavior. Moreover, "regardless of whether motivation is considered as attenuating the achievements of retarded individuals (Zigler, 1973) or actually shaping them, it is important to study the impact of motivation, both in its own right and as a determinant of the performance deficit" (Kreitler & Kreitler, 1989).

Thus, *both* IQ and personality–motivational factors are important determinants in life success. Personality–motivational factors may exert more influence when IQ is at or above moderate levels of mental retardation, and higher IQ still may facilitate adjustment. More work is needed on the relationship between IQ, personality–motivation, and life success.

Assessment and intervention techniques

Despite the wealth of data on motivational variables, there has been little translation of research findings into comprehensive assessment and intervention techniques that can be used outside the lab. To bring empirical findings into the real world (e.g., the classroom), special attention must be paid to the practical applications of the study. For example, we said earlier that retarded children in general are more likely to display outerdirected behavior than are nonretarded children of the same MA. Bybee and Zigler (1988) looked at factors influencing an outerdirected approach to problem solving and concluded that the difficulty of the preceding task greatly affected the subsequent performance of the retarded children. This finding has many practical implications. In view of the strong effect an initial task can have on the performance of a retarded child, attending to the degree of difficulty and complexity of a set of tasks (e.g., easier first, difficult last) can influence the child's problem-solving behavior. Moreover, by allowing a retarded child to experience success and accomplishment in the early stages of a task, the probability of success on subsequent stages is greatly enhanced. By fostering initial success on a new task, the teacher will also help the child develop a sense of accomplishment that will be reflected in other domains.

The relationship between IQ and psychiatric disorders

The third area needing further study is that of dual diagnosis – that is, mentally retarded individuals who also suffer from mental illness. For years, the areas of mental retardation and mental illness were treated as independent phenomena. Linking mental retardation and mental illness has generated strong negative reactions from advocacy groups such as parent organizations, although several investigators (e.g., Zigler, 1971) have long anticipated a relation between these two areas.

Recent work in the area of dual diagnosis has illuminated possible emotional factors that influence retarded persons. Zigler and Burack (in press) addressed these issues and contended that "Researchers in mental retardation have traditionally focused on cognitive aspects of the disorder and ignored social and personality factors. One consequence is that little attention has been paid to the mental health of mentally retarded persons." It is important to acknowledge that the lives of retarded persons are very much affected by the same emotions and life events (e.g., fear, anxiety, death of loved ones) that affect nonretarded individuals.

Further, in the case of retarded persons, certain motivational styles such as outerdirectedness and negative-reaction tendency may lead to personality profiles that display higher than average levels of dependency, or even avoidance. In addition, having a past history of consistent failure and limited social praise can lead to depression. Recent work using self-report scales of depression has shown that in fact some mentally retarded persons do manifest feelings that meet the criteria for a formal diagnosis of depression (Reynolds & Baker, 1988).

These findings point to the need for clinical diagnoses by mental health professionals to determine the incidence of emotional problems among mentally retarded individuals. At present helpful treatment is not available because the link between motivational variables and personality disorders has been largely unexplored.

The role of etiology

A fourth area of motivational influence concerns the effect of etiology. Until recently, little attention had been given to the effect of different organic etiologies among the mentally retarded population. Given that more than 200 different forms of mental retardation are currently documented, it would be myopic for researchers to conclude that differences in etiology have no influence on adjustment. Burack, Hodapp, and Zigler (1988; see also chapter 2 of this book) support this view, and state that "Although an undifferentiated view may have been a helpful theoretical framework for earlier work in mental retardation, it is our contention that continuing to ignore etiological variables will adversely impact both research and intervention in this field" (p. 766). This renewed attention to etiology might also be important as concerns the effect of personality–motivational variables on the functioning of mentally retarded individuals. As an example, Yando, Seitz, and Zigler (1988) found that differences emerged on measures of imitativeness between groups of noninstitutionalized organic and familial retarded children at two CA levels. Findings of this sort begin to demonstrate that etiology, independent of IQ, has an impact on the functioning of retarded individuals. See chapter 2 for a more complete analysis of this issue.

The emergence of the area of motivational influences in the behavior of retarded persons has enhanced our knowledge as well as generated many new avenues of inquiry. The issues of motivational influences on different levels of retardation, research-based intervention work, dual diagnosis, and etiology are only a few of the areas that merit investigation. As we continue to expand our knowledge of motivational, personality, and mental health factors that affect the functioning of retarded persons, the closer we will come to understanding the retarded individual not as a cognitive system but as a whole person.

References

Achenbach, T., & Zigler, E. (1963). Social competence and self-image disparity in psychiatric and nonpsychiatric patients. *Journal of Abnormal and Social Psychology*, *67*, 197–205.

Achenbach, T., & Zigler, E. (1968). Cue-learning and problem-learning strategies in normal and retarded children. *Child Development*, *3*, 827–848.

Balla, D., Butterfield, E., & Zigler, E. (1974). Effects of institutionalization on retarded children: A longitudinal, cross-institutional investigation. *American Journal of Mental Deficiency*, *78*, 530–549.

Balla, D., Kossan, N., & Zigler, E. (1980). *Effects of preinstitutional history and institutionalization on the behavior of the retarded*. Unpublished manuscript, Yale University, New Haven, CT.

Balla, D., Styfco, S., & Zigler, E. (1971). Use of the opposition concept and outer-directedness in intellectually average, familial retarded, and organically retarded children. *American Journal of Mental Deficiency*, *75*, 863–880.

Balla, D., & Zigler, E. (1975). Pre-institutional social deprivation, responses to social reinforcement, and IQ change in institutionalized retarded individuals: A six-year follow-up study. *American Journal of Mental Deficiency*, *80*, 228–230.

Balla, D., & Zigler, E. (1979). Personality development in retarded persons. In N.R. Ellis (Ed.), *Handbook of mental deficiency* (2nd ed.). Hillside, NJ: Erlbaum.

Burack, J.A., Hodapp, R.M., & Zigler, E. (1988). Issues in the classification of mental retardation: Differentiating among organic etiologies. *Journal of Child Psychology and Psychiatry*, *29*(6), 765–779.

Butterfield, E.C., & MacIntyre, A. (1969). Cognitive and motivational factors in concept switching among the retarded. *American Journal of Mental Deficiency*, *74*, 235–241.

Butterfield, E.C., & Zigler, E. (1965b). The influence of differing social climates on the effectiveness of social reinforcement in the mentally retarded. *American Journal of Mental Deficiency*, *70*, 48–56.

Butterfield, E.C., & Zigler, E. (1970). Preinstitutional social deprivation and IQ changes among institutionalized retarded children. *Journal of Abnormal Psychology*, *75*, 83–89.

Bybee, J.A., & Zigler, E. (1988). *Is outerdirectedness harmful or beneficial to normal and mentally retarded children?* Manuscript submitted for publication..

Clarke, A.D.B., & Clarke, A.M. (1954). Cognitive changes in the feeble-minded. *British Journal of Psychology*, *45*, 173–179.

Dobbs, V. (1967). *Motivational orientation and programmed instruction achievement gains of educable mentally retarded adolescents*. Unpublished doctoral dissertation, George Peabody College, Nashville, TN.

Fernald, G. (1919). The defective delinquent since the war. *Journal of Psycho-Asthenics*, *24*, 55–64.

Glick, M., & Zigler, E. (1985). Self-image: A cognitive–developmental approach. In R.L. Leahy (Ed.), *The development of the self* (pp. 1–53). New York: Academic Press.

Gordan, D.A., & MacLean, W.E. (1977). Developmental analysis of outerdirectedness in institutionalized EMR children. *American Journal of Mental Deficiency, 81*, 508–511.

Gorlow, L., Butler, A., & Guthrie, G. (1963). Correlates of self-attitudes of retardates. *American Journal of Mental Deficiency, 67*, 549–554.

Granat, K., & Granat, S. (1973). Below-average intelligence and mental retardation. *American Journal of Mental Deficiency, 78*, 27–32.

Granat, K., & Granat, S. (1978). Adjustment of intellectually below-average men not identified as mentally retarded. *Scandinavian Journal of Psychology, 19*, 41–51.

Gruen, G., Ottinger, D., & Zigler, E. (1970). Level of aspiration and the probability learning of middle- and lower-class children. *Developmental Psychology, 3*, 133–142.

Harrell, T.W., & Harrell, M.S. (1945). Army general classification test scores for civilian occupations. *Educational and Psychological Measurement, 5*, 229–239.

Harrison, R.H., & Budoff, H. (1972). Demographic, historical and ability correlates of the Laurelton self-concept scale in an EMR sample. *American Journal of Mental Deficiency, 76*, 460–480.

Harter, S. (1967). Mental age, IQ, and motivational factors in the discrimination learning set performance of normal and retarded children. *Journal of Experimental Child Psychology, 5*, 123–141.

Harter, S., & Zigler, E. (1968). Effectiveness of adult and peer reinforcement on the performance of institutionalized and noninstitutionalized retardates. *Journal of Abnormal Psychology, 73*, 144–149.

Harter, S., & Zigler, E. (1974). The assessment of effectance motivation in normal and retarded children. *Developmental Psychology, 10*, 169–180.

Haywood, H.C. (1968a). Motivational orientation of overachieving and underachieving elementary school children. *American Journal of Mental Deficiency, 72*, 662–667.

Haywood, H.C. (1968b). Psychometric motivation and the efficiency of learning and performance in the mentally retarded. In B.W. Richards (Ed.), *Proceedings of the First Congress of the International Association for the Scientific Study of Mental Deficiency* (pp. 276–283). Reigate, England: Michael Jackson.

Haywood, H.C., & Switzky, H.N. (1985). Work response of mildly mentally retarded adults to self versus external regulation as a function of motivational orientation. *American Journal of Mental Deficiency, 90*, 151–159.

Haywood, H.C., & Wachs, T.D. (1966). Size discrimination learning as a function of motivation-hygiene orientation in adolescents. *Journal of Educational Psychology, 57*, 279–286.

Haywood, H.C., & Weaver, S.J. (1967). Differential effects of motivational orientation and incentive conditions on motor performance in institutionalized retardates. *American Journal of Mental Deficiency, 72*, 459–467.

Kaplun, D. (1935). The high-grade moron. *Proceedings of the American Association on Mental Deficiency, 40*, 68–89.

Katz, P., & Zigler, E. (1967). Self-image disparity: A developmental approach. *Journal of Personality and Social Psychology, 5*, 186–195.

Kier, R.J., Styfco, S.J., & Zigler, E. (1977). Success expectancies and the probability learning of children of low and middle socioeconomic status. *Developmental Psychology, 13*, 444–449.

King, R.D., Raynes, N.V., & Tizard, J. (1971). *Patterns of residential care: Sociological studies in institutions for handicapped children.* London: Routledge and Kegan Paul.

Kounin, J. (1941a). Experimental studies of rigidity: I. The measurement of rigidity in normal and feebleminded persons. *Character and Personality, 9*, 251–272.

Kounin, J. (1941b). Experimental studies of rigidity: II. The explanatory power of the concept of rigidity as applied to feeble-mindedness. *Character and Personality, 9,* 273–282.

Kreitler, S., & Kreitler, H. (1989). The cognitive approach to motivation in retarded individuals. *International review of research in mental retardation* (Vol. 15, pp. 81–123). New York: Academic Press.

Kreitler, S., & Zigler, E. (1988). *Motivational determinants of children's probability learning.* Manuscript submitted for publication.

Leahy, R., Balla, D., & Zigler, E. (1982). Role taking, self-image, and imitation in retarded and nonretarded individuals. *American Journal of Mental Deficiency, 86,* 372–379.

Luthar, S., & Zigler, E. (1988). Motivational factors, school atmosphere, and SES: Determinants of children's probability task performance. *Journal of Applied Developmental Psychology, 9,* 477–494.

MacMillan, D.L. (1969). Motivational differences: Cultural–familial retardates vs. normal subjects on expectancy for failure. *American Journal of Mental Deficiency, 74,* 254–258.

MacMillan, D.L., & Keogh, B.K. (1971). Normal and retarded children's expectancy for failure. *Developmental Psychology, 4,* 343–348.

MacMillan, D.L., & Knopf, E.D. (1971). Effect of instructional set on perceptions of event outcomes by EMR and nonretarded children. *American Journal of Mental Deficiency, 76,* 185–189.

MacMillan, D.L., & Wright, D.L. (1974). Outerdirectedness in children of three ages as a function of experimentally induced success and failure. *Journal of Educational Psychology, 68,* 919–925.

Ollendick, T., & Gruen, G. (1971). Level of achievement and probability in children. *Developmental Psychology, 4,* 486.

Penrose, L.S. (1963). *The biology of mental defect.* London: Sidgwick & Jackson.

Phillips, D.A., & Zigler, E. (1980). Children's self-image disparity: Effects of age, socioeconomic status, ethnicity, and gender. *Journal of Personality and Social Psychology, 39,* 689–700.

Plenderleith, M. (1956). Discrimination learning and discrimination reversal learning in normal and feebleminded children. *Journal of Genetic Psychology, 88,* 107–112.

Potter, H. (1922). The relationship of personality to the mental defective with a method for its evaluation. *Journal of Psycho-Asthenics, 27,* 27–38.

Reynolds, W.M., & Baker, J.A. (1988). Assessment of depression in persons with mental retardation. *American Journal on Mental Retardation, 93,* 93–103.

Rosenberg, M. (1979). *Conceiving the self.* New York: Basic Books.

Rosenberg, M., & Simmons, R. (1971). *Black and white self-esteem: The urban school child* (Monograph: Arnold and Caroline Rose Series in Ecology). Washington, DC: American Sociological Association.

Ross, T.T., Begab, M.J., Dondis, E.H., Giampiccolo, J.S., & Meyers, C.E. (1985). *Lives of the mentally retarded: A forty-year follow-up study.* Stanford, CA: Stanford University Press.

Ruble, D.N., & Nakamura, C. (1973). Outerdirectedness as a problem-solving approach in relation to developmental level and selected task variables. *Child Development, 44,* 519–528.

Sanders, B., Zigler, E., & Butterfield, E.C. (1968). Outer-directedness in the discrimination learning of normal and mentally retarded children. *Journal of Abnormal Psychology, 73,* 368–375.

Sarason, S.B. (1953). *Psychological problems in mental deficiency.* New York: Harper & Row.

Shultz, T., & Zigler, E. (1970). Emotional concomitants of visual mastery in infants: The effects of stimulus movement on smiling and vocalizing. *Journal of Experimental Child Psychology, 10,* 390–402.

Stevenson, H.W., & Zigler, E. (1957). Discrimination learning and rigidity in normal and feebleminded individuals. *Journal of Personality, 25,* 699–711.

Switzky, H.N., & Haywood, H.C. (1974). Motivational orientation and the relative efficacy of self-monitored and externally imposed reinforcements schedules. *Journal of Personality and Social Psychology, 30,* 360–366.

Tizard, J. (1953). The prevalence of mental subnormality. *Bulletin of the World Health Organization, 9,* 423–440.

Trowbridge, N. (1972). Self-concept and socio-economic status in elementary school children. *American Educational Research Journal, 4,* 525–537.

Turnure, J.E. (1970a). Reactions to physical and social distractors by moderately retarded institutionalized children. *Journal of Special Education, 4,* 283–294.

Turnure, J.E. (1970b). Distractibility in the mentally retarded: Negative evidence for an orienting inadequacy. *Exceptional Children, 37,* 181–186.

Turnure, J.E., & Zigler, E. (1964). Outer-directedness in the problem-solving of normal and retarded children. *Journal of Abnormal and Social Psychology, 69,* 427–436.

Weaver, T.R. (1946). The incident of maladjustment among mental defectives in military environments. *American Journal of Mental Deficiency, 51,* 238–246.

White, R. (1959). Motivation reconsidered: The concept of competence. *Psychological Review, 66,* 297–333.

Windle, C. (1962). Prognosis of mental subnormals. *American Journal of Mental Deficiency, 66* (Monograph Supplement to No. 5).

Wooldrige, R. (1966). *Motivation–hygiene orientation and school achievement in mentally subnormal children.* Unpublished Ed. D. study, George Peabody College, Nashville, TN.

Yando, R., Seitz, V., & Zigler, E. (1988). *Imitation, recall, and imitativeness in organic and familial retarded children.* Manuscript submitted for publication.

Yando, R., & Zigler, E. (1971). Outerdirectedness in the problem-solving of institutionalized and noninstitutionalized normal and retarded children. *Developmental Psychology, 4,* 277–288.

Zigler, E. (1958). *The effect of preinstitutional social deprivation on the performance of feebleminded children.* Unpublished doctoral dissertation, University of Texas, Austin, TX.

Zigler, E. (1961). Social deprivation and rigidity in the performance of feebleminded children. *Journal of Abnormal and Social Psychology, 62,* 413–421.

Zigler, E. (1962). Social deprivation in familial and organic retardates. *Psychological Reports, 10,* 370.

Zigler, E. (1966a). Mental retardation: Current issues and approaches. In L.W. Hoffman & M.L. Hoffman (Eds.), *Review of child development research* (Vol. 2). New York: Russell Sage.

Zigler, E. (1966b). Motivational determinants in the performance of feebleminded children. *American Journal of Orthopsychiatry, 36,* 848–856.

Zigler, E. (1971). The retarded child as a whole person. In H.E. Adams & W.K. Boardman (Eds.), *Advances in experimental clinical psychology.* New York: Pergamon.

Zigler, E. (1973). Why retarded children do not perform up to the level of their ability. In R.M. Allen, A.D. Cortazzo, & R. Toister (Eds.), *Theories of cognitive development: Implications for the mentally retarded.* Coral Gables, FL: University of Miami Press.

Zigler, E., & Balla, D. (1972). Developmental course of responsiveness to social reinforcement in normal children and institutionalized retarded children. *Developmental Psychology, 6,* 66–73.

Zigler, E., Balla, D., & Butterfield, E.C. (1968). A longitudinal investigation of the relationship between preinstitutional social deprivation and social motivation in institutionalized retardates. *Journal of Personality and Social Psychology, 10,* 437–445.

Zigler, E., Balla, D., & Kossan, N. (1986). Effects of types of institutionalization on some non-intellective correlates of retarded persons' behavior. *American Journal of Mental Deficiency, 91*, 10–17.

Zigler, E., Balla, D., & Watson, N. (1972). Developmental and experimental determinants of self-image disparity in institutionalized and noninstitutionalized retarded and normal children. *Journal of Personality and Social Psychology, 23*, 81–87.

Zigler, E., & Burack, J.A. (in press). Personality development and the dually diagnosed person. *Journal of Developmental Disabilities.*

Zigler, E., Butterfield, E.C., & Capobianco, F. (1970). Institutionalization and the effectiveness of social reinforcement: A five- and eight-year follow-up study. *Developmental Psychology, 3*, 255–263.

Zigler, E., Butterfield, E.C., & Goff, G.A. (1966). A measure of preinstitutional social deprivation for institutionalized retardates. *American Journal of Mental Deficiency, 70*, 873–885.

Zigler, E., & deLabry, J. (1962). Concept-switching in middle-class, lower-class, and retarded children. *Journal of Abnormal and Social Psychology, 65*, 267–273.

Zigler, E., & Harter, S. (1969). Socialization of the mentally retarded. In D.A. Goslin & D.C. Glass (Eds.), *Handbook of socialization theory and research.*. New York: Rand McNally.

Zigler, E., & Hodapp, R.M. (1984). *Understanding mental retardation.* New York: Cambridge University Press.

Zigler, E., Levine, J., & Gould, L. (1967). Cognitive challenge as a factor in children's humor appreciation. *Journal of Personality and Social Psychology, 6*, 332–336.

Zigler, E., & Unell, E. (1962). Concept-switching in normal and feebleminded children as a function of reinforcement. *American Journal of Mental Deficiency, 66*, 651–657.

Zigler, E., & Williams, J. (1963). Institutionalization and the effectiveness of social reinforcement: A three year follow-up study. *Journal of Abnormal Social Psychology, 66*, 197–205.

Zigler, E., & Yando, R. (1972). Outerdirectedness and imitative behavior of institutionalized and noninstitutionalized younger and older children. *Child Development, 43*, 413–425.

Part 2

**Applying developmental theory to
different types of retarded individuals**

7   Cultural–familial mental retardation: A developmental perspective on cognitive performance and "helpless" behavior

John R. Weisz

The developmental position – to which this volume is devoted – has proven to be a theory-rich enterprise. This position is associated most directly with theories of cognitive functioning in mentally retarded persons. However, the developmental position has also stimulated a wealth of theory on the role of extracognitive (e.g., motivational and personality) factors that influence the behavior of mentally retarded people. In keeping with that tradition, this chapter will address both cognitive and extracognitive processes, delving into theory and research on how both processes may shape the observed behavior of mentally retarded people.

Cultural–familial retardation

The chapter will focus specifically on cultural-familial retardation, a condition that describes approximately 75% of all retarded people. Individuals suffering from this form of retardation have also been labeled "retarded due to psychosocial disadvantage" in an American Association on Mental Deficiency publication on classification (Grossman, 1983, p. 149).

Characteristics of cultural–familial retarded people

The cultural–familial group includes those individuals whose mental retardation does not result from specific, identifiable organic or genetic anomalies (e.g., Down syndrome or focused brain damage); excluded from the cultural–familial group are "those whose intellectual apparatus has been damaged, thus altering the biological side of the formula" (Zigler, 1987, p. 4). Accordingly, unusual physical characteristics such as those associated with Down syndrome or phenylketonuria are not likely to be present; instead, cultural–familial retarded persons tend to look very much like their nonretarded peers. To fit a strict definition of cultural–familial retardation, the individual must have at least one other immediate family member who is also mentally retarded. Finally, the level of retardation is usually mild, with IQs rarely lower than 45–50.

Prevalence

Exact figures on the prevalence of cultural–familial retardation in the United States are not available. However, it is possible to generate a reasonable estimate. If we assume a U.S. population of 240 million and a prevalence rate of 3% for all forms of mental retardation combined, we can estimate the prevalence to be 7,500,000 – the approximate number of mentally retarded people in the United States. Of these, approximately 75% – 5,625,000 – can be expected to suffer from cultural–familial mental retardation.

Etiology: Resurgence of the nature–nurture debate

What causes cultural–familial retardation? Efforts to answer this question have fanned the flames of the nature–nurture controversy. Some experts emphasize the possible role of environmental factors. Indeed, recent American Association on Mental Deficiency manuals (Grossman 1977, 1983) appear to assume a heavily environmental etiology. In stressing environmental factors, some note that cultural–familial retardation is most prevalent in lower SES groups; they suggest that environmental factors associated with low SES – factors such as relatively poor prenatal care, poor childhood nutrition, and poor educational opportunity – may inhibit intellectual development, thus increasing the likelihood of cultural–familial mental retardation.

Some evidence supporting an environmental view comes from various early intervention projects focused on children thought to be at risk for mental retardation (because of such risk factors as low parental IQ, low parental educational attainment, and low family income). In general, the best known of these studies (some described by Zigler and Hodapp, 1986) suggest that various educational and social support procedures may enhance intellectual development (or prevent declines in intellectual development), at least in the years immediately following the interventions. In some cases, the effects of these interventions on IQ may well have been sufficient to prevent some youngsters from being classified as cultural–familial mentally retarded. It should be added, though, that IQ effects of the early interventions are often found to fade substantially over the years after termination of the interventions (Bronfenbrenner, 1975).

Other researchers have emphasized the role of genetic factors. Even the linkage between cultural–familial retardation and low SES could be consistent with this emphasis: Genetic factors could limit intellectual development, thus inhibiting educational and occupational attainment, which in turn would lead to low SES ratings.

The expanding body of evidence from studies of twins and adopted children casts serious doubt on any claim that IQ scores reflect exclusive or predominant effects of environment. For example, the correlation between the IQs of siblings increases markedly with increases in their genetic similarity. Vernon (1979) reported an average intelligence test score correlation coefficient of .24 for unrelated siblings (i.e., one or both adopted) reared together, .56 for dizygotic twins reared together, .74 for monozygotic twins reared apart, and .87 for monozygotic twins reared together. Note that monozygotic twin pairs showed strongly correlated IQs even when they were reared apart.

Although such evidence tends to highlight the role of genetic factors, we should add three qualifications. First, we should not overlook the fact that being reared in the same home slightly enhanced the correlation for monozygotic twins; this supports the notion that environment does play a role. Second, adoption agencies do not place children randomly; instead, agencies tend to place children in environments similar to those of their biological families. This means that monozygotic twins reared apart may often be reared in similar environments. So, comparison of monozygotic twins reared together and apart may underestimate the effects of environment. Third, monozygotic twins, because they resemble one another so closely, may be treated more similarly by parents and others than are dizygotic twins; this tendency might partially explain the finding that monozygotic twins were more highly correlated in IQ than were dizygotic twins.

Finally, it is useful to bear in mind the relativity of our assessments of heritability of intelligence or any other human characteristic. If all individuals under study lived within exactly the same environment (obviously an impossibility), all the variance in intelligence across those individuals would be attributable to genetic factors. With other factors held constant, (1) the proportion of variance in intelligence that is attributable to environmental factors increases with the variability of the environments studied, and (2) the proportion of variance in intelligence that is attributable to genetic factors increases with the variability of the genetic endowments studied.

Despite these caveats, many experts agree that the overall pattern of findings from studies of twins and adopted children makes a convincing case for the role of genetic factors. According to Zigler (1987), "Many heritability studies indicate that approximately 60 percent of the variation in IQ scores is due to genetic factors" (p. 4). In my view, given the current state of knowledge, the most valid etiological model for cultural–familial retardation includes both environmental and genetic factors, with the latter apparently contributing somewhat more than the former, at least in most populations and environments studied thus far.

Development of cognitive functioning among cultural–familial retarded people and nonretarded people

Cultural–familial retarded people are unquestionably different from nonretarded people in their cognitive functioning. But *how* are they different? As the following review suggests, the answer to this question may turn out to be surprisingly complex.

The developmental–difference controversy

The review is organized around a theoretical debate that has come to be called the "developmental–difference controversy." The debate, discussed throughout this volume, involves several theories that cluster around two poles.

At one pole is the "developmental position," articulated by Edward Zigler and his colleagues (e.g., Zigler, 1969; Zigler & Balla, 1982). This position applies specifically to cultural–familial retarded persons. This limitation seems appropriate in that the population of retarded people who have specific physiological deficits and genetic anomalies may have a more heterogeneous array of cognitive processes that are difficult to encompass within a single cognitive theory. Retarded people without such specific deficits – i.e., the cultural–familial group – are thought to represent the natural lower end of the normal distribution of intelligence. As such, they are subject to the provisions of the general theory.

Retarded individuals in this cultural–familial group, according to the developmental position, pass through stages of cognitive development in the same order as nonretarded individuals. But the two groups are said to differ in two respects – retarded people pass through the stages at a slower pace, and cease their cognitive development at a lower level than do the nonretarded. Zigler (for example, 1969) does not explicitly define the "stages" to which he refers, but he appears to construe them in largely Piagetian terms. The developmental position also holds that familial retarded and nonretarded people who are similar in level of cognitive development (typically, operationally defined as mental age) will also be similar in the formal cognitive processes they employ in reasoning and solving problems (similar-structure hypothesis).

At the other pole in the controversy is a heterogeneous group of theories, each differing from the developmental position in some important aspect (see, for example, Ellis & Cavalier, 1982; Milgram, 1973). Because of his perception that these theories emphasize differences between retarded and nonretarded groups more than does his own, Zigler (for example, 1969) has labeled them collectively the "difference position." Such theories may emphasize retarded–nonretarded differences in stages of cognitive development, or in the cognitive processes employed by retarded and nonretarded people at similar levels of cognitive development. Thus, two separable hypotheses may be discussed within the developmental position, either or both of which may be opposed by a difference theorist. Our survey of the evidence is organized around these two hypotheses.

Tests of the similar-sequence hypothesis

First, we consider what Zigler and I (Weisz & Zigler, 1979) have labeled the similar-sequence hypothesis. This is the view that nonretarded and cultural–familial retarded individuals traverse the same general sequence of cognitive-developmental stages, in the same order, differing only in their rate of development and in the ceiling at which their cognitive development ultimately terminates.

Some theoretical support for this hypothesis can be found in the Piagetian literature. Piaget (1956), for example, argued that "the minimum program for establishment of stages is the recognition of a distinct chronology, in the sense of a constant order of succession" (p. 13). Kohlberg (1969, 1971), building on Piaget's perspective, argued that certain cognitive developmental stage sequences might well be similar across individuals because the stages are rooted in certain invariant characteristics of the environment and of the nervous system. Kohlberg also maintained that the stages of understanding described by Piaget might partake of certain "inherent orderings" dictated by logic, and independent of differences among developing individuals. As Kohlberg put it, "The invariance of sequence in the development of a concept or category is not dependent upon a prepatterned unfolding of neural patterns; it must depend upon a logical analysis of the concept itself" (p. 355). To the extent that a given sequence of cognitive stages does depend upon a logical order (e.g., stage 3 involves reorganizing a network of thought patterns that first developed in stage 2), one might predict that the order of cognitive stages would be similar for retarded and nonretarded youngsters. Moreover, it could even be argued that if an inherent logic dictates the order of stages, the similar-sequence hypothesis might well apply to all mentally retarded people, not just the cultural–familial population.

It is possible, however, to derive quite a different hypothesis from the Piagetian literature. Milgram (1973) has done so. After reviewing Piagetian research with the mentally retarded (Inhelder, 1968) and discussing Piaget's perspective with Piaget himself, Milgram concluded that the stages or levels of the retarded person's cognitive development may be different from those of the nonretarded person in some important ways. For example, Milgram argued that "when a retardate moves from one cognitive level to the next, traces of the previous level persist much longer, and the retardate is more likely to regress to earlier, long-practiced modes of thought" (p. 206). This apparent difference position differs from the similar sequence hypothesis in two ways: (1) It implies that the cognitive stages of retarded and nonretarded groups may be qualitatively different, and (2) it implies that, in contrast to the monotonic sequences described by Piaget for nonretarded youngsters, retarded individuals may under some conditions move backward from more mature to less mature levels of thought.

The conflicting hypotheses advanced by Zigler (1969) and Milgram (1973) are both linked to the Piagetian literature. This is reasonable, because Piagetian theory and research are cast explicitly in terms of cognitive stages. Moreover, the Piagetian research literature includes numerous tasks designed to assess those stage levels. Thus, Piagetian research provides an especially valuable base of evidence to use in testing the similar-sequence hypothesis against conflicting views. In what follows, I will offer a brief review of the Piagetian evidence. Robert Hodapp provides a more detailed treatment in chapter 3.

Cross-sectional and order-of-difficulty evidence: Studies using only retarded samples. One general way of testing the similar-sequence hypothesis is with cross-sectional research in which groups of mentally retarded children at more than one developmental level are tested with multiple Piagetian tasks. If the direction of performance differences between developmental levels is the same for the mentally retarded as for the nonretarded, the similar-sequence hypothesis is supported. A second general approach is to compare the relative difficulty levels of the various tests or items. The assumption is that the item passed by the largest number of subjects reflects the process that develops earliest, the item passed by the fewest subjects reflects the process that develops latest, and so forth. If the rank-ordering of difficulty levels among a nonretarded population matches the rank-ordering among the retarded, the similar-sequence hypothesis receives support. One may also apply formal scaling procedures (e.g., Green, 1956) to such ordinal data. Developmental sequences can be inferred from the pattern of passes and failures for each individual subject. If retarded subjects show pass–fail patterns fitting the same stage sequence that has been demonstrated for nonretarded subjects in other samples, the similar-sequence hypothesis is supported.

Numerous investigators have employed some type of cross-sectional research, order-of-difficulty research, or combination of the two. In several of the studies involved, it is difficult to determine whether the samples included only cultural–familial retarded individuals. However, the studies generally support the hypothesis that the order of cognitive developmental stages in groups of retarded persons closely resembles the order identified among nonretarded groups. This conclusion has been supported in studies of conservation of mass, weight, and volume (Marchi, 1971); qualitative identity, quantitative identity, and equivalence conservation (Roodin, Sullivan, & Rybash, 1976); identity and equivalence conservation (McManis, 1969); numerical concepts (see Mannix, 1960, Singh & Stott, 1975; for an exception to this pattern, see Lister, 1972); concepts of space (Houssiadas & Brown, 1967; Stearns & Borkowski, 1969); the logic of relations (e.g., "Show me your right hand, your left; show me my right hand, my left," Lane & Kinder, 1939); and moral judgment (Abel, 1941).

Other cross-sectional and order-of-difficulty evidence: Studies in which retarded and nonretarded samples are directly compared. Unlike the research reviewed earlier, some studies have directly compared the performance of retarded and nonretarded groups in the same experiment. In these studies, too, method descriptions often leave open the question of whether the samples may have included non-cultural–familial retarded persons. The question may be academic, however, because the findings rather consistently indicate that the order of difficulty of various Piagetian tasks is the same for retarded and nonretarded groups.

This is the case in studies of conservation concepts (Achenbach, 1969; Gruen & Vore, 1972) and concepts of time (Lovell & Slater, 1960; Montroy, McManis, & Bell, 1971). It is also true for diverse collections of Piagetian concepts, including (1) generic and gender identity, various conservations, magic and dream concepts, class inclusion, role taking, and the logic of relations (see DeVries, 1970, 1973a, b, 1974), and (2) additive classification, multiplicative classification, seriation, and multiplication of asymmetrical transitive relations (i.e., coordinating size and color seriation in a two-dimensional array; see Lovell, Healey, & Rowland, 1962; Lovell, Mitchell, & Everett, 1962).

Longitudinal evidence. Longitudinal research, in principle, affords the most powerful test of the similar-sequence hypothesis. However, repeated assessments of retarded and nonretarded individuals over time tend to be expensive, logistically difficult, and thus relatively rare. For these reasons, when such a study is carried out it is of special interest, particularly when the retarded sample appears to consist primarily or exclusively of cultural–familial retarded persons. Such a study was conducted by Stephens and colleagues (see Stephens, Mahaney, & McLaughlin, 1972; Stephens, Stephens, & McLaughlin, 1974; Stephens, McLaughlin, Hunt, Mahaney, Kohlberg, Moore, & Aronfreed, 1974) over the late 1960s and early 1970s. The research team tested 75 retarded and 75 nonretarded persons on multiple Piagetian tasks at two points in time, 2 years apart.

Some 11 measures were used to assess various aspects of moral judgment. On nine of the measures, the direction of change over 2 years was the same for both the retarded and nonretarded subjects. However, Mahaney and Stephens (1974) reported oscillations, defined as instances when "the improvement which occurred in one area of moral judgment was not maintained when opinions were solicited on another, but similar, situation" (1974, p. 137). These oscillations evidently occurred more often among retarded than nonretarded subjects. This finding is difficult to interpret, given Kohlberg's (1974) criticism of the measures of Stephens et al. "Empirical research confirms the fact that Piaget's moral stage measures do not meet the criteria of structural stages" (p. 142).

Stephens et al. used 29 additional measures of cognitive development across four conceptual domains (conservation, logic and classification, operativity and symbolic imagery, and combinatory logic). Over the 2-year longitudinal period, both the retarded and nonretarded groups showed significant improvement on nearly all of the measures. Evidently, the direction of development on these tasks was similar among the retarded and nonretarded groups.

Status of evidence on the similar-sequence hypothesis. With a few exceptions, the bulk of the evidence reviewed here is consistent with the similar-sequence hypothesis. However, the conclusion is tempered by the irregular quality of the evidence. The cross-sectional data reviewed here have most often been presented in ways that offer weak inferential power. Information on the percentage of subjects at each age level that pass each Piagetian item is not nearly as useful as information on individual pass–fail patterns, subjected to a scaling analysis (e.g., Green, 1956; Guttman, 1950). But such procedures were not often used in these studies.

By the same token, most of the longitudinal data discussed here were presented in such relatively weak forms as mean differences between experimental groups, or changes in group means or percentages over time (the one exception is the moral judgment data). As Hunt (1974) has noted, reporting only group summary statistics at time 1 and time 2 can mask the fact that some individuals progressed, whereas others regressed over time. Although it is useful to know that the time 1 and time 2 means differed in the same direction for retarded and nonretarded groups, such information is less persuasive than data on the number of individuals in each group showing specific developmental patterns over time.

In conclusion, whereas most of the evidence to date is consistent with the similar-sequence hypothesis, there is considerable room for improvement in the quality of that evidence.

The similar-structure hypothesis and opposing difference positions

Next, we consider the cognitive performance of cultural–familial mentally retarded groups and nonretarded groups that are similar in level of development. The developmental position (e.g., Zigler, 1969) includes the hypothesis that familial retarded and nonretarded individuals who are similar in developmental level will also be similar in the kinds of cognitive structures described by Piaget (see Zigler, 1969, pp. 537–541) – that is, the intellectual structures with which they reason and solve problems. This notion has been labeled the *similar-structure hypothesis* (Weisz & Zigler, 1979; Weisz & Yeates, 1981). It generates the prediction that retarded and nonretarded groups matched for developmental level (operationally defined as MA) will manifest similar performances on a variety of cognitive measures, provided that certain procedural requirements (detailed later) are satisfied.

The similar-structure hypothesis is opposed by two quite dissimilar "difference" positions. One of these is the view that retarded people will show cognitive skills inferior to those of nonretarded people of similar developmental level. An example of such a position – that of Milgram (1973) – is rooted in Piagetian theory. Milgram, as noted earlier, holds that at any given level of development, the retarded person's reasoning is especially likely to contain traces of more primitive developmental stages and especially prone to show regression to those earlier stages. Consequently, Milgram argues, retarded groups are likely to score lower on cognitive measures than are MA-matched nonretarded groups. As

Milgram put it, "Given tasks without a ceiling or floor effect for the general MA of the subjects being used, the retarded will dependably demonstrate an equal-MA deficit" (1973, p. 209). Milgram appears to be arguing that retarded groups will perform at lower levels than nonretarded groups of equal MA, provided that the experimental tasks being used are not so simple *or* so difficult that there is little variability in the groups' performance.

In contrast to Milgram, Kohlberg (1968) has argued that mentally retarded people should be *more* advanced cognitively than their non-retarded MA peers. His reasoning is that cognitive development depends heavily upon the child's "general experience" in the world. Because retarded people of a given MA have lived longer than nonretarded people of the same MA, those who are retarded should have a more extensive base of general experience and thus be more advanced cognitively.

To summarize, three theoretical positions differ sharply on what will be found when retarded and nonretarded groups are matched for MA and given tests of cognitive performance. One position (Zigler, 1969) maintains that no reliable group differences will be found; another (Milgram, 1973) holds that the retarded will prove to be inferior; still another (Kohlberg, 1968) predicts that the retarded will prove to be superior.

How to test the similar-structure hypothesis. To provide a context for evaluating tests of the similar-structure hypothesis, it is useful to specify some characteristics of the "ideal" experiment in this area. First, retarded and nonretarded groups have to be matched closely for developmental level via some psychometrically acceptable measure. Some workers (e.g., Zigler, 1969) would prefer a theoretically derived measure (e.g., one based on Piaget's work); however, all the theorists discussed appear to consider the MA generated by conventional intelligence tests an acceptable operational definition of developmental level.

As noted, the developmental position applies only to familial retarded persons. Thus, a second feature of the ideal experiment is systematic exclusion from the retarded sample of those individuals suffering from specific organic or genetic anomalies.

A third feature of the ideal experiment was suggested by Milgram (1973): the use of measures that do not have marked ceiling or floor effects for the MA level being sampled. Pronounced floor or ceiling effects might result, of course, in artifactual findings of "no difference" that would constitute spurious support for the similar-structure hypothesis.

A final feature of the ideal experiment is an effort to provide experimental conditions that optimize motivation to perform well. A substantial body of research (see Cromwell, 1963; Heber, 1964; Stevenson, 1965; Zigler, 1971) suggests that certain motivational and personality factors may often undermine the performance of retarded subjects on cognitive tasks. It follows that efforts to gauge the cognitive skills of retarded individuals should, where possible, minimize the effects of such noncognitive factors.

Of the preceding four features of the "ideal" experiment, only the first (MA matching) has been made a requirement for the review that follows. The other three features provide useful criteria for evaluating the research reviewed, however, and I will illustrate how such evaluations may be made.

Piagetian tests of the similar-structure hypothesis

In this section, I will summarize the findings of a review that Keith Yeates and I carried out (Weisz & Yeates, 1981). We surveyed the findings of 32 experiments comparing the performance of MA-matched retarded and nonretarded groups on various Piagetian tasks. The 32 studies included 113 different comparisons across the following areas of conceptual development: additive composition, animism, artificialism, causality, classification, class inclusion, conservation (of area, color, continuous quantity, discontinuous quantity, length, mass, number, two-dimensional space, volume, and weight), dream concepts, extensive qualities, generic identity, gross qualities, identity concepts, intensive qualities, logical contradiction, magic concepts, moral judgment, perceptual decentering, perspective taking, probability, realism, relative thinking, role taking, seriation, time concepts, and transitivity.

The concepts and age groups studied provided reasonably broad coverage of the preoperational and concrete operational periods. The findings as a whole showed a rather mixed picture concerning the similar-structure hypothesis. Of the 113 group comparisons, 82 (73%) yielded results consistent with the hypothesis. Some 26 comparisons (23%) generated findings consistent with the difference position taken by Milgram (1973); and 5 of the comparisons (4%) supported Kohlberg's (1968) view that retarded groups would prove to be superior to their nonretarded MA peers.

We took a closer look at the studies, however, trying to distinguish between those studies in which an effort was made to include in the retarded sample only those individuals who were not suffering from some specific organic impairment or genetic anomaly. Certainly, the present state of diagnosis of such problems is primitive at best; but investigators who at least attempt to select their sample with attention to such factors appear to be doing a better job than other investigators who test the similar-structure hypothesis by focusing on cultural–familial retarded groups. Of the 113 total comparisons, only 39 appeared to have involved some effort to control for organicity and/or genetic anomalies. Of these 39, only 4 (10%) yielded results inconsistent with the similar-structure hypothesis.

The "null hypothesis" issue. This apparent support for the similar-structure hypothesis needs to be examined more closely. One reason is that some of the studies involved were relatively low in statistical power. Low power in some of the experiments may have resulted in a spuriously high number of "no difference" findings – findings consistent with the similar-structure hypothesis, which is essentially a "null" hypothesis. In contrast, one might argue that there is an inherent bias against the similar-structure hypothesis precisely because it is a null hypothesis. Many trained psychologists have been taught to be prejudiced against null findings, and to consider findings of "no difference between groups" as an experimental failure that proves nothing.

Some prominent statisticians maintain that if the null hypothesis can be tested, it can also be accepted as valid (for detailed discussion of this issue, see Binder, 1963; Grant, 1962). Nonetheless, Greenwald (1975) has argued that prejudice against the null persists, and that such prejudice can inhibit publication in areas for which the null hypothesis is actually a reasonable approximation to truth. It is possible, then, that findings supporting the similar-structure hypothesis may, because of their inherent "nullness," have been underrepresented in the population of published reports. It is difficult to gauge or correct for biases that might work for or against the similar-structure hypothesis. However, the possibility of such biases suggests the need for a more critical scrutiny of the evidence than a simple "box score" survey.

Comparing the actual distribution with the expected distribution. One approach to such critical scrutiny is to fashion an overall test of the similar-structure hypothesis by pooling the results of the various studies. Methods that involve pooling exact significance levels and their corresponding Z scores could not be used with these data because too few of the articles included the necessary data (e.g., exact significance levels; written requests for such data yielded too few responses to permit pooling). Instead, we used a counting method. We relied on the fact that if a null hypothesis is true, differences between any two groups across independent studies should approximate a normal distribution. Accordingly, the proportion of significant differences in either direction should be equal to the alpha level that has been selected. The array of differences actually obtained across the studies can be compared with the hypothetical distribution by means of the Chi-square test. Table 7.1 shows the result obtained when such a test is applied to the data of the 113 retarded–nonretarded comparisons.

The calculations reflected in Table 7.2 involved an alpha level of 0.05 for both tails of the hypothetical normal distribution. The expectation, assuming a normal distribution around a "no difference" mean, would be that 10% of the studies would yield significant group differences (i.e., 5% on each tail) and that 90% would yield no reliable group differences. This means that the similar-structure hypothesis would be supported by a distribution of findings in which 90% of the comparisons showed no reliable retarded–nonretarded group difference, 5% showed significant differences in the direction predicted by Milgram (1973), and 5% showed significant differences in the direction predicted by Kohlberg (1968). In Table 7.2, this expected distribution of studies is compared with the obtained distribution via Chi-square tests (for qualifications on the use of Chi-square with such data, see Weisz & Yeates, 1981, p. 171). When the tests are calculated separately for studies that excluded organically impaired retarded subjects (the "etiology controlled" studies) and studies that did not (the "etiology uncontrolled" studies), two rather different patterns are obtained. In the etiology-uncontrolled studies, more comparisons than expected by chance supported Milgram's (1973) difference position ($p < .001$). Among the etiology-controlled studies, by contrast,

Table 7.1. *Directional comparisons of MA-matched retarded and nonretarded groups, summed across various Piagetian tasks*

Group	Direction of Difference		
	MR > NMR	MR = NMR	MR < NMR
Etiology controlled[a]			
Actual total	1	35	3
Expected total	1.95	35.10	1.95
Etiology uncontrolled[b]			
Actual total	4	47	23
Expected total	3.70	66.60	3.70

Note: MR = mentally retarded, NMR = non-mentally retarded.
Source: Data from Weisz and Yeates (1981).
[a] Chi-square ($df = 2$) = 1.02, $p > 0.50$.
[b] Chi-square ($df = 2$) = 106.46, $p < 0.001$.

Table 7.2. *Comparisons of MA-matched retarded and nonretarded groups on Piagetian and information-processing tasks*

Tasks	Direction of difference			Statistical test
	MR > NMR	MR = NMR	MR < NMR	
Piagetian				
Actual totals	0	30	3	$\chi^2 = 2.76, p > .25$
Expected totals	1.65	29.70	1.65	
Information processing				
Actual totals	2	31	26	$\chi^2 = 185.77,$
Expected totals	2.95	53.10	2.95	$p < .001$

Note: MR = mentally retarded, NMR = non-mentally retarded.
Source: Data from Weisz & Yeates (1981) and Weiss, Weisz, & Bromfield (1986).

the distribution is not significantly different from the distribution that would be expected if the similar-structure hypothesis were valid ($p > 0.50$).

Critique of the Piagetian evidence. This pattern of findings appears to support the similar-structure hypothesis, at least for studies that involve screening for organic and genetic deficits. These studies could be improved in a number of ways. Few included any explicit attempt to counter motivational and personality problems that may interfere with the performance of retarded people. Several of the studies included institutionalized retarded subjects – and there is considerable evidence that institutionalization may depress cognitive performance in this population (see, e.g., Balla & Zigler, 1982; Lyle, 1959). A number of the studies can be faulted for imprecise MA-matching procedures. Finally, it is important to note that we have focused thus far on only those domains of cognitive performance addressed by Piaget and investigators in the Genevan tradition. In the next section, the focus shifts to non-Piagetian cognitive processes.

Information-processing tests of the similar-structure hypothesis

The last cognitive domain that we have systematically surveyed is a broad one: cognitive processes that fall not within the Piagetian tradition but rather within the tradition of information-processing research. The survey was originally reported by Weiss, Weisz, and Bromfield (1986). It includes 24 studies, involving 59 comparisons of retarded and nonretarded groups on such cognitive processes as selective attention, input organization, memory, paired-associate learning, incidental learning, discrimination learning and learning set information, concept usage and matching, hypothesis testing behavior, and even humor. To be included in this review, studies had to meet three methodological criteria, reflecting concerns raised in the preceding critique. The retarded samples had to be (1) matched on MA with a nonretarded group, (2) screened to exclude organically impaired individuals, and (3) noninstitutionalized. Studies that meet all three criteria are relatively rare in this field. This is reflected in the fact that our initial pool included 227 studies; of these, 203 (89%) were eliminated for failure to meet one or more of the criteria.

A gross examination of findings across the 59 retarded–nonretarded group comparisons suggests the possibility of an empirical standoff: whereas 52% of the 59 comparisons revealed no significant retarded–nonretarded difference, another 45% revealed significant differences favoring the nonretarded group. Only 3% (two comparisons) revealed significant differences favoring Kohlberg's (1968) prediction, with the retarded group outperforming the nonretarded group. Thus, about half the findings supported the similar-structure hypothesis, and about half ran counter to it. However, as noted (see also Weisz & Yeates, 1981), box score tallies of this sort are not the most appropriate means of testing the similar-structure hypothesis.

Because the similar-structure hypothesis is essentially a null hypothesis, it is most appropriately tested against an expected normal distribution of group differences, the distribution one would expect if the hypothesis were in fact valid. We carried out such a test with these data, first using a Chi-square test (as in Weisz & Yeates, 1981), then using a meta-analysis.

Results of the Chi-square test are shown in Table 7.2. The table summarizes the findings of the information-processing studies, together with the findings of the Piagetian studies from the Weisz–Yeates (1981) review. To enhance the comparability of the two data sets, the table includes only those studies from the Piagetian review that included procedures for screening organically impaired subjects (because such procedures were required for all studies included in the information processing review). As noted earlier, the distribution of findings of the Piagetian studies did not differ significantly from the hypothetical normal distribution that would be expected if the similar-structure hypothesis were valid. By contrast, the Chi-square test for the information-processing studies showed a highly significant deviation from the distribution expected under the null hypothesis:

$$\chi^2 (2, n = 59) = 185.77, p < 0.001$$

Many more comparisons than would be expected under the null showed nonretarded groups outperforming the retarded comparison groups.

A meta-analysis of information-processing findings. Next, we carried out a meta-analysis of the information-processing findings. For each of the studies reviewed, we computed the Z-score equivalent (Rosenthal, 1978) for the probability of the group effect (the retarded–nonretarded comparison): F and t values for each group effect were converted to p values, and hence to Z scores. We then computed a mean of these Z-score equivalents, averaging across the various group comparisons. The similar-structure hypothesis would have been supported by a mean Z of 0 (or a figure not significantly different from 0). The hypothesis was clearly *not* supported. The meta-analysis revealed a highly significant difference between the performance of the retarded and nonretarded groups, mean Z = 1.32; test that mean

$$Z = 0: t (52) = 5.37, p < 0.0001$$

Retarded subjects performed significantly worse than nonretarded subjects, averaged across tasks and subject samples.

Comparing findings across information-processing domains. We sought to delineate the cognitive domains in which retarded and nonretarded groups differed most significantly. The results of this effort are shown in Table 7.3. In the table, we report the mean Z statistic for each domain in which there were at least three group comparisons. As the table shows, performance differences between retarded and nonretarded groups were most signifi-

Table 7.3. *Meta-analytic findings within seven cognitive domains*

Domain	No. of comparisons	Mean Z	p value
Concept usage	3	0.58	.16
Discrimination and learning-set formulation	6	2.64	.0001
Distractibility and selective attention	3	− 0.97	.05
Verbal explanations	3	1.09	.03
Hypothesis-testing behavior	3	0.73	.10
Incidental learning	4	0.14	.39
Memory	21	1.93	.00001

Note: Significance levels in this table are a function of both the mean probability level and the number of comparisons.

cant in the areas of (1) memory and (2) discrimination learning and learning-set formation. We next took a closer look at the findings in these two areas.

In the area of discrimination learning and learning-set formation, a Chi-square test for homogeneity of group differences revealed that retarded–nonretarded differences were not consistent across studies. Two of the most striking group differences were in the area of learning-set formation. In the area of memory, our test for homogeneity of differences again revealed that inferior performance by retarded subjects was not uniform across studies. Deficits were found in the performance of retarded groups on visual short-term memory (STM), nonserial auditory STM, cross-modal STM, and visual paired-associate learning. By contrast, retarded and nonretarded groups did not differ on serial STM, verbal paired-associate learning, or susceptibility to the von Restorff effect (improved recall on memory items that differ from others along a salient dimension – for example, items that are louder than others on a list).

One area in which nonretarded groups showed consistent superiority was verbal explanation of the strategies they used in the various tasks. By contrast, retarded and nonretarded groups performed equally well in tests of incidental learning, and retarded groups tended to outperform their nonretarded MA peers on tests of distractibility and selective attention. Of special interest, retarded groups failed to show performance deficits on most tests of more integrated or higher-order cognitive behaviors such as concept usage and matching, and hypothesis testing. This finding seems to run counter to Spitz's (1976) hypothesis that retarded individuals are particularly deficient in cognitive areas that have developed relatively recently in human evolution.

Summarizing the information-processing findings. The information-processing findings, taken together, do not appear to support the similar-structure hypothesis. The meta-analysis of findings indicated that, overall, the performance of retarded groups was significantly inferior to that of MA-matched nonretarded groups. The inferiority appeared most pro-nounced in the areas of memory, discrimination learning, and discrimina-tion-set learning. Although these findings are not consistent with the similar-structure hypothesis, it is premature to dismiss the hypothesis. Instead, what appears to be warranted is a careful analysis of possible interpretations of the *full* array of findings bearing on the similar-structure hypothesis – the information-processing findings and the Piagetian find-ings, considered together.

Interpreting the Piagetian and information-processing evidence

What can we conclude from the findings just reviewed? The most obvious possibility would be that the similar-structure hypothesis may be generally valid for the conceptual domains studied by Piagetian investigators, but not for at least some of the cognitive domains in the information-processing tradition. On the other hand, several alternative interpretations should be considered.

Artifactual explanations. Various artifacts might possibly explain the discrepancy between the Piagetian findings and the information-processing findings. One such artifact might be a subtle form of experimenter selectivity and bias. Investigators who carry out Piagetian studies may be more likely than those who conduct information-processing studies to favor the developmental hypothesis, which is, after all, closely linked to Piagetian theory (see Zigler, 1969; Zigler & Balla, 1982). Through various inadvertent forms of experimenter bias – for example, influencing, sampling, task administration (see Rosenthal, 1966) – the two groups of investigators might have tended to find results supporting their respective a priori points of view. Such bias might help explain some of the inconsistencies across studies; however, it does not seem likely that the bias could fully account for the strong consistency in the Piagetian research literature.

Other artifactual explanations may merit consideration. For instance, it could be argued that Piagetian tasks are more susceptible than information-processing tasks to ceiling and floor effects (see Milgram, 1973), or that the information-processing tasks used inferior procedures for screening out organically impaired retarded persons. Such explanations, while potentially plausible, do not seem any better equipped than the experimenter bias explanation to account for the strong consistency within the Piagetian evidence and the sharp contrast between that evidence and the information-processing findings. Thus, it seems that other interpretations have to be considered.

Interpretations favoring the difference position. One set of interpretations favors the general difference position. It could be argued that the kinds of cognitive tasks most likely to reveal true cognitive deficits in mentally retarded people are those within the information-processing tradition. Information-processing research, after all, developed out of a search for individual and group differences. The Piagetian tradition, by contrast, grew out of a search for commonalities that underlie development. Thus,

Piagetian research may have evolved toward the use of tasks that are sensitive to developmental change but not to differences between individuals or groups at similar levels of development. This might help to explain why a review of Piagetian evidence would support the similar-structure hypothesis, whereas a review of information-processing evidence would not. Even this explanation, though, would not explain why some information-processing domains showed marked retarded–nonretarded differences, whereas other information-processing domains showed similar performance by retarded and nonretarded groups. To account for this aspect of the findings, we may have to consider the types of information-processing tasks that revealed significant group differences.

One impression that we and others (e.g., Keith Yeates, personal communication, July 10, 1984) shared was that tasks requiring substantial amounts of verbal processing were especially likely to yield significant retarded–nonretarded group differences. We had independent ratings made of whether stimuli used in each information-processing experiment were predominantly verbal or nonverbal; a Chi-square test revealed that a marginally higher proportion of the comparisons showed retarded–nonretarded group differences when verbal stimuli were used than when nonverbal stimuli were used ($p < 0.07$). This, in turn, suggested the possibility that tasks requiring substantial activity in the left cerebral hemisphere might reveal the most pronounced deficit in mentally retarded persons. Certainly, there is a rather widely held view that retarded persons are particularly deficient in verbal skills (see, e.g., Clarke & Clarke, 1965; Ingalls, 1978) and that the left hemisphere is more efficient than the right at verbal processing (Bradshaw & Nettleton, 1981). Could it be true that cultural–familial retarded people are particularly deficient in left hemisphere processing? Such a deficit might even help to explain the fact that retarded–nonretarded performance differences were found on information-processing tasks but not Piagetian tasks, because there is some evidence suggesting that processing of most Piagetian tasks occurs primarily in the right hemisphere.

We also considered several relatively comprehensive difference theories as possible explanations for the pattern of findings just reported. For example, *verbal mediation theory* (Borkowski & Wanschura, 1974) proposes that retarded persons are deficient in the production of verbal mediators. The theory could account for some but not all of the findings we reviewed. We also considered *inhibition theory*, which holds that retarded persons are often unable to properly inhibit learned responses or suppress extraneous stimulus input when such actions would be adaptive. This theory, too, could account for only some of the information-processing findings. After weighing several promising theoretical accounts, we concluded that no single difference position seems well equipped to explain our findings in a comprehensive fashion. If the findings are ultimately interpreted as supporting a difference position, that position may well be an amalgam of multiple difference theories – one that could encompass multiple deficits (perhaps as suggested by Fisher & Zeaman, 1973; Heal & Johnson, 1970).

Interpretations favoring the developmental position. Another set of interpretations of the information-processing and Piagetian findings can be offered, those favoring the developmental position. One such interpretation is concerned with the issue of ecological validity. A case could be made for the notion that most Piagetian tasks are more "lifelike" or ecologically valid than most information-processing tasks. Consider, for example, the contrast between the task of making moral judgments about lifelike dilemmas and that of learning to discriminate between colored shapes. Even the manner in which Piagetian tasks are administered tends to be more conversational and natural than the more academic approach that is typically used to assess memory skills, discrimination learning, and so forth. It is possible that the retarded groups were outperformed on the information-processing tasks in part because they found those tasks relatively unengaging. Moreover, the academic nature of the tasks may have reminded retarded subjects of the school tasks with which they all had a history of difficulty.

A related interpretation favoring the developmental position is that retarded and nonretarded children differ significantly on some extracognitive variable such as motivation or expectancy of success that may influence performance on some types of tasks (e.g., information-processing) more than others (e.g., Piagetian). Some reviews (e.g., Zigler & Balla, 1982; Zigler & Hodapp, 1986) indicate that retarded and nonretarded individuals of similar MA appear to differ in motivational and other extracognitive characteristics. Of course, such evidence alone is not sufficient to validate a motivational explanation for observed group differences on cognitive tasks. Motivational differences might exist concurrently with group differences in cognitive ability. To rule out a cognitive ability explanation, one needs to show that when motivational differences are controlled, differences between retarded and nonretarded subjects on cognitive task performance are no longer significant.

Information available in the information-processing studies permitted a rough test of the motivational interpretation. In several of the studies, subjects were told they would receive some form of reward for good performance. We (Weiss et al., 1986) tested whether the presence or absence of such motivational manipulations affected the retarded–nonretarded group comparisons. We found that whether or not studies included motivational manipulations did not significantly predict whether they would find retarded–nonretarded group differences ($p < 0.25$). Studies that included such manipulations were somewhat less likely to show group differences, but not significantly so. Whether such short-term reward-for-good-performance manipulations could be expected to counter a lifetime of experience is a question that this analysis cannot answer.

This limitation underscores the need for those theorists who emphasize the role of extracognitive factors to generate more specific hypotheses. Several potentially important variables (e.g., motivation – Zigler, 1969; outerdirectedness – Yando & Zigler, 1971; see also chapter 6 in this volume) have been suggested as possible causes of performance differences between MA-matched retarded and nonretarded groups. It would be useful at this point for specific hypotheses to be advanced as to which of these variables will be most important for which subject groups and on which tasks. Moreover, it would be useful to have specific proposals on how the effects of these variables can most fairly be assessed and controlled within an experimental situation.

A final interpretation relates to one finding of the meta-analyis that I have not yet mentioned. We found a significant interaction of IQ and MA, such that as the average MA of subjects in the information-processing experiments increased, so did the likelihood of significant retarded–nonretarded performance differences. What factor or factors might change with increasing MA that might, in turn, be related to increasing performance deficits in mentally retarded youngsters? One possibility is that the propensity to develop learned helplessness (and concomitant performance deficits) is positively related to cognitive developmental level or MA (see Weisz, 1979).

Some findings appear consistent with this notion. For example, Rholes, Blackwell, Jordan, and Walters (1980) found that susceptibility to learned helplessness increased among nonretarded children as the age of the children increased from the kindergarten through late elementary years. In addition, in an earlier study of learned helplessness among retarded and nonretarded children, I found that as MA increased (over the range of 5–9 years) the helplessness of the retarded youngsters relative to that of the nonretarded youngsters increased. I argued that this trend might reflect the tendency of retarded youngsters to accumulate failure experiences and low-ability feedback over years of development. It is possible that the IQ × MA interaction in our meta-analysis of information-processing studies might be partly explained by MA-related increments in the susceptibility of mentally retarded youngsters to helplessness and a tendency to give up in the face of difficult problems. I will return to the topic of helplessness in the final section of this chapter.

Summarizing evidence on the similar-structure hypothesis

To summarize, the findings from Piagetian research generally offer strong support for the similar-structure hypothesis, indicating that MA-matched retarded and nonretarded groups show similar levels of task performance. By contrast, the evidence from information-processing experiments reveals a highly significant overall group difference, with nonretarded subjects outperforming retarded subjects of similar MA. Even within the pool of information-processing studies, the pattern is not consistent across domains; tasks involving memory, discrimination learning, and learning set revealed highly significant retarded–nonretarded group differences; tasks involving concept usage and incidental learning did not reveal group differences. Moreover, a significant IQ × MA interaction revealed that as subjects increased in MA the likelihood of significant retarded–nonretarded performance differences increased. A number of possible interpretations of the various findings were discussed, but no final conclusion was reached as to which might be the most valid.

Performance deficits and extracognitive factors

Because cultural–familial retardation is defined largely in terms of cognitive functioning, it is certainly important to learn what we can about the cognitive development and abilities of those who suffer from this condition. It is also important to recognize that the cognitive performance of cultural–familial retarded persons (and of the rest of us) is likely to be influenced by factors other than cognitive ability alone. Indeed, efforts to identify such extracognitive factors and trace their impact have generated one of the richest legacies of the developmental–difference controversy. Edward Zigler and his colleagues have spearheaded these efforts, demonstrating the impact of such factors as outerdirectedness, low expectancy of success, wariness of adults, and atypical reward preference (see chapter 6 of this volume).

As my mentor, Edward Zigler has inspired vigilance on my part as to the impact of extracognitive factors. One result has been a series of studies by my students and me on the possible role of learned helplessness in the lives of retarded youngsters. I mentioned this work briefly in discussing alternative interpretations of the earlier information-processing findings. Now I will return to the topic for a more detailed discussion.

Learned helplessness and the mentally retarded person

The learned helplessness syndrome has been conceptualized in a number of different ways (see e.g., Abramson, Seligman, & Teasdale, 1978; Garber & Seligman, 1980; Seligman, 1975), but most accounts applied to humans include the following two components: (1) a subjective perception by individuals that they cannot exert control over certain salient outcomes, and (2) corresponding deficits in response initiation or perseverance. My own interactions with mentally retarded youngsters in and out of school have led me to suspect that the helplessness construct may hold some explanatory power for this population. I suspect that mentally retarded youngsters often do anticipate low levels of control over outcomes in the school-achievement domain, and that they often show deficits in the application of their cognitive abilities in school – for example, in problem-solving situations.

Studies of helplessness-like performance deficits. Studies designed to explore this possibility have been few in number and preliminary in nature. Nonetheless, they do provide a point of departure for helplessness research on the retarded, and they may help to suggest useful directions for future empirical efforts. The initial studies dealt primarily with performance deficits. My first effort was a study of learned helplessness in cultural–familial retarded and nonretarded children who were matched at three levels of ability: MA levels 5½, 7½, and 9½ years (Weisz, 1979). The sample included not only retarded and intellectually average children, but groups of high-IQ children as well.

I used four operational definitions of helplessness. To gauge perseverance following failure, children were presented with a puzzle and allowed to complete it successfully; then they were presented with a second puzzle and stopped before completing it – in an apparent failure. They were then asked to decide whether to repeat the failure puzzle or to repeat the one at which they had just succeeded. Using a similar procedure, Dweck and Bush (1976) had found that children who ascribed their failures to uncontrollable factors (a defining characteristic of learned helplessness) were less likely to persevere at the failed task than children who believed their failures were due to controllable factors.

A second operational definition was a set of response-initiation measures. For example, children were trained to turn off a buzzer in a reaction-time task; later, the experimenter left the child alone and activated the buzzer with a remote control switch. The length of time the child tolerated the unpleasant noise before initiating a controlling response (i.e., shutting off the buzzer) was scored, together with other measures, to form an overall response initiation score.

Two questionnaires were also used. In one, teachers estimated each child's likelihood of initiating controlling responses in a variety of class-room situations – for example, when the child faced a new activity that looked difficult. In a second questionnaire, the children selected causal attributions for various favorable and unfavorable outcomes at school and at home. On a similar measure, Diener and Dweck (1978) had found that children who attributed unfavorable outcomes to their own insufficient effort (presumably regarding their failures as reversible through increased effort) showed low levels of helplessness.

Results with all three children's measures (but not the teacher ques-tionnaire) involved IQ × MA interactions. All showed the retarded chil-dren to be more helpless than the nonretarded children, but only at one or both of the upper MA levels. One interpretation of this pattern, suggested earlier, is that retarded children may learn helplessness gradually, over years of development.

These data suggest that retarded children at relatively mature MA levels may be more susceptible to helplessness than their nonretarded MA peers. The data, though, must be regarded as preliminary, given the experimental nature of the measures employed. A more commonly used procedure for the assessment of learned helplessness involves the creation of a series of uncontrollable aversive experiences, often problem-solving activities involving a series of failures. The way people respond to these failures, especially their perseverance at the same or subsequent tasks, is read as an indication of their resistance to helplessness.

In a second study (Weisz, 1981a), I used such a procedure in an effort to learn whether retarded children might be more susceptible to a "helpless" response pattern than would MA-matched nonretarded children. In the study, retarded and nonretarded children with average MAs of about 9½ years were taken through a series of concept-formation problems, then given feedback indicating that they had the wrong answers during four successive test problems. These problems followed a series of similar training problems involving veridical feedback that was frequently positive.

The two groups performed similarly on the training problems, suggest-ing that they were similar not only in MA but also in their ability to solve problems of this type. Yet the groups diverged markedly when the performance feedback became negative. Under the "failure feedback" condition, retarded children showed a highly significant decline in their use of effective strategies, from early to late test problems. Nonretarded children, by contrast, did not show a significant decline, and in fact showed a slight increase in their use of effective strategies over the course of the "failure" problems. The pattern of results suggests that there is at least one situation in which negative feedback may indeed provoke a kind of "giving up" on the part of mentally retarded youngsters. The study also included a new means of assessing teachers' ratings of their pupils' helplessness in the classroom. In this Helpless Behavior Checklist, teachers were presented with a series of brief behavior descriptions and asked to indicate whether each was "not true," "somewhat or sometimes true," or "very true or often true" of the target child. Some of the items involved helpless attributions (e.g., "Says 'I can't do it,' when having trouble with the work"); some involved helpless behavior (e.g., "When running into difficulty, gives up and quits trying"). On both attributions and behavior, teachers rated retarded subjects significantly more helpless than their nonretarded peers.

Probing the etiology of helplessness: Classroom feedback. If retarded youngsters do develop a tendency toward helplessness, why is this? Our research has generated several possible answers. First, our observations in classrooms (Raber & Weisz, 1981) have suggested that retarded children may receive feedback patterns that foster a helpless orientation. They receive relatively frequent negative feedback. This could lead them to begin a variety of school-like tasks with a readiness to anticipate failure (see Zigler & Balla, 1982); this readiness may be activated when the problems get tough, or when early errors begin to pile up. A high proportion of the negative feedback that mentally retarded children do receive appears to be performance-related and relevant to their cognitive abilities. This pattern has been linked to helplessness in earlier research with nonretarded youngsters (see Dweck, Davidson, Nelson, & Enna, 1978). The pattern can foster a tendency to attribute failures to low ability – a stable, uncontrollable cause. Evidently as a result, children who receive such feedback patterns have been found to show performance debilitation in response to feedback suggesting failure (see Dweck et al., 1978).

Probing the etiology of helplessness: Judgments and attributions of nonretarded persons in response to the "mentally retarded" label. It is also possible that helplessness is fostered in mentally retarded people by the judgments and attributions that are made about them by nonretarded people. Specifically, nonretarded people may interpret failure by a retarded person in ways that lead them to tolerate or even encourage deficits in perseverance. To explore this possibility, we have carried out several studies of how the judgments and attributions of nonretarded people are influenced by the "mentally retarded" label.

To illustrate the reasoning underlying our research, let us consider attributions that nonretarded people might make for failure by a child labeled mentally retarded. A defining characteristic of mental retardation is low ability. Because low ability is such a salient attribute of retarded children, it may be emphasized in causal attributions for such children even when they are being compared with nonretarded children of similar ability. Such reasoning would illustrate *attributional overextension*, the extension of a salient causal ascription (e.g., low ability) beyond its logical limits (see Weisz, 1981b). If such overextension were to occur when adults make judgments about a retarded child, the resulting emphasis on the causal importance of low ability might (following Kelley, 1973) lead the adults to discount the role of other plausible causal factors such as insufficient effort. Adults who believe that a child's failure at a task resulted primarily from low ability and not from insufficient effort are not likely to encourage that child to persist at the task. Instead, they might well allow the child to give up – that is, they might condone helpless behavior.

In an initial effort to explore this line of reasoning, I carried out a series of three studies (Weisz, 1981) in which college students made judgments about a problem-solving failure by a mentally retarded child and an unlabeled child of equal MA. In one study, the students made judgments about either the retarded or the unlabeled child (i.e., a between-groups design). In the second study, all judgments were made about both children (i.e., a repeated-measures design). In both studies, low ability was rated as a significantly more important cause of failure for the retarded than for the unlabeled child, insufficient effort was rated more important for the unlabeled child, and the unlabeled child was rated as more likely to succeed at the task in future attempts. In the third study, college students were given both the "retarded child" pattern of expectancies and attributions and the unlabeled child pattern, derived from studies 1 and 2. After reading both descriptions, applied to hypothetical children, the students were asked to indicate how likely it was that they would urge each child to persevere following failure. As expected, the students reported that the retarded child pattern would make them less likely to urge perseverance than would the unlabeled child pattern.

The attributional pattern identified in Weisz (1981a) was further supported in a study by Bromfield (1983) using a videotaped experience of child failure. The tape showed a "teacher" and a young girl interacting for about five minutes. The child succeeded at one block design problem, but then struggled with the next block design problem throughout the remainder of the tape, never succeeding. Half the college students who viewed the tape were told that the child was mentally retarded; half were not. All students were given identical information about the child's MA, achievement test performance, *and* ability at block design problems. Despite this fact, the students who thought they were viewing a mentally retarded child made markedly different judgments about what they had seen than did the other students. Subjects in the retarded child condition were significantly more likely than the other subjects to (1) attribute the child's failure to insufficient ability, (2) predict future failure at the block design problem with the same teacher, and (3) predict future failure at the block design problem even with a more experienced teacher. In fact, subjects in the retarded child condition actually rated the child as lower in block design ability than did the other subjects, despite the fact that all subjects had been given exactly the same block design ability scores. The two groups did not differ, though, in their attributions to low effort or in their judgments as to how much they would have encouraged the child to persist at the block design problem. With these two exceptions, though, the results replicated the findings of Weisz (1981a).

Are some groups of nonretarded people more susceptible than others to effects of the mentally retarded label? We explored this question in two studies. In one, Keith Yeates and I (Yeates & Weisz, 1982) used vignettes to compare the susceptibility of various adult groups to label effects. We found that adults who had limited experience with mentally retarded people (i.e., university undergraduates and regular classroom teachers) showed relatively strong label effects of the sort discussed here; more experienced adults (i.e., graduate students in special education and special education teachers) did not. Interestingly, we also found that adults who endorsed the similar-structure hypothesis on a separately administered questionnaire were less susceptible to label effects than were adults who rejected the hypothesis.

In a related study, Bromfield, Weisz, and Messer (1986) used the video-tape described earlier to assess susceptibility to effects of the mentally retarded label by nonretarded third, sixth, and ninth graders. Consistent with developmental literature on person perception and social cognition, we found that label effects were negligible among the youngest group, strong among sixth graders, and even stronger among ninth graders. This suggests that the attributional and other judgmental processes of interest here may take shape over the course of development in nonretarded people.

Taken together, our vignette and videotape attributional research suggests that some of the adults in the retarded youngster's world, and even some of the retarded child's older peers, may be influenced by the mentally retarded label. That label, applied to a child who has failed a problem-solving task, may lead nonretarded people into a potentially helplessness-promoting pattern of attributions and behavior with respect to the labeled child. I do not suggest that this is the sole cause of the helpless behavior sometimes shown by mentally retarded individuals, but if it is one of the causes, it may be one of the most remediable. If nonretarded people who directly influence the lives of mentally retarded people – for example, teachers, parents, siblings, and classmates – were aware of the ways retarded people do and do not differ cognitively from nonretarded people, the judgmental patterns we have identified might be less pronounced. This notion is supported by the finding (Yeates & Weisz, 1982) that helplessness-fostering judgmental patterns are generally not found among adults who believe that retarded and nonretarded groups at similar cognitive developmental levels are similar in cognitive ability.

Concluding comment: cognitive and extracognitive processes

The findings reviewed here – in the three somewhat distinct areas of cognitive processes, helplessness, and labeling effects – may ultimately converge in a potentially useful way. Considered together, they may help sharpen our picture of (1) the cognitive capabilities of retarded people, (2) circumstances in which retarded people may perform below the level of those capabilities, and (3) judgments and behavior by nonretarded people in the retarded person's environment that might contribute to such subability performance. The picture assembled here is probably best viewed as a set of hypotheses to be explored in further research. I suspect that there can be real value in such research, that weaving together the study of cognitive abilities and such extracognitive factors as helplessness can enrich our understanding of why cultural–familial retarded people behave as they do. If so, the research will fit nicely into the tradition now associated with the venerable developmental position on cultural–familial mental retardation.

References

Abel, T.M. (1941). Moral judgments among subnormals. *Journal of Abnormal and Social Psychology, 36*, 378–392.

Abramson, L.Y., Seligman, M.E.P., & Teasdale, J.D. (1978). Learned helplessness in humans: Critique and reformulation. *Journal of Abnormal Psychology, 87*, 49–74.

Achenbach, T.M. (1969). Conservation of illusion-distorted identity: Its relation to MA and CA in normals and retardates. *Child Development, 40*, 663–679.

Balla, D., & Zigler, E. (1982). Impact of institutional experience on the behavior and development of retarded persons. In E. Zigler & D. Balla (Eds.), *Mental retardation: The developmental–difference controversy* (pp. 41–60). Hillsdale, NJ: Erlbaum.

Binder, A. (1963). Further consideration on testing the null hypothesis and the strategy and tactics of investigating theoretical models. *Psychological Review, 70*, 107–115.

Borkowski, J.G., & Wanschura, P.B. (1974). Mediational processes in the retarded. In N.R. Ellis (Ed.), *International review of research in mental retardation* (Vol. 7, pp. 1–54). New York: Academic Press.

Bradshaw, J.L., & Nettleton, N.C. (1981). The nature of hemispheric specialization in man. *Behavioral and Brain Sciences, 4*, 51–91.

Bromfield, R.N. (1983). *Effects of the "mentally retarded" label on perceptions of a child's failure.* Unpublished masters thesis, University of North Carolina at Chapel Hill.

Bromfield, R., Weisz, J.R., & Messer, T. (1986). Children's judgments and attributions in response to the "mentally retarded" label: A developmental approach. *Journal of Abnormal Psychology, 95*, 81–87.

Bronfenbrenner, U. (1975). Is early intervention effective? In M. Guttentag & E.L. Struening (Eds.), *Handbook of evaluation research* (Vol. 2). Beverly Hills, CA: Sage.

Clarke, A.M., & Clarke, A.D.B. (1965). *Mental deficiency: The changing outlook.* New York: Free Press.

Cromwell, R.L. (1963). A social-learning theory approach to mental retardation. In N.R. Ellis (Ed.), *Handbook of mental deficiency.* New York: McGraw-Hill.

DeVries, R. (1970). The development of vote taking as reflected by behavior of bright, average, and retarded children in a social guessing game. *Child Development, 41*, 759–770.

DeVries, R. (1973a). *Performance on Piaget-type tasks of high-IQ, average-IQ, and low-IQ children.* Chicago: University of Illinois at Chicago Circle (ERIC Document Reproduction Service No. ED086, 374/PS007 129).

DeVries, R. (1973b). *The two intelligences of bright, average, and retarded children.* Chicago: University of Illinois at Chicago Circle (ERIC Document Reproduction Service No. ED079/102/SE 016 419).

DeVries, R. (1974). Relationships among Piagetian, IQ, and achievement assessments. *Child Development, 45*, 746–756.

Diener, C.S., & Dweck, C.S. (1978). An analysis of learned helplessness: Continuous changes in performance, strategy, and achievement cognitions following failure. *Journal of Personality and Social Psychology, 36*, 451–462.

Dweck, C.S., & Bush, E.S. (1976). Sex difference in learned helplessness: I. Differential debilitation with peer and adult evaluators. *Developmental Psychology, 12*, 147–156.

Dweck, C.S., Davidson, W., Nelson, S., & Enna, B. (1978). Sex differences in learned helplessness: II. The contingencies of evaluative feedback in the classroom. III. An experimental analysis. *Developmental Psychology, 14*, 268–276.

Ellis, N.R., & Cavalier, A.R. (1982). Research perspectives in mental retardation. In E. Zigler & D. Balla (Eds.), *Mental retardation: The developmental–difference controversy* (pp. 121–152). Hillsdale, NJ: Erlbaum.

Fisher, M.A., & Zeaman, D. (1973). An attention–retention theory of retardate discrimination learning. In N.R. Ellis (Ed.), *International review of research in mental retardation* (Vol. 6, pp. 171–257). New York: Academic Press.

Garber, J., & Seligman, M.E.P. (Eds.). (1980). *Human helplessness: Theory and application.* New York: Academic Press.

Grant, D.H. (1962). Testing the null hypothesis and the strategy and tactics of investigating theoretical models. *Psychological Review, 69*, 54–61.

Green, B.F. (1956). A method for scalogram analysis using summary statistics. *Psychometrika, 21*, 79–88.

Greenwald, A.G. (1975). Consequence of prejudice against the null hypothesis. *Psychological Bulletin, 82*, 1–20.

Grossman, H.J. (1977). *Manual on terminology and classification in mental retardation* (rev. ed.). Washington, DC: American Association on Mental Deficiency.

Grossman, H.J. (1983). *Classification in mental retardation*. Washington, DC: American Association on Mental Deficiency.

Gruen, G.E., & Vore, D.A. (1972). Development of conservation in normal and retarded children. *Developmental Psychology, 6*, 146–157.

Guttman, L. (1950). The basis of scalogram analysis. In S.A. Stouffer et al. (Eds.), *Measurement and prediction* (Vol. 4). Princeton, NJ: Princeton University Press.

Heal, L.W., & Johnson, J.T., Jr. (1970). Inhibition deficits in retardate learning and attention. In N.R. Ellis (Ed.), *International review of research in mental retardation* (Vol. 4, pp. 107–150). New York: Academic Press.

Heber, R.T. (1964). Personality. In H.A. Stouffer et al. (Eds.), *Measurement and prediction* (Vol. 4). Princeton, NJ: Princeton University Press.

Houssiadas, L., & Brown, L.B. (1967). The coordination of perspectives by mentally retarded children. *Journal of Genetic Psychology, 110*, 211–215.

Hunt, J.McV. (1974). Discussion: Developmental gains in reasoning. *American Journal of Mental Deficiency, 79*, 127–133.

Ingalls, R.P. (1978). *Mental retardation: The changing outlook*. New York: Wiley.

Inhelder, B. (1968). *The diagnosis of reasoning in the mentally retarded*. New York: Day (originally published in 1943).

Kelley, H.H. (1973) The process of causal attribution. *American Psychologist, 28*, 107–128.

Kohlberg, L. (1968). Early education: A cognitive-developmental view. *Child Development, 39*, 1013–1062.

Kohlberg, L. (1969). Stage and sequence: The cognitive-developmental approach to socialization. In D. Goslin (Ed.), *Handbook of socialization theory and research*. Chicago: Rand McNally.

Kohlberg, L. (1971). From is to ought: How to commit the naturalistic fallacy and get away with it in the study of moral development. In Kohlberg, L. (1974). Discussion: Development gains in moral judgment. *American Journal of Mental deficiency, 79*, 142–146.

Lane, E.B., & Kinder, E.F. (1939). Relativism in the thinking of subnormal subjects as measured by certain of Piaget's tests. *Journal of Genetic Psychology, 54*, 107–118.

Lister, C. (1972). The development of ESN children's understanding of conservation in a range of attribute situations. *British Journal of Educational Psychology, 42*, 14–22.

Lovell, K., Healey, D., & Rowland, A.D. (1962). Growth of some geometric concepts. *Child Development, 33*, 751–767.

Lovell, K., Mitchell, B., & Everett, I.R. (1962). An experimental study of the growth of some logical structures. *British Journal of Psychology, 53*, 175–188.

Lovell, K., & Slater, A. (1960). The growth of the concept of time: A comparative study. *Child Psychology and Psychiatry, 1*, 179–190.

Lyle, L. (1959). The effects of an institutional environment upon the verbal development of imbecile children. I. Verbal intelligence. *Journal of Mental Deficiency Research, 3*, 122–128.

McManis, D.L. (1969). Conservation of identity and equivalence of quantity by retardates. *Journal of Genetic Psychology, 115*, 63–69.

Mahaney, E.J., & Stevens, B. (1974). Two-year gains in moral judgment by retarded and nonretarded persons. *American Journal of Mental Deficiency, 79,* 139–141.

Mannix, J.B. (1960). The number concepts of a group of E.S.N. children. *British Journal of Educational Psychology, 30,* 180–181.

Marchi, J.U. (1971). *Comparison of selected Piagetian tasks with the Wechsler Intelligence Scale for Children as measures of mental retardation.* Doctoral dissertation, University of California, Berkeley. *Dissertation Abstracts International, 31,* 6442A (University Microfilms No. 71–51, 833).

Milgram, N.A. (1973). Cognition and language in mental retardation: Distinctions and implications. In D.K. Routh (Ed.), *The experimental psychology of mental retardation.* Chicago: Aldine.

Montroy, P., McManis, D., & Bell, T. (1971). Development of time concepts in normal and retarded children. *Psychological Reports, 28,* 895–902.

Piaget, J. (1953). *The origins of intelligence in the child.* London: Routledge & Kegan Paul.

Piaget, J. (1956). The general problem of the psychobiological development of the child. *Discussions on Child Development, 4,* 3–27.

Raber, S.M., & Weisz, J.R. (1981). Teacher feedback to mentally retarded and nonretarded children. *American Journal of Mental Deficiency, 86,* 148–156.

Rholes, W.S., Blackwell, J., Jordan, C., & Walters, C. (1980). A developmental study of learned helplessness. *Developmental Psychology, 16* (6), 616–624.

Roodin, P.A., Sullivan, L., & Rybash, J.M. (1976). Effects of a memory aid on three types of conservation in institutionalized retarded children. *Journal of Genetic Psychology, 129,* 253–259.

Rosenthal, R. (1966). *Experimenter effects in behavioral research.* New York: Appleton-Century-Crofts.

Rosenthal, R. (1978). Combining results of independent studies. *Psychological Bulletin, 85,* 185–193.

Rosenthal, R., & Rubin, D.B. (1979). Comparing significance levels of independent studies. *Psychological Bulletin, 86,* 1165–1168.

Rosenthal, R., & Rubin, D.B. (1982). Comparing effect sizes of independent studies. *Psychological Bulletin, 92,* 500–504.

Seligman, M.E.P. (1975). *Helplessness: On depression, development, and death.* San Francisco: Freeman.

Singh, N.N., & Stott, G. (1975). The conservation of number in mental retardates. *Australian Journal of Mental Retardation, 3,* 215–221.

Spitz, H.H. (1976). Toward a relative psychology of mental retardation, with a special emphasis on evolution. In N.R. Ellis (Ed.), *International review of research in mental retardation* (Vol. 8, pp. 35–56). New York: Academic Press.

Stearns, K., & Borkowski, J.G. (1969). The development of conservation and horizontal-vertical space perception in mental retardation. *American Journal of Mental Deficiency, 73,* 785–790.

Stephens, B., Mahaney, E.J., & McLaughlin, J.A. (1972). Mental ages for achievement of Piagetian reasoning tasks. *Education and Training of the Mentally Retarded, 7,* 124–128.

Stephens, B., McLaughlin, J.A., Hunt, J., Mahaney, E.J., Kohlberg, L., Moore, B., & Aronfreed, J. (1974). Symposium: Developmental gains in the moral reasoning, moral judgment, and moral conduct of retarded and nonretarded persons. *American Journal of Mental Deficiency, 79,* 113–161.

Stephens, B., & McLaughlin, J.A. (1974). Two-year gains in reasoning by retarded and nonretarded persons. *American Journal of Mental Deficiency, 79,* 116–126.

Stevenson, H.W. (1965). Social reinforcement of children's behavior. In L.P. Lipsitt & C. Spiker (Eds.), *Advances in child development* (Vol. 2). New York: Academic Press.

Vernon, P.E. (1979). *Intelligence, heredity and environment.* San Francisco: Freeman.

Weiss, B., Weisz, J.R., & Bromfield, R. (1986). Performance of retarded and nonretarded persons on information-processing tasks: Further tests of the similar structure hypothesis. *Psychological Bulletin, 100*, 157–175.

Weisz, J.R. (1979). Perceived control and learned helplessness among mentally retarded and nonretarded children: A developmental analysis. *Developmental Psychology, 15*, 311–319.

Weisz, J.R. (1981a). Effects of the "mentally retarded" label on adult judgments about child failure. *Journal of Abnormal Psychology, 90*, 371–374.

Weisz, J.R. (1981b). Learned helplessness in black and white children identified by their schools as retarded and nonretarded: Performance deterioration in response to failure. *Developmental Psychology, 17*, 499–508.

Weisz, J.R., & Yeates, K.O. (1981). Cognitive development in retarded and nonretarded persons: Piagetian tests of the similar structure hypothesis. *Psychological Bulletin, 90*, 153–178.

Weisz, J.R., & Zigler, E. (1979). Cognitive development in retarded and nonretarded persons: Piagetian tests of the similar sequence hypothesis. *Psychological Bulletin, 86*, 831–851.

Yeates, K.O., & Weisz, J.R. (1985). On being called mentally retarded: Do developmental and professional perspectives limit labeling effects? *American Journal of Mental Deficiency, 90*, 349–352.

Yando, R., & Zigler, E. (1971). Outerdirectedness in the problem-solving of institutionalized and noninstitutionalized normal and retarded children. *Developmental Psychology, 4*, 277–288.

Zigler, E. (1969). Development versus difference theories of mental retardation and the problem of motivation. *American Journal of Mental Deficiency, 73*, 536–556.

Zigler, E. (1971). The retarded child as a whole person. In H.E. Adams, & W.K. Boardman (Eds.), *Advances in experimental clinical psychology*. Oxford: Pergamon.

Zigler, E. (1987). The definition and classification of mental retardation. *Upsala Journal of Medical Science, Supplement, 13*, 1–10.

Zigler, E., & Balla, D. (Eds.) (1982). *Mental retardation: The developmental–difference controversy*. Hillsdale, NJ: Erlbaum.

Zigler, E., & Hodapp, R.M. (1986). *Understanding mental retardation*. New York: Cambridge University Press.

8 The organization and coherence of developmental processes in infants and children with Down syndrome

Dante Cicchetti and Jody Ganiban

Goals of this chapter

In this chapter, we examine the applicability òf an organizational developmental perspective to the study of infants and children with Down syndrome. Specifically, we review the knowledge base on temperament and socioemotional, cognitive, and representational development, focusing on whether children with Down syndrome proceed through the same sequences, stages, and structures in these domains as nonhandicapped children. Moreover, we explore both qualitative and quantitative differences, in addition to similarities, in the development of children with Down syndrome and normal youngsters. Finally, we determine whether, despite the differences that do exist, the development of children with Down syndrome is organized, meaningful, and lawful – in short, coherent.

Introduction

Over the past several decades, research on Down syndrome from a developmental perspective has burgeoned (see Cicchetti and Beeghly, in

Dante Cicchetti would like to acknowledge the grants he received from the John D. and Catherine T. MacArthur Foundation Network on Early Childhood, the March of Dimes Birth Foundation, and the Spencer Foundation. We would like to thank the many individuals who played important roles in conducting the research reported herein – most notably, Marjorie Beeghly, Mary Breitenbucher, Michelle Gersten, Dan Nichols, Bedonna Weiss-Perry, Alan Sroufe, and Linda Mans-Wagener. We wish to acknowledge the comments and feedback provided on this manuscript by Sheree Toth and Sheldon Wagner. We also extend our thanks to Victoria Gill for typing the manuscript.

Finally, we want to send our appreciation and affection to the parents and to the children with Down syndrome who have participated in our research projects over the course of the past two decades. We have grown immeasurably as a result of our association with them, and hope that our work can result in a more accurate and sensitive understanding of the Down syndrome condition. Furthermore, we believe that the application of research on Down syndrome from a developmental perspective can result in improved educational and intervention programs.

169

press). Prior to these efforts, theoreticians and researchers had primarily conceptualized the developmental process of children with Down syndrome as being qualitatively different from that of MA-matched non-handicapped children (Cicchetti & Pogge-Hesse, 1982; Gibson, 1978). Historically, this issue has been examined within the context of the developmental–difference controversy in the field of mental retardation (Zigler, 1969; Zigler & Balla, 1982).

According to the classic developmental model, explicated most lucidly by Zigler (1969, 1973) and intended to apply only to retarded persons free from organic involvement (i.e., individuals with cultural–familial mental retardation), the retarded child is thought to progress through the cognitive-developmental stages in the same sequence as the nonhandicapped child, albeit at a slower pace and with a lower asymptote. This viewpoint generates the testable hypothesis that the performance of children of varying levels of intelligence who are functioning at the same developmental stage (and who are therefore of different chronological ages) should be identical on cognitive tasks. The differences in rate and ultimate level of developmental attainment are thought to be dictated by the normal variability inherent in the gene pool. In essence, Zigler believes that cultural–familial mentally retarded persons are "normal" individuals whose intelligence is at the low end of the polygenic distribution.

Although a detailed review of the experimental findings emanating from the research of Zigler and his colleagues is beyond the scope of this chapter, in the main the three predictions that Zigler has articulated about cultural–familial mentally retarded children have been confirmed. Specifically, Weisz and Zigler (1979), in their review of the literature, concluded that the vast majority of the studies were congruent with the *similar-sequence hypothesis* – that is, that familial retarded and nonhandicapped persons progress through the developmental stages in the same order, diverging only in the rate at which they advance and in the ultimate level they attain. Likewise, Weisz and Yeates (1981) stated that the literature supported the *similar-structure hypothesis* – namely, that children with cultural–familial mental retardation manifest the same structures in their performance on a variety of experimental tests. Finally, Zigler and Balla (1977) have demonstrated that familially retarded children respond similarly to MA-matched normal individuals when experiencing failure and institutionalization – the *similar-response hypothesis*.

As originally formulated, Zigler's developmental approach applied only to those mentally retarded children who manifest no demonstrable organic etiology for their retardation. Zigler believed that because organically retarded persons have identifiable physiological, biochemical, and/or anatomical deficits contributing to their retardation, they may traverse a divergent set of developmental pathways of cognition and manifest a different kind of cognitive functioning at a given point in time than non-handicapped individuals or persons with cultural–familial mental retardation (Zigler, 1969, 1973).

Beginning with the publication of several early studies on the perceptual-cognitive and socioemotional development of infants and toddlers with Down syndrome (Cicchetti & Sroufe, 1976, 1978; Fantz, Fagan, & Miranda, 1975; Miranda & Fantz, 1974; Serafica & Cicchetti, 1976), a number of researchers have investigated the developmental process of Down syndrome individuals (see reviews in Cicchetti & Beeghly, in press). Drawing on the existing empirical literature on Down syndrome and the organismic theoretical approach to the study of normal development, Cicchetti and Pogge-Hesse (1982) advocated the application of a more liberal organizational developmental perspective to individuals with Down syndrome and to additional groups of organically retarded persons. Subsequently, the scope of the empirical work on Down syndrome has burgeoned such that virtually every key developmental issue and ontogenetic domain has been examined in one or more research laboratories across the United States.

The organismic/organizational perspective

An organismic model of development underscores the active role an individual plays in his or her own development and conceptualizes the individual as an organized whole. Principles of behavior are seen in terms of the organization between parts and wholes and of the dynamic relationship between the individual and the environment (Reese & Overton, 1970; Werner, 1957; Werner & Kaplan, 1963).

An important component of this organismic model is the organizational approach. This perspective on development (Cicchetti & Pogge-Hesse, 1982; Cicchetti & Sroufe, 1978; Sroufe, 1979a) is comprised of a set of regulative principles that can guide research and theorizing on human behavior (Werner, 1957; Werner & Kaplan, 1963). In calling these principles "regulative" we follow Werner (1948), who denied that they are themselves to be taken as empirical laws, or that in research and theory one should necessarily attempt to find laws that can be seen as simple translations of these principles into empirical terms. Rather, these regulative principles are to be taken as heuristic tools, by means of which one can look for meaningful patterns in the great variety and quantity of data often accumulated in contemporary studies of human development and developmental psychopathology (Cicchetti, 1984b; Sroufe & Rutter, 1984). With the aid of this heuristic, investigators may formulate empirical laws with greater confidence that they have uncovered lawful relations than merely accidental correlations.

According to the organizational approach, development may be conceived of as a series of qualitative reorganizations among and within behavioral and biological systems that take place by means of differentiation and hierarchical integration. Variables at many levels of analysis determine the character of these reorganizations: genetic, constitutional, neurobiological, biochemical, behavioral, psychological, environmental, and sociological. Moreover, these variables are conceived as being in dynamic transaction with one another.

Normal development is defined in terms of a series of interlocking social, emotional, and cognitive/representational competencies. Competence at one period of development, which tends to make the individual broadly adapted to his or her environment, prepares the way for the formation of competence at the next (Sroufe & Rutter, 1984). Moreover, normal development is marked by the integration of earlier competencies into later modes of functioning. It follows then that early adaptation tends to promote later adaptation and integration.

Pathological development, in contrast, may be conceived of as a lack of integration of the social, emotional, and cognitive/representational competencies that are important to achieving adaptation at a particular developmental level (Cicchetti & Schneider-Rosen, 1986; Kaplan, 1966; Sroufe, 1979a). Because early structures are often incorporated into later structures, an early deviation or disturbance in functioning may ultimately cause much larger disturbances to emerge later on.

In the organizational approach, the qualitative reorganizations characteristic of development are conceived of as proceeding in accordance with the *orthogenetic principle* (Werner, 1948), which states that the developing organism moves from a relatively diffuse and globally undifferentiated state, by means of *differentiation* and *hierarchical integration*, to a state of greater articulation and organized complexity. The orthogenetic principle may be seen as a solution to the problem of the individual's continuous adaptation to the environment and to the question of how integrity of function may be maintained in the face of change. Continuity in functioning can be maintained via hierarchical integration despite rapid constitutional changes and biobehavioral shifts (Block & Block, 1980; Sackett, Sameroff, Cairns, & Suomi, 1981; Sroufe, 1979a).

In addition to orthogenesis, several related principles characterize the organizational framework: (1) With development, there is change in structure–function relationships over time; (2) the change that occurs is both qualitative and quantitative; and (3) developmental change is best conceived of as a move toward increasing cortical control over the more diffuse, automatic behavioral centers.

Children with Down syndrome are a particularly interesting population for developmentalists. As an "experiment in nature" (Bronfenbrenner, 1979), Down syndrome presents an excellent opportunity to answer critical questions in developmental theory that on ethical grounds alone would be impossible to manipulate experimentally. In addition, unlike most other groups of mentally retarded youngsters, children with Down syndrome are etiologically homogeneous and their condition is detectable at birth; therefore, their developmental progress can be charted virtually from the beginning. Although their development unfolds at a slower pace than for non-Down syndrome children, children with Down syndrome are quite heterogeneous, ranging from severely mentally retarded to approximately normal intellectual functioning. This combination of delayed, yet variable, development permits a more careful examination of the nature of developmental stages and sequences across different developmental domains and of the interrelations among behavioral and biological systems at a particular point in development. In essence, the study of Down syndrome, as is true for cross-cultural research, can inform us about what stages, sequences, and structures are logically necessary and what alternate pathways of ontogenesis are possible, and can provide us with evidence about which factors contributing to the developmental process are most critical.

Temperament

The concept of temperament describes the characteristic manner in which an individual responds to the world. Qualities such as emotionality, activity, tendency to approach or withdraw from interactions, and intensity of reactions are all components of temperament profiles, which shape the way in which individuals engage the world. One approach to examining temperament has been put forward by Rothbart and Derryberry (1981). In this approach, temperament is determined by one's physiological reactivity, ability to self-regulate, emotionality, and evaluative capacity. Individual differences in temperament arise from variation within each capacity across people, as well as from variation in their interactions. Thus, at different stages of development, changes in the expression of temperament characteristics are dependent upon the reorganization and interaction of cognitive abilities, self-regulation, and reactivity.

Most studies that have examined differences in temperament characteristics between individuals with and without Down syndrome have relied
upon parent's ratings of their children along various response dimensions.
In these studies, the Carey Infant Temperament Questionnaire (ITQ;
Carey, 1973) or the Toddler Temperament Scale (TTS; Fullard, McDevitt,
& Carey, 1978, 1984) are most often used. Both questionnaires ask parents
to rate the behavior of their children across ten dimensions: activity
level, rhythmicity, willingness to approach new situations, adaptability,
threshold of stimulation, reaction intensity, quality of mood, distractibility, attention span, and persistence. These ratings are also used to classify
infants as "easy" or "difficult" in temperament. In addition, a third questionnaire, the Infant Behavior Questionnaire (IBQ, Rothbart, 1981) has
also been used to assess parental perceptions of temperament. In contrast
to the other instruments, the IBQ contains questions about six behavioral
dimensions: activity level, positive affect (smiling and laughter), negative
affect (fear), distress to limitations, soothability, and duration of orienting.

Studies of this type have taken two approaches. In the first, children with
Down syndrome are selected with the same CA as the normally developing
standardization sample of children. In the second approach, attempts are
made to match both groups of children on the basis of developmental level
(as measured by standardized infant tests such as the Bayley Scales of
Infant Development; Bayley, 1969). No research groups have administered
temperament questionnaires to both normally developing children and
children with Down syndrome. Thus, all profile comparisons are based on
similarities to and differences from the means and standard deviations of
the original standardization samples.

Comparisons between the temperament characteristics of infants with
Down syndrome and normally developing infants of the same CA have
suggested that differences in parental perceptions of temperament exist
between the two groups. Rothbart and Hanson (1983), using the IBQ
in addition to laboratory measurements of motor development, vocal
activity, and startle to stimulation, examined the temperament characteristics of both groups of infants at 6, 9, and 12 months of age. In general,
the infants with Down syndrome demonstrated less positive and negative
affect and startles than normally developing infants across the first year of
life. However, decreased affect does not indicate that these infants were
generally perceived as less responsive to stimulation. The infants with
Down syndrome were also rated as more attentive than normally developing infants of the same age, and average in their activity level, soothability, and distress to limitations at all ages tested.

Bridges and Cicchetti (1982) and Gunn, Berry, and Andrews (1981) have used the ITQ to assess maternal perceptions of temperament in Down syndrome infants. In both studies, the developmental levels of the infants with Down syndrome were approximately equivalent to those of the normally developing standardization sample of infants. In addition, both groups of researchers asked mothers to complete an additional questionnaire that was designed to measure the overall impressions parents have of their children (General Impressions Inventory, GII; Carey, 1973).

Gunn et al. found that mothers of infants with Down syndrome generally rated their children as average on the ten dimensions of the ITQ. In addition, they found that the distribution of temperament types (i.e., easy versus difficult) was similar for the normally developing and Down syndrome groups. In contrast, however, Bridges and Cicchetti found that mothers of infants with Down syndrome rated their children as less approaching, lower in threshold to stimulation, and high in persistence relative to the ratings provided by mothers of the standardization sample. Moreover, when Bridges and Cicchetti classified infants as easy or difficult based upon the distribution of characteristics of the standardization sample, approximately 40% of the infants with Down syndrome fit the difficult temperament profile, while only 25% of the standardization sample fell into this classification.

Thus, in infancy, CA comparisons have suggested that children with Down syndrome are perceived as less intense in their expression of affect than normally developing infants. Studies that are based upon MA comparisons have yielded equivocal results that may reflect interactive qualities, parent perceptions, or problems in comparing children with Down syndrome with standardization norms, rather than the temperament characteristics of the child.

Studies with toddlers with Down syndrome have also compared groups of infants matched for CA or developmental level. Within their continuing study of individuals with Down syndrome, Gunn et al. (1981, 1983) examined the stability of temperament characteristics from infancy to early childhood. In a cross-sectional study, Gunn and his colleagues (1981) noted that more infants with Down syndrome received difficult ratings on specific dimensions than the toddlers. Although this effect was small, Gunn et al. argue that this difference reflects a transition in temperament characteristics from easy to difficult. In a previous study, Bridges and Cicchetti (1982) failed to find significant trends in the direction of change.

In a longitudinal study, Gunn et al. again addressed the issue of transition from difficult to easy temperament characteristics in infants with Down syndrome. Gunn and his colleagues found little stability or clear patterns in change of clusters of temperament characteristics from infant ratings of temperament to toddler ratings. Despite this, Gunn et al. claim that at the level of the individual, when changes in a particular dimension occurred, they were usually in the direction of difficult to easy characteristics, rather than easy to difficult. Generally, Gunn and his collaborators argue that these changes reflect the creation of appropriate expectations by the care givers for the development of their children, rather than true, objective changes in the characteristics of infants with Down syndrome. The effect of age noted by Gunn et al. also may be due to the use of different questionnaires in the infancy and toddler periods.

In recent years, only a few studies have focused on temperament in toddlers with Down syndrome. Gunn and Berry (1985) asked mothers to use the TTS to rate the temperament of their toddlers. In this study, the children with Down syndrome were approximately 30 months old, and had reached an average developmental level of 18 months. In their analyses, Gunn and Berry compared these ratings with ratings of normally developing toddlers of the same CA and with normally developing toddlers at the same developmental level. Comparisons based on CA showed that toddlers with Down syndrome were relatively high in rhythmicity, low in response intensity, predominantly positive in mood, low in persistence, and high in threshold relative to the standardization sample. Comparisons with normally developing infants of the same developmental age, however, indicated that the toddlers with Down syndrome were high in approach and adaptability, low in response intensity, positive in mood, and low in threshold. Therefore, the comparisons yielded different patterns of results. For both comparisons, however, threshold, mood, and intensity were important distinguishing characteristics. These findings suggest that differences along these parameters may be particularly salient.

In addition, studies have examined the temperament of individuals with Down syndrome along with other groups of children with developmental delays of unknown etiology and neurological impairments. Heffernan, Black, and Poche (1982) obtained TTS ratings for a group of toddlers with various neurological impairments, and Marcovitch, Goldberg, MacGregor, and Lojkasek (1986) compared TTS ratings of toddlers with Down syndrome and neurological disorders, in addition to toddlers with developmental delay of unknown etiology. Heffernan and her colleagues failed to find significant differences between the different groups of delayed infants. In contrast, significant differences in the temperament characteristics between the various groups studied by Marcovitch and colleagues did emerge. Comparisons of the different groups indicated that toddlers with Down syndrome were slightly more active than the other delayed groups, less distractible and approaching than the neurological impairment group, but more approaching and distractible than the unknown etiology group. When the ratings of the toddlers with Down syndrome were compared with those of the normally developing, standardization sample, the children with Down syndrome seemed to be more approaching, less persistent, and had higher thresholds to stimulation than the average child.

These differences were similar to those found when Marcovitch and collaborators combined the various groups of delayed children to compare their overall temperament characteristics with the standardization sample. Again, the delayed children, on average, were rated as more approaching, less intense, less persistent, and higher in sensory threshold than the standardization sample. Thus, overall, the delayed children seemed to engage in interactions; however, they seemed to be less reactive than the normally developing children. However, when Heffernan combined both groups of handicapped children, she found that they were rated, on average, as less active, low in attention and persistence, withdrawing from stimulation, and having a high sensory threshold. These findings suggest that the delayed group is perceived as less interactive than the nondelayed group.

Thus, studies with toddlers also have provided equivocal results. Chronological age comparisons noted differences in approach, intensity, mood, and threshold. Similarly, MA comparisons also suggest differences between toddlers with Down syndrome and normally developing children in intensity, mood and threshold, in addition to rhythmicity and persistence. Differences in intensity of responsiveness are similarly found in infancy. Likewise, differences in level of threshold are also apparent during infancy. The persistence of differences across both age groups suggests, therefore, that such perceptions truly may reflect temperament differences between normally developing infants and infants with Down syndrome. Studies that have compared toddlers with Down syndrome with other groups of children with neurological impairments have also been conducted. In these studies, inconsistent differences have been noted. These differences may arise, however, from variations in the nature, cause, and extent of neurological impairments of the delayed comparison groups.

Another line of research relevant to temperament is the examination of the interaction of abilities and physiological functioning that might account for differences in temperament between individuals with and without Down syndrome. Weinshilbaum, Thoa, Johnson, Kopin, and Axelrod (1971) found an enzyme that facilitates the formation of noradrenaline, a neurotransmitter important to the activation of the sympathetic nervous system (SNS), to be deficient in the blood of individuals with Down syndrome. Likewise, Keele, Richards, Brown, and Marshall (1969) have found decreases in levels of the metabolites of another neurotransmitter (adrenalin), which is usually released when the SNS is activated. Both cholinergic systems (Casanova, Walker, Whitehouse, & Price, 1975; Yates, Simpson, Maloney, Gorden, & Reid, 1980) and serotonergic systems (Scott, Becker, & Petit, 1983) are also influenced by Down syndrome.

In addition to finding abnormalities in the functioning and activity of neurotransmitter systems, some studies have also found that Down syndrome affects the maturation of the brain (Becker, Armstrong, & Chan, 1986; Purpura, 1975; Takashima, Becker, Armstrong, & Chan, 1981). These studies have examined the growth of neuronal networks throughout the brains of infants and children with Down syndrome. Their basic findings suggest that after a short period of growth within the first few months of life, the maturation of the brains of individuals with Down syndrome seems to decrease relative to the normally developing networks. Neuronal networks appear to be less differentiated and less elaborate in the brains of children with Down syndrome by comparison with the normally developing population as the rate of maturation of the Down syndrome children decreases by comparison with the others.

The implications of decreases or cessation in the maturation and development of the brain are widespread. First, one would expect development in general to be delayed as the brain slowly develops the neuronal networks capable of quickly and efficiently synthesizing information. Second, decreased maturation may also inhibit the full development of important inhibitory tracts that control behavioral systems. This may account for the persistence of primitive reflexes beyond the neonatal period in individuals with Down syndrome (Cicchetti & Sroufe, 1978; Cowie, 1970). In addition, biological constraints on the maturation of the brain may influence developmental changes in temperament (Rothbart & Derryberry, 1981; Wilson & Matheny, 1986). If changes in temperament across time reflect the maturation of the central nervous system (CNS), as prescribed by the qualities of the system, individuals with Down syndrome would not be expected to demonstrate the same shifts or changes in temperament characteristics at the same time as the normal population. Further research must be conducted in order to determine whether these differences in dendritic maturation are an effect of mental retardation or a consequence of Down syndrome per se.

Thus, briefly, neuroanatomical studies also suggest that differences in the maturational components of temperament exist between individuals with Down syndrome and normal individuals. These studies have pointed toward possible restrictions on the growth and maturation of capacities that underlie and guide temperament. These restrictions may place restraints on the rate of development and the onset of transition and changes in temperament characteristics.

Differences in the reactivity of arousal systems and neurological maturation constitute the most basic level of temperament. However, these characteristics establish only a possible range of responses by influencing the perception of events and arousal level. In this sense, following Werner's (1957) conception of development, biological predispositions for reactivity or emotionality and maturation may be viewed as the undifferentiated state from which the characteristic behavior of the individual will be fashioned. The ultimate response emitted by the individual will be shaped by the development, refinement, and reorganization of additional abilities.

Within the Rothbart and Derryberry (1981) framework of temperament, one ability that modifies reactivity and shapes responses to the world is the capacity to interpret and analyze an event. Studies that have examined the evaluative capacities of individuals with Down syndrome have primarily used selective visual attention as an index of information processing (see Wagner, Ganiban, & Cicchetti, in press). Implicit in this approach is the assumption that one's evaluation of an event or stimulus directs and drives attention. For example, novelty may motivate one's attention, whereas familiarity has little impact on the interest or attention of the infant. Thus, in terms of temperament, one's evaluation of an event will determine, to some extent, approach and orientation to an event.

Current research has shown that infants with Down syndrome are delayed in their ability to process visual information (Fantz et al., 1975; Miranda & Fantz, 1973, 1974); to develop complex voice features (Glenn & Cunningham, 1983); to compare information across two modalities (Lewis & Bryant, 1982); and to develop recognition memory (Fantz et al., 1975). These difficulties in processing complex information may be reflected in the approach or orientation of Down syndrome infants to the world. For example, infants with Down syndrome may need more time to focus, comprehend, and form appropriate responses to their environment. Or difficulties in evaluating their experiences may make such infants very directed in their attention to the world in order to reduce complexity. In free-play situations, Vietze, McCarthy, McQuiston, MacTurk, and Yarrow (1983) have noted that infants with Down syndrome have a greater tendency to attend visually to objects rather than to interact actively with them. Their visual attention in these cases is greater than normally developing infants of both the same chronological and developmental age. Similarly, MacTurk, Vietze, McCarthy, McQuiston, and Yarrow (1985) claim that during free play, interactions for infants with Down syndrome center on visual attention, whereas interactions for normally developing infants center on social interactions. Consequently, to the observer, infants with Down syndrome may seem reticent and less interested in engaging their environment. This temperament difference, however, may partially stem from the facility with which individuals with Down syndrome process information and evaluate their experiences.

The capacity of individuals to understand the world may affect approach and engagement of the world. Studies of infants with Down syndrome have indicated that these children are delayed in their ability to process information. In turn, difficulties in this area may make Down syndrome children seem less interactive with their environment. Behaviorally, they may be extremely visually attentive, but they take longer to approach a situation and to interact actively with the world than nonhandicapped infants.

One's evaluative capacity is also expected to affect the emotional qualities of interactions with the world. Thus, temperament characteristics also reflect the interchange between affect (emotionality) and cognition. For example, the evaluation of an event as positive or negative may set the affective tone of a response. In addition, one's interpretation of an event may provide the "psychological tension" necessary to fuel expressions of joy or fear by accentuating one's arousal level (Cicchetti & Sroufe, 1978).

Within this area, Cicchetti and his colleagues have completed the most extensive research. For individuals with Down syndrome, affect and cognition appear to be intimately related. Studies that have examined positive affect (Cicchetti & Sroufe, 1976; 1978) and negative affect (Cicchetti & Sroufe, 1978) have revealed interactions between developmental level and the expression of affect (see the next section on socioemotional development). Infants at the highest level of cognitive functioning also demonstrate the greatest differentiation of emotion.

Therefore, infants and children with Down syndrome differ from normal youngsters along several dimensions relevant to temperament. As the individual with Down syndrome develops, his or her ability to respond to the environment is likewise affected by the interaction of cognitive ability and reactivity, again given restrictions specified by genetic makeup. Thus, changes in temperament – or responsivity – are due to a myriad of factors. The studies of Cicchetti and Sroufe (1976, 1978) suggest that the manifestation of affect seems to be related to the extent to which a person can appropriately evaluate an event. Consequently, at different periods of development, the manner in which abilities are organized is similar for infants with Down syndrome and normally developing infants. However, the intensity of expression (e.g., blinking versus crying) seems related to noncognitive factors. Given possible constitutional and maturational differences between Down syndrome infants and normal infants at different points in development, the inherent reactivity of Down syndrome may affect the sensitivity to stimulation and the intensity qualities of emotions as well (Thompson, Cicchetti, Lamb, & Malkin, 1985). These relationships between appraisal processes, reactivity, and constitution are central to Rothbart and Derryberry's (1981) theory of temperament.

The Rothbart and Derryberry (1981) conceptualization describes temperament as reflective of the development and organization of reactive capacities, emotionality, cognitive, and self-regulatory abilities. Therefore, one's current perceptions of temperament are determined by the status of capacities in various domains.

Parent-report measures suggest that infants with Down syndrome differ from nonhandicapped, normally developing infants along several dimensions: affect intensity, threshold attention, and threshold level. Similarly, biological studies have indicated that individuals with Down syndrome may be inherently less reactive to stimulation and possess higher threshold levels than individuals without Down syndrome. Studies with neurotransmitters have pointed toward decreased function of both the parasympathetic and sympathetic branches of the peripheral nervous system, and decreases in serotonergic activity, thought to affect consciousness. These biological differences may predispose infants with Down syndrome to be more passive or less reactive than other children of their CA.

In addition, neuroanatomical studies have provided evidence for delayed or arrested neurological maturation. Thus, the timing of shifts and changes in temperament characteristics is expected to differ both for children with and without Down syndrome. Another effect of delayed neurological development might be the development of forebrain inhibitory tracts that are important for the development of self-regulation. Behaviorally, this may be expressed in long periods of attention fixation, in which the individual has difficulty redirecting and refocusing his or her attention.

Temperament research on children with Down syndrome has just started. Further research that concurrently measures physiological differences in reactivity in addition to the expression of affect or cognitive development is needed before conclusions about the structures that underlie temperament and the course of development for children with Down syndrome can be drawn. However, given organismic theory, in which the individual characteristics of the child interact with the environment to shape development, temperament is an important area for research.

Socioemotional development

Affect development

The study of emotional phenomena has important implications for understanding the organization of the developmental process of Down syndrome individuals – in particular, the relationship between emotion and cognition (Hesse & Cicchetti, 1982). Emotions may be regarded as developing ontogenetically earlier than cognition, thereby providing the context within which cognitive development may occur (*cognitive epiphenomenalism*). The emergence of new emotions may be dependent on cognitive advances that must be made before various emotions may be expressed (*emotional epiphenomenalism*). Emotions may develop along a separate pathway from cognitive advances, so that the sequence, rate, and quality of change must be considered distinctly within each domain (*parallelism*). Finally, emotions may emerge in interaction with cognitive advances, thereby suggesting a progression that necessitates a consideration of developmental changes that occur across domains and that exert a reciprocal influence on each other (*interactionism*).

In fact, children with Down syndrome provide an important test of the nature of the relationship between emotional and cognitive development. In contrast to the rapid development of the normal infant, in whom the simultaneous emergence of behaviors may be viewed as coincidental, the slower advances of children with Down syndrome through the same progression of stages as normal babies allow us to observe and demonstrate true convergences and discontinuities in development. Because of the slower cognitive development in infants with Down syndrome, it is possible to separate the early prototypes of what will later be affective expression from genuine emotional reactions that are dependent on psychological processes (Cicchetti & Sroufe, 1978). Finally, the developmental heterogeneity of Down syndrome infants allows specification of the interdependence of the relationship between affect and cognition.

Studies of positive affect

The ontogenesis of smiling and laughter in infants with Down syndrome provides a good illustration of the intimate connection that underlies emotional and cognitive development. Previous research with several samples of nonretarded infants between the ages of 4 and 12 months found that changes in laughter were associated with advancing cognitive development (Sroufe & Wunsch, 1972). Whereas infants in the first half year of life laughed mostly in situations that were physically intense or vigorous – and increasingly so during the second year of life – infants laughed at progressively more subtle and complex social and visual stimulation and were less likely to laugh at simpler stimuli.

In a study of 25 infants with Down syndrome between 4 and 24 months of age, the subjects were presented with the standard series of 30 laughter items used in studies of normal infants (Cicchetti & Sroufe, 1976, 1978), as well as psychometric scales (Bayley, 1969) and Piagetian-based cognitive scales (Uzgiris & Hunt, 1975). Results showed that even though infants with Down syndrome showed a later onset of laughter, they laughed at the incongruous stimulus items in the same order as normal infants – initially at intrusive auditory and tactile items, later at the more complex social and visual items. This ordering suggests an interrelation between cognitive and affective development. Furthermore, as is the case with nonretarded infants, with development it appears that it is the "effort" of infants with Down syndrome in processing the stimulus content or "participation" in the event that produces the tension necessary for smiling and laughter, rather than stimulation per se (Kagan, 1971; Sroufe & Waters, 1976). That is, as schema formation becomes increasingly important in the elicitation of positive affect, it is no longer stimulation that produces the affective response, but the infant's effort in processing the stimulus content.

Down syndrome infants and nonretarded infants develop toward an ever more active participation in producing affectively effective stimulation. In this example of the development of smiling and laughter in infants with Down syndrome, the similarity in the ordering of the responsivity to the laughter items to that demonstrated in nonretarded infants suggests that the development of the emotional domain is inextricably interwoven with changes within the cognitive arena.

Moreover, evidence from the results of the cognitive tests strengthens this interactive conceptualization of the relationship between affective and cognitive development. It was found that the level of cognitive development as measured by performance on the Uzgiris-Hunt and Bayley scales correlated highly with the level of affective development as measured by the smiling and laughter items.

Studies on the development of negative affect

The organizational perspective assumes a close relationship between strong positive and strong negative affect in that they are linked by degree of cognitively produced arousal (Sroufe & Waters, 1976). Because the same event can produce the range of affective reactions, factors beyond information inherent in the event are seen as influencing the direction of and thresholds for affective reactions (Cicchetti & Sroufe, 1976, 1978; Sroufe & Waters, 1976).

Cicchetti and Sroufe (1978) have compared the responses of infants with Down syndrome and nonretarded infants to looming objects at 4, 8, and 12 months, and studied responses of infants with Down syndrome at 16 months. Although there were no differences in the amount of crying displayed at 4 months, significantly more normal infants than those with Down syndrome cried at 8 and 12 months. Actually, it was not until 16 months that infants with Down syndrome showed any substantial crying. Moreover, the infants with Down syndrome who cried had significantly higher scores on the Bayley scales of mental and motor development than those who did not. Therefore, those infants with Down syndrome who had high Bayley scales and showed fear and distress reactions early were more differentiated in their cognitive and emotional development.

A close relationship between cognitive and emotional development was also found in the study of the reactions of infants with Down syndrome to being placed atop the visual cliff. It was found that far fewer infants with Down syndrome than normal infants exhibited fear reactions (for example, crying, heart rate acceleration, behavioral freezing) when placed directly atop the deep side. Just as was found for the looming data, the infants with Down syndrome who manifested negative reactions on the visual cliff were more cognitively mature, with significantly higher scores on the Bayley scales of development than those with Down syndrome who did not show fear.

The organization of affect, motivation, cognition, and play

Studies examining the play behavior of children with Down syndrome have revealed more about the role of emotional development in Down syndrome. Researchers have noted that although emerging cognitive abilities may underlie the structure of children's play, the force behind play is often affective in nature (Cicchetti & Hesse, 1983; Piaget, 1962). Studies of the play of nonretarded children have yielded information about the interrelations among affect, cognition, and symbolic development. Children's enthusiasm and persistence in object play have been found to be correlated significantly with the complexity and maturity of object play in these studies (Bretherton, 1984; Matas, Arend, & Sroufe, 1978). Similar interrelations between cognitive and affective dimensions of object play have been observed in children with Down syndrome (Beeghly & Cicchetti, 1987; Hill & McCune-Nicolich, 1981).

For example, in a longitudinal study of 31 children with Down syndrome, Motti, Cicchetti, and Sroufe (1983) found that both symbolic play maturity and affective play behavior at 3–5 years were significantly correlated with indices of affective and cognitive development assessed during the first and second years of these children's lives, respectively. Marked individual differences existed for these children such that children with higher levels of cognitive development engaged in more mature levels of symbolic and social play, explored toys more actively and thoroughly, were more enthusiastic during play, and exhibited more positive affect than less cognitively advanced children.

In a study conducted by Beeghly and Cicchetti (1987), results of correlational analyses revealed that affective–motivational play style (enthuiasm, persistence, positive affect) was significantly correlated both with level of cognitive development and with symbolic play maturity in children with Down syndrome and in cognitively matched normal children. These findings indicate that affective, motivational, and cognitive aspects of symbolic development apparent in the play of children with Down syndrome are organized similarly to those of normal children at a comparable level of cognitive development.

The relationship between emotion and cognition

These studies of infants with Down syndrome suggest that cognitive factors alone are not sufficient to account for the affective behavior of these infants. Analysis of the data indicates that the slower cognitive development of Down syndrome infants only partially accounts for the reduced incidence of extreme forms of affect expression (for example, laughter and crying). In the laughter studies, even after comparing the infants with Down syndrome with their MA-matched normal counterparts, less laughter was found than with the normal infants. Likewise, even when cognitive-developmental level was comparable between infants with Down syndrome and nonretarded infants, normal infants showed more negative reactions to the visual cliff and to looming objects. Fewer infants with Down syndrome were fearful of being placed directly on the deep side of the visual cliff than their cognitive-developmental level would have led us to predict. Even taking developmental level into account, infants with Down syndrome manifested less crying than normal infants (Cicchetti & Sroufe, 1978). We interpret these data to mean that affect and cognition are indeed separate developmental systems and that both of the epiphenomenalist positions on the relationship between cognition and emotion (Hesse & Cicchetti, 1982) are thus refuted in infants with Down syndrome.

Because a focus on cognitive factors is insufficient to explain these results, individual differences in the strength of external stimulation necessary to produce a given amount of physiological stimulation must be simultaneously considered. Perhaps the differing rates and levels of maturation of the neuroendocrinological system, in combination with the slowed rate of cortical development, account in part for the decreased intensity and the muted affect systems of infants and children with Down syndrome (see Ganiban, Wagner, & Cicchetti, in press, for an elaboration).

We think that the data on the development of positive and negative affect, as well as the investigations on affect, motivation, and play, support an interactional interpretation of the relationship between affect and cognition (Hesse & Cicchetti, 1982).

Attachment

The development of a secure, adaptive attachment relationship with the primary care giver is a stage-salient issue that has generated considerable research (Ainsworth, Blehar, Waters & Wall, 1978; Bowlby, 1969/1982). It is marked by increased attention and attunement to interpersonal interaction (Stern, 1985). Whereas the capacity for attachment originates in earlier stages, overt manifestations of this issue reach ascendancy in the latter half of the first year of life in normal infants (Sroufe, 1979a). During this period, the infant learns to coordinate a broad variety of behavioral responses into an adaptive and flexible goal-corrected response repertoire. Dyadic interactions, marked by relatedness and synchrony, resiliency to stress, and appropriate affective interchange, are associated with successful adaptation during this stage (Sroufe, 1979b). Also critical is the knowledge that a care giver is reliable and responsive. Inadequate response-contingent stimulation is likely to exert a negative impact on the infant's ability to master the tasks of this stage. In the absence of regular contingent responsivity, neither infant nor care giver develops feelings of efficacy, and the development of a secure attachment relationship may be impeded (Ainsworth et al., 1978; Belsky, Rovine, & Taylor, 1984; Lamb, Thompson, Gardner, Charnov, & Estes, 1984).

Despite their constitutional anomalies, the attachment system of infants with Down syndrome is organized similarly to that of MA-matched non-handicapped youngsters. The majority of these children form secure attachment relationships with their care givers (Thompson, Cicchetti, Lamb, & Malkin, 1985). Research on infants with Down syndrome also demonstrates that a relationship similar to that exhibited in normal infants may be found between early attachment with the primary care giver and the control of emotions. Cicchetti and Serafica (1981) found the attachment, affiliation, and fear/wariness systems of infants with Down syndrome to be organized similarly to those in normal infants (Bretherton & Ainsworth, 1974), In particular, the intensity of emotional responses in the infants with Down syndrome varied with the context and the behaviors of both mother and stranger, thereby suggesting an awareness of and sensitivity to different eliciting conditions, and a capacity for the modulation and control of emotional states.

Cicchetti and Serafica's (1981) analysis of qualitative and quantitative differences in responsiveness to mother and stranger for the fear/wariness, affiliation, and attachment behavioral systems allowed for a better understanding of the complexity of the potential conclusions that could be drawn about the emotional control of the infants with Down syndrome. For example, the increased latency to crying during separation from the mother, and the greater difficulty in soothing and calming the distressed infant with Down syndrome, reflects the influence of the higher arousal threshold in these infants. This psychophysiological disturbance mediates the overt display of affective responsiveness, but does not minimize the need for attributing importance to the control that infants with Down syndrome must learn to exert over their emotional displays. Berry, Gunn, and Andrews (1980) found that Down syndrome babies observed in a sequence of episodes similar to the "strange situation" (Ainsworth et al., 1978) displayed greater distress upon separation from the mother than those infants studied by Cicchetti and Serafica (1981). However, the infants in the investigation conducted by Berry and his colleagues (1980) were younger in mental and chronological age than those included in Cicchetti and Serafica's (1981) sample, thereby indicating the potential influence of increased socialization experiences upon the capacity for emotional control.

Although the organization of behavioral systems may be similar for normal infants and infants with Down syndrome, qualitative differences in the emotionality of each group do exist (Thompson, Cicchetti, Lamb, & Malkin, 1985). Infants with Down syndrome demonstrate less intense separation distress, longer response latencies, briefer recoveries, and a smaller range of affect lability in their responses compared with normal infants of the same CA or MA.

Self-development

The toddler's emerging acquisition of a sense of self, seen as encompassing both affective and cognitive dimensions, is a significant developmental task

(Lewis & Brooks-Gunn, 1979; Stern, 1985). The evolution of this ability enables the toddler to understand environmental occurrences more fully. Moreover, a well-differentiated sense of self provides the toddler with greater comprehension of personal functioning as a separate and independent entity. Issues of body management begin to emerge from the context of the mother–infant relationship into the realm of autonomous function. The infant becomes increasingly invested in self-managing as a result of new cognitive and motor achievements, as well as in more sophisticated notions about self and other. Empathic acts also begin to emerge at this time, again a manifestation of the realization that the self can have an impact on others (Zahn-Waxler & Radke-Yarrow, 1982). Caretaker sensitivity and ability to tolerate the toddler's strivings for autonomy, as well as the capacity to set age-appropriate limits, are integral to the successful resolution of this issue. In contrast, intolerance for infant initiative may impede the development of autonomy. Caretakers who tend to feel rejected by the infants' increasing independence and/or overwhelmed by the infant's actively initiated demands may inhibit the emergence of age-appropriate independence (Mahler, Pine, & Bergman, 1975).

Toddlers with Down syndrome evidence visual self-recognition in the mirror-and-rouge paradigm (Lewis & Brooks-Gunn, 1979) when they reach a mental age of approximately 2 years (Hill & Tomlin, 1981; Loveland, 1987; Mans, Cicchetti, & Sroufe, 1978). In normal infants at approximately 18 to 24 months, visual self-recognition and the development of shame have been found to coincide with the emergence of the autonomous self and positive valuation of the self (Lewis & Brooks-Gunn, 1979). When shown their rouge-marked noses in a mirror, most normal infants evidence their self-knowledge by touching their own noses while examining their reflections in the mirror. The emergence of self-directed behaviors is first observed at 15–18 months and is common by 21–24 months of age.

Mans and her colleagues (1978) found that when infants with Down syndrome achieved the appropriate cognitive developmental level, they too showed the emergence of self-recognition. Thus, self-recognition was not the coincidental result of a particular CA, but rather was closely tied to and emerged with cognitive development. Moreover, the positive affect accompanying their visual self-recognition suggests that children with Down syndrome feel positive about themselves. In contrast, the affective responses of abused/neglected toddlers (Schneider-Rosen & Cicchetti, 1984) and autistic youngsters (Spiker & Ricks, 1984) to their mirror self-reflections are predominantly neutral or negative in nature.

In a related study to that of Mans and collaborators, Hill and Tomlin (1981) observed the responses of two groups of preverbal retarded toddlers to watching marked or unmarked television images of themselves. One group was comprised of toddlers with Down syndrome, whereas the other was a multihandicapped group, including toddlers with anoxia, rubella, and seizure disorders. Hill and Tomlin (1981) found that the toddlers with Down syndrome all showed the curiosity and self-conscious behaviors that characterize nonhandicapped babies during the second year of life. Moreover, 11 of the 12 toddlers with Down syndrome recognized their television images. In contrast, fewer than half the multiply handicapped group evinced self-recognition, and their affective reactions were like those of normal 1 year olds. Among both groups of toddlers, Hill and Tomlin (1981) reported that all those who could recognize themselves had reached mental ages comparable with normal toddlers who manifested that aspect of self-knowledge.

Similarly, Loveland (1987) found that young children with Down syndrome learned to find things in a mirror – including themselves – in a manner that paralleled strikingly that of normally developing children of similar developmental levels. Loveland observed many similarities between the normal and Down syndrome groups, including the use of "incorrect strategies," behavioral reactions to the mirror, and pattern of task solution. In addition, Loveland concluded that children with Down syndrome may not proceed along this developmental pathway the same way as normal youngsters. She reached this conclusion because the children with Down syndrome employed different means, strategies, or exploratory tendencies than did the normal children in front of the mirror.

In normally developing children, the use of language and play to represent early conceptions of relationships is an age-appropriate manifestation of children's growing awareness of self and other (Bretherton, 1984). This awareness typically emerges and becomes more elaborated during the second and third years of life. For example, self-descriptive utterances are used more frequently as children provide verbal accompaniments to their ongoing behavior (Kagan, 1981). In addition, children become increasingly able to label the emotional states, intentions, and cognitions of both themselves and others (Bretherton & Beeghly, 1982), and begin to use their own name and personal pronouns appropriately. Moreover, the use of self-related language becomes increasingly decontextualized, with children first speaking primarily about themselves in the here-and-now, then discussing the actions and internal states of other nonpresent individuals or of hypothetical contexts.

Beeghly and Cicchetti (1987) found that children with Down syndrome showed similar but delayed sequences in their conceptions of self and other development as assessed through language and play to the sequences observed in nonhandicapped children. In both language and play, these children first represented *themselves* symbolically. With increasing age and cognitive maturity, the language and play of children with Down syndrome became more decentered, integrated, and decontextualized. Only the most cognitively mature children used language and play to represent self and other hypothetical situations. Children with Down syndrome were significantly more advanced in symbolic play maturity than their MLU-matched controls (but not their MA-matched controls). However, the children with Down syndrome did differ from their language controls when *linguistic* representatives of self and other were analyzed. These results suggest that despite the similarity in developmental sequence in both domains, children with Down syndrome may be more advanced in nonlinguistic domains of symbolic representation. However, both linguistic and nonlinguistic variables are significantly correlated with MA for children with Down syndrome. These findings attest to the coherence of symbolic development in children with Down syndrome (for an elaboration, see the discussion on symbolic play that follows).

Finally, children with Down syndrome show increasingly differentiated concepts of self and other in play. During play, their self-related language (e.g., talking about their ongoing activities and internal states, using personal pronouns, etc.) was related to advances in both symbolic and cognitive development. In addition, parallel advances were found in their ability to use language as a communicative social tool (Beeghly & Cicchetti, 1987).

In many of the ontogenetic domains examined to this point, the development of individuals with Down syndrome is similar to that of nonhandicapped, normal infants. Children with Down syndrome seem to follow similar sequences of development, acquiring and demonstrating increasingly more complex behaviors. Additionally, the developmental process occurs in an orderly fashion in which the child's various capacities are coherently organized.

Changes observed in the socioemotional development of individuals with Down syndrome, however, seem to be related to concomitant changes in cognitive skills, rather than to CA. As these children develop intellectually, the manner in which they respond to and interact with the world also changes. In this sense, affect and cognition interact greatly through development to shape the responses of individuals to their environment. In the next section, the discussion will turn to studies that have focused upon the cognitive development of individuals with Down syndrome.

Pre-representational cognitive development

Attention and information processing

Attention is necessary to the careful examination and understanding of one's environment. In many ways attention is a state of preparedness, in which people orient themselves toward an object, enabling them to assess, interpret, and create mental representations of their experiences. Initially, however, infants have little control over their own attention. Through the first months of life, infants gradually acquire the ability to self-regulate states of alertness and attentiveness (Olson & Sherman, 1983). Thus, infants move from having little control over their arousal states to being able to orient their own attention selectively to attractive, interesting, or important events in the environment.

The development of selective attention is dependent on two factors: neurological maturation and motivation. As children develop, the forebrain inhibitory systems necessary to control reflexes and arousal levels undergo increasing differentiation. This development enables individuals to exert control over their states of arousal and attention. As this occurs, attention also becomes selective, motivated and directed by the infant's interest and appraisals of the environment. Consequently, at later ages, level of attention and selective attention reflect one's information-processing abilities as well as one's more general ability to control attention states neurologically.

Reports on various areas of development have noted that youngsters with Down syndrome generally have long attention spans, appearing to be less distractible than nonhandicapped, normally developing infants of the same age (Berger, in press; Ganiban et al., in press; Gibson, 1978; Loveland, 1987). For example, utilizing a habituation task, Cohen (1981) noted that by 19 weeks of age, infants with Down syndrome fixate on a target stimulus for longer periods of time than do same-age, normally developing infants. Likewise, Miranda and Fantz (1973, 1974), in preferential looking and recognition memory tasks, observed that infants with Down syndrome attended to the test stimuli for longer periods of time than normal infants. In these studies, significant differences in visual attention were apparent by 17–29 weeks of age, and persisted through the last age group studied. Additional studies by MacTurk, Vietze, McCarthy, McQuiston, and Yarrow (1985) and Vietze, McCarthy, McQuiston, MacTurk, and Yarrow (1983) have noted that infants with Down syndrome are more visually attentive in their interactions than normally developing infants.

Loveland (1987) has speculated that differences in attention level are due to poorly developed forebrain inhibitory mechanisms that diminish one's ability to control states and actions (see Cicchetti & Sroufe, 1978; Cowie, 1970). Thus, if such inhibitory mechanisms are impaired, a person's ability to disengage from a task or to redirect attention may suffer simply because the physical ability to self-regulate is impaired. If such impairments are present in infants with Down syndrome (as suggested by Cicchetti and Sroufe, 1978, and Cowie, 1970), these individuals may have difficulty in disengaging from an object, appearing more attentive and less distractible than normally developing infants. This difference should become particularly apparent by the end of the first year of life, when most infants start to demonstrate selective attention to their environment.

However, the impact of Down syndrome on attention is not uniform, nor easily definable. Lewis and Brooks-Gunn (1984), in a habituation study including infants with disorders thought to affect the CNS (i.e., Down syndrome, cerebral palsy, developmental delay of unknown origin, and multiple handicaps), found that the influence of neurological disorders on attention is varied. In this study, the infants with Down syndrome did not demonstrate a specific attention pattern and were not distinguishable from the other groups of organic mentally retarded infants. However, pattern of attention, independent of an infant's group membership, was significantly related to developmental level (as assessed by the Bayley Scales of Infant Development; Bayley, 1969). The lack of a specific relationship between type of disorder and pattern of attention suggests that the developmental outcome varies for each group of infants. Nevertheless, patterns of attention are sensitive to or reflective of cognitive skills. Unfortunately, Lewis and Brooks-Gunn did not include a group of normally developing, nonhandicapped children in their analyses. Thus, whether these patterns of attention represent similar mental abilities within the handicapped and nonhandicapped populations cannot be answered.

In general, studies that have used selective attention as an index of information processing have shown delays in development when tasks required higher-level processing skills. In one review, Wagner, Ganiban, and Cicchetti (in press) concluded that infants with Down syndrome are not distinguishable from normally developing infants when fundamental abilities are assessed. Rather, differences emerge only when higher-level processing of information is required. In these cases, infants with Down syndrome generally demonstrate delay in the onset of certain behaviors (such as selective attention) that are thought to be motivated and directed by higher-level information processing skills.

Within the domain of vision, Fantz, Fagan, and Miranda (1975) have shown that infants with Down syndrome selectively attend to various black and white patterns approximately 2 to 4 months after nonhandicapped, normally developing infants. These delays, however, are not related to perceptual abilities or to lack of general attention to the stimuli. The configurations the infants with Down syndrome had most difficulty in "solving" required either the use of experience or the perception and understanding of whole configurations, instead of distinct parts. Evaluation of stimuli on these dimensions requires higher-level processing abilities than simply perceiving and distinguishing between two patterns on the basis of a single dimension such as stripe width. Consequently, Fantz and collaborators propose that the difficulties the infants with Down syndrome experienced in discriminating patterns relative to the other infants reflect deficiencies in higher perceptual and cognitive processes that are not tied to the development of basic sensory capacities.

Similarly, Glenn, Cunningham, and Joyce (1981) have found that basic tasks involving selective attention do not distinguish infants with Down syndrome from normally developing infants within the auditory domain. In these studies, infants with Down syndrome and normally developing infants of the same MA were provided with a toy that could produce either a human voice or an instrument (Glenn, Cunningham, & Joyce, 1981) or baby talk or adult speech (Glenn & Cunningham, 1983). When both groups of infants attained a developmental level of 9 months, they selectively attended to and attempted to elicit the sound of a human voice over a musical instrument. By this point in their development, both groups of infants also selectively attended to and preferred baby talk over adult speech. However, by the time both groups of infants reached a developmental level of 18 months, the preference for baby talk decreased for the subjects with Down syndrome, whereas it increased for the nonhandicapped infants. Glenn and Cunningham argue that the older infants with Down syndrome were less motivated to attend to the baby talk because of deficits in receptive language skills. The exaggerated features of baby talk did not enhance speech comprehension for the infants with Down syndrome, whereas baby talk facilitated the nonhandicapped infants' understanding of speech features. Consequently, the normally developing infants selectively attended to and preferred baby talk over normal adult speech because it provided meaningful and useful information. Like Fantz and colleagues (1975), therefore, Glenn and Cunningham argue that infants with Down syndrome have the perceptual capacity to distinguish between the different stimuli, but that they may lack the motivation to direct their attention because of failures in appreciating the complex or novel qualities of the stimuli. Similar findings of delays, even when matching on MA, have been found for intermodal and intramodal matching tasks by Lewis and Bryant (1982).

Selective attention also has been used to assess the development of recognition memory in infants. In general, infants with Down syndrome, despite perceptual skills comparable to the normal infants, are delayed by approximately 2 months in their visual discrimination between novel and familiar patterns. These results imply that divergences between the performances of infants with and without Down syndrome are due to the development of higher-level information processing skills such as recognizing previously experienced events or patterns rather than perceptual difficulties.

This brief description of selective attention suggests that the appearance of some higher-level information processing skills that motivate and direct attention of nonhandicapped infants is delayed in the Down syndrome population. Although individuals with Down syndrome possess the basic ability to perceive information accurately, they appear to be delayed in their ability to utilize and interpret their experiences to the same extent as normally developing infants.

Difficulties in information processing also may interact with additional difficulties in focusing or redirecting attention to various aspects of the environment (Cicchetti & Sroufe, 1978). Individuals with Down syndrome may be susceptible to varying degrees to becoming fixated on a single dimension or event in their environment to the exclusion of other important qualities of the environment. Such directed attention coupled with difficulties in processing information may limit these individuals' experience with the world, thereby diminishing the richness of their interactions with the world compared with nonhandicapped, normally developing infants (MacTurk et al., 1985). In turn, failure to take full advantage of their experiences may further accentuate difficulties in information processing. Krakow and Kopp (1983), in a study of the play interactions of infants and toddlers with Down syndrome and developmental delay of unknown etiology, have underscored this point and concluded that for both groups of delayed infants:

> The reduction in simultaneous monitoring, the occurrence of primitive activity, and the presence of time spent unoccupied all point to systematic problems in processing stimuli and taking full advantage of the experience at hand. These, in turn, undoubtedly have significant developmental ramifications and may have rippling effects such that these

subtle behavioral differences lead to more exaggerated problems with learning.
(Krakow & Kopp, 1983; p. 1153)

Consequently, delays in the attainment of cognitive skills may be ex-acerbated and perpetuated by the nature of interactions with both the world that children with Down syndrome create for themselves and experience.

Although these findings differentiate individuals with Down syndrome from those without Down syndrome, they do not support the difference hypothesis. Each study reports a main effect for mental retardation or Down syndrome, rather than examining the organization of processes that form selective attention or intermodal matching. To illustrate this point, Wagner and colleagues (in press), utilizing the information-processing framework described by Stanovitch (1978), have argued that processing of visual information in preferential looking or recognition memory tasks can be broken down into components such as perception, encoding, storage, and retrieval. To support the difference position, one needs to demon-strate that individuals with Down syndrome are either selectively deficient in one of these capacities or that they organize these processes differently from individuals without Down syndrome. Such an investigation would elucidate whether the development of information-processing skills in individuals with Down syndrome is different or delayed.

Sensorimotor development

Within Piagetian theory, sensorimotor development represents the growth of prerepresentational thought and skills. Cognitive development within this period and subsequent periods is commonly perceived as occurring in various structured stages. Individuals are expected to progress through such stages in a fixed order as they mature. When regressions in abilities occur, individuals are thought to be undergoing periods of transition, in which specific abilities have not been completely internalized.

Studies of sensorimotor development in children and infants with Down syndrome have explored similarities and differences in the structure of sensorimotor stages and the developmental course adopted by these in-dividuals. These studies have examined the extent to which children with Down syndrome progress through each stage as they grow older and the extent to which they follow the same sequences as nonhandicapped in-dividuals. In addition, researchers have explored the coherence of the development of different skills within each stage of sensorimotor develop-ment and the transition from one stage to the next.

In terms of the ordinality of development, individuals with Down syndrome, as well as other groups of retarded individuals, follow the same stage sequence within different domains as normally developing, nonhandicapped infants. Both retarded and nonretarded children acquire more complex skills and abilities as they progress through the different stages of sensorimotor development. Dunst (in press), applying scalogram analyses to the scores obtained by the infants with Down syndrome on the Uzgiris-Hunt scales of sensorimotor development, found that infants with Down syndrome progress through the same sequence of skill attainment as nonhandicapped, normally developing infants.

Likewise, Cicchetti and Mans-Wagener (1987) also noted that infants with Down syndrome within the first 2 years of life consistently attained higher levels of cognitive development as they grew older. Each domain of the sensorimotor period develops in a parallel fashion, as the child acquires increasingly more complex skills in different sensorimotor areas. Cicchetti and Mans-Wagener point out that development in each domain does not always occur at the same rate. Rather, when one compares the stages of development attained by children with Down syndrome within each domain, congruence between stages decreases between 13 and 19 months of age. However, between 19 and 24 months of age, Cicchetti and Mans-Wagener observed an increase in congruence. Similarly, Dunst (in press), in a review of existing studies, has found that stage congruence over time represents a U-function. In this case, Dunst reports that the highest stage congruence is apparent in the 2–6 month and 18–22 month age ranges, and the lowest congruence between stages of development is found in the 6–18 month age range. In addition, Dunst also reports that stage congruence is greater for normally developing children than for children with Down syndrome during the sensorimotor period. However, the stage congruence of children with Down syndrome is generally greater than for other retarded children without Down syndrome.

Cicchetti and Mans-Wagener claim that the decrease in stage congruence reflects a period of transition for the infants in which they are acquiring, consolidating, and assimilating new skills. By the end of the sensorimotor period – 24 months of age – however, the transition phase has ended, and new skills have been assimilated, prompting movement to the next phase of development. This type of developmental pattern is similar to that proposed by Piaget, and thought to characterize the development of nonhandicapped, normally developing children.

Within the sensorimotor period, researchers also have examined stage stability and structure for both children with Down syndrome and normally developing children. Stage instability – or regressions from one stage to a previous stage of less complex abilities – are thought to appear when a child has not fully acquired or assimilated a particular cognitive skill. Consequently, they represent periods of transition during which children consolidate and refine their abilities. In one study, Dunst (1981) examined the appearance and persistence of regressions in skills in the sensorimotor development of individuals with Down syndrome. The children with Down syndrome were found to have twice as many regressions as non-handicapped, normally developing children. Likewise, Morss (1983) has found that the test−retest reliability for the expression of sensorimotor skills over a short period of time is lower for children with Down syndrome than for nonhandicapped, normally developing infants.

Dunst (in press), however, argues that such regressions by individuals with Down syndrome may be due to their pace of development. Because the development of Down syndrome children occurs more slowly, regressions that are not commonly seen in children without Down syndrome become accentuated and more salient to observers. When Dunst attempted to control statistically for rate of development in comparing the children with Down syndrome and the normally developing children, the children with Down syndrome still appeared to have more regressions than the nonhandicapped infants and children. Consequently, the children with Down syndrome may have more difficulty mastering and assimilating new skills than normally developing infants. "Regressions" in development, however, may not be true reversions to a more primitive level of functioning, but rather "false equilibriums" in development (Inhelder, 1966). Here, regressions reflect extended periods of transition in which the expressions of ability are unstable and do not reach the same level of stability found in the normally developing populations. Inhelder referred to this lack of attainment of skills as "premature closure."

In order to examine the internal structure of stages during sensorimotor development, several studies have used factor analysis to determine which skills develop concurrently or covary to the greatest extent. Overall, normally developing infants, retarded infants without Down syndrome, and infants with Down syndrome show similar shifts and changes in their patterns of organization of their sensorimotor skills. For example, the factor structures of each age group tested (0−4 months, 4−8 months, 8−12 months, 12−16 months, 16−20 months, and 20−24 months) differed significantly, indicating shifts and changes in the organization of skills. The factor structures obtained from the infants with Down syndrome also differed from those of normally developing infants, whereas some similarities emerged for retarded children without Down syndrome. However, Dunst (in press) points out that further research needs to be conducted before conclusions may be drawn about similarities or differences in stage structures based on factor analyses. For the normally developing and retarded populations, there is little stability and consistency of factor structures across studies. Thus, the intercorrelations between abilities that emerge in factor analyses may be related more to the studies (i.e., age of subjects) than to true differences between the populations.

Another related area of investigation is the difficulty with which individuals with Down syndrome move from one stage of development to the next. Mervis and Cardoso-Martins (1984) and Dunst (in press) have explored this question. In each case, the Uzgiris-Hunt scales were used as indexes of sensorimotor development. Mervis and Cardoso-Martins suggested that there were no differences in the facility with which individuals with and without Down syndrome moved from one stage of development to the next. In this study, Mervis and Cardoso-Martins tested six infants with Down syndrome and six normally developing infants every 6 to 12 weeks. A ratio based on the difference between the ages at which infants attained landmark abilities in stage V and stage VI of sensorimotor functioning was calculated, and used as a measure of movement across the stages. Both groups received similar average scores.

In an additional study, Dunst (in press) also examined the issue of stage transitioning in children with Down syndrome. The Dunst study differed from that of Mervis and Cardoso-Martins (1984) in several important ways. First, Dunst used a different index of stage transitioning. Second, Dunst attempted to control statistically for the slower rate of development of the individuals with Down syndrome. When rate of development was taken into account, the individuals with Down syndrome, for the most part, still moved more slowly from stage to stage than the nonhandicapped, normally developing infants.

Therefore, children with Down syndrome may have more difficulty in moving through the stages of development, as implied by their slower rate of stage transition. In addition, children with Down syndrome appear to regress more, indicating that they have less stable skills than nonhandicapped children (see also the discussion in Cicchetti & Pogge-Hesse, 1982).

Representational development

Play

In recent years, investigators have adopted a developmental approach to the study of play behavior in children with Down syndrome. The results of such studies have suggested that the course and content of play development in children with Down syndrome is markedly similar to that observed in normal children.

In support of the findings of play research conducted on normal children, researchers have reported that the *sequence* of early play development in children with Down syndrome mirrors that of normal children (Beeghly & Cicchetti, 1987; Hill & McCune-Nicolich, 1981; Motti et al., 1983). For example, sequences in object use that *precede* the emergence of true symbolic play also appear to be similar to the sequences in children with Down syndrome. For example, in normally developing children, qualitative, age-graded changes in play behavior have been observed during the first year of life that are thought to form the foundation for true symbolic play that emerges during the second year of life. During infancy (up to 8–9 months), play is characterized primarily by visual–tactual object exploration and manipulation. Near the end of the first year, infants begin to manipulate objects in relational and combinatorial ways. At the start of the second year of life, infants start to use objects in functionally appropriate ways. During the second year, true symbolic use of objects emerges and becomes elaborated (Belsky & Most, 1981; Nicolich, 1977; Piaget, 1962). Beeghly, Weiss-Perry, and Cicchetti (1989) have demonstrated that children with Down syndrome, when compared with normal youngsters on MA, progress through the same sequences in the development of presymbolic play.

Although emerging at a delayed pace, the symbolic play of children with Down syndrome progresses through the same developmental sequences of decentration, decontextualization, and integration in object and social play that characterize the play development of normal children in early childhood (see Bretherton, 1984, and Rubin, Fein, & Vandenberg, 1983, for reviews). Additionally, investigators of play development in children with Down syndrome have replicated studies in the normal play literature documenting a significant relationship between level of cognitive development and symbolic play maturity (see, for example, Beeghly & Cicchetti, 1987; Hill & McCune-Nicolich, 1981; Motti et al., 1983). Similarly, Wing, Gould, Yeates, and Brierly (1977), in a study of handicapped children of varying etiology and degree of handicap, reported that no child with an MA under 20 months engaged in symbolic play. Moreover, among the organically retarded subgroups studied by Wing and her colleagues (1977), children with Down syndrome exhibited the most fluent and flexible symbolic play.

Several studies on play behavior in children with Down syndrome that were conducted in our laboratory merit elaboration. In studies of the longitudinal course of various aspects of play in children with Down syndrome and MA-matched nonhandicapped youngsters, we examined changes in the structure and content of play (Beeghly & Cicchetti, 1987; Beeghly et al., 1989).

Beeghly and colleagues (1989) examined age-related changes in the proportion of time children were engaged in different categories of object and social play. These investigators studied two cohorts of children – a younger and an older group of children with Down syndrome, each of which was matched to a cognitively comparable group of normal children.

Results indicated that similar MA-related changes in the distribution of categories of object and social play occurred for both cohorts of children with Down syndrome and the cognitively comparable normal children. As children increased in level of cognitive development, the time engaged in simple object manipulation decreased significantly, whereas the reverse trend was observed for time engaged in decontextualized symbolic play and in structured social interaction. Children with Down syndrome in both cohorts did not differ significantly from their MA-matched controls on any object play category, although children with Down syndrome in both cohorts engaged in significantly fewer structured turn-taking games with their mothers. These developmental trends in object play are similar to those reported in previous studies of play development in normal young-sters (e.g., Belsky & Most, 1981).

Dimensions of social play (turn taking) and social interaction (e.g., responsiveness, dyadic harmony, initiating behavior) also were correlated significantly with both level of play maturity and cognitive development. These results were observed despite the fact that children with Down syndrome as a group engaged in significantly less social play and were rated as being less responsive and initiating than their cognitively matched controls during social interaction. Comparable unique characteristics have been reported in other studies of children with Down syndrome (Berger, in press). These similar correlational findings suggest that aspects of child-ren with Down syndrome's cognitive, affective, and social behavior relevant to symbolic functioning are organized similarly to equivalent aspects of normal children at a corresponding level of cognitive development.

In a second study, we examined the structure and content of four different aspects of symbolic play in greater detail on the same two cohorts of children with Down syndrome and MA-matched normal children used in the investigation of Beeghly and colleagues just described. Children's play was coded from transcripts of mother–child interactions using four developmental play scales derived from empirical data reported in the play literature. Two scores were derived from each play scale: the highest level of symbolic play observed and the average level observed. In addition, the density (number of connected symbolic play schemes per play episode) and the complexity (number of different connected symbolic schemes per play episode) were assessed.

The children with Down syndrome and their MA controls did not differ significantly on the highest level of play observed for each play scale (with the exception of the object substitution scale for children with Down syndrome in the older cohort). Nor did they differ in the density and complexity of symbolic play exhibited. For all children, MA was significantly correlated with play maturity (both highest and average levels) on each of the four scales, as well as with play density and complexity. These findings support those reported in previous studies of both normal and delayed populations and attest to the developmental validity of the play scales.

However, several important differences in play development emerged. Children with Down syndrome had significantly lower average scores on each of the four play scales, although their highest scores achieved on each scale (except the object substitution scale) did not differ from those obtained by their controls. This latter finding may be explained by the tendency of children with Down syndrome to perseverate and to repeat the same scheme more often (see Wagner et al., in press). It also is likely that the different strategies used by the children with Down syndrome reflect their slower information-processing abilities (Lincoln, Courchesne, Kilman, & Galambos, 1985). However, the fact that the children with Down syndrome were able to achieve similar play performances, based on highest levels of play, as the normal children, suggests that their unique aspects of play did not interfere drastically with their ultimate play achievement (cf. Werner, 1937).

Another important difference that emerged was the observation that children with Down syndrome in the older cohort performed at a significantly less mature level (both average and highest) on the play scale measuring children's decontextualization of object use. This difference suggests that children with Down syndrome play more concretely than do nonhandicapped children. Group differences on the scale also might be explained by the significantly delayed expressive language of the children with Down syndrome compared with their controls. (Recall that the highest levels of this play scale generally require verbal transformation of objects or verbal ideation.) Nevertheless, the delayed expressive language abilities of the children with Down syndrome did not preclude their engaging in complex episodes of multischemed and multithemed symbolic play. Moreover, the nature of these episodes did not differ from those of the nonhandicapped controls.

Conceptual development

Throughout the first year of life, as children develop the capacity to categorize their experiences, objects are no longer viewed as single and unique, but rather as exemplars of broader categories. Rosch and Mervis (1975) have argued that normally developing, nonhandicapped children initially construct basic-level categories in which objects within a category have similar overall attributes (i.e., shape, size and function). Through development, concepts may become more finite and define categories on the basis of minute, specialized features of objects rather than their overall appearance (subordinate level). Or, basic-level concepts may become subsumed under broader concepts in which the similarities between objects within a specific category decrease (superordinate level).

Inclusion in categories at each level, however, is not determined by a list of necessary and sufficient characteristics specified by the underlying concepts. Rather the internal structure of categories is considered to be defined by a continuum of acceptable attribute types. Thus, categories are thought to include a range of objects, some of which are good, or easily recognized, prototypical exemplars of the category, whereas others are poor exemplars that may have only a few attributes that are similar to the other exemplars.

Although category and concept formation have been studied extensively in normally developing infants and children using a variety of paradigms (i.e., Cohen & Strauss, 1979; Fagan, 1976; Reznick & Kagan, 1981; Rosch & Mervis, 1975), little research has been conducted with infants and children with Down syndrome. In the studies that do exist, as in studies of nonretarded children (Mervis, in press), receptive and productive language skills have been used to infer the structure and development of concepts.

In one study, Gillham (1979) recorded the early vocabularies of toddlers with Down syndrome. In this study, Gillham generated a list of the first words used by one group of 4 children with Down syndrome and by another group of 14 nonhandicapped children. When both lists were compared, several similarities in category composition and level of organization emerged. First, both groups of children tended to use only words to refer to whole objects. Thus, although the referents for words may sometimes be ambiguous, both groups of children assumed that the words they learned corresponded to whole objects rather than part objects. Second, the words produced by the children with and without Down syndrome formed similar subsets of objects (i.e., food, people, toys; Mervis, in press). Finally, the early vocabularies of both groups of children referred to categories at the basic level of organization.

Taken together, these findings suggest that both groups of children organize their experiences in a similar manner and construct concepts and categories that attend to similar features and principles. Children with Down syndrome and normally developing, nonhandicapped children construct categories that are comprised of whole objects rather than distinct parts of objects, and use basic-level relationships to organize these objects. In addition, the presence of similar-object subsets in the categories of both groups of children implies that within the basic level of categorization, the children might be attracted to and attending to similar features in their environment (for example, saliency of features or novelty) and using these features to construct concepts of the world.

Another explanation for these results, however, may lie in the manner in which mothers of both groups of children interacted with their children as they started to learn words and categorize objects. For example, parents may have communicated basic-level categories to their children by the way they presented and labeled objects for their children. Mervis (in press) has recently completed a longitudinal study of children with Down syndrome that addresses this criticism. In this study, Mervis concurrently examined the early vocabulary development of six children with Down syndrome and six nonhandicapped children and the labeling techniques their mothers employed. At the beginning of the study, the nonhandicapped children were 9 months old and the children with Down syndrome were between 17 and 19 months old. The children in both groups were unable to produce or comprehend language.

To examine concept formation, Mervis, over a period of several months, introduced each child to a set of toys that exemplified three categories of objects: kitty, ball, and car. Some toys were predicted to be classed together based on their appearance (child-category), whereas other toys were chosen because they were considered to be poor examples of the adult categories for these objects. In the first interactions, Mervis provided children with exemplars of each category. In subsequent visits, the children were given additional toys to play with that were similar in shape and potential function to the initial exemplars of each category. The children were able to play with the toys, and were tested for their ability to name the objects (production skills) or the ability to select the objects that corresponded to a word (comprehension). Mervis recorded the children's reactions, use of each object, and spontaneous categorizations of objects, as well as all the words used by mothers and children.

The results of this longitudinal study showed that although the rate of development for children with Down syndrome is slower than that of the nonhandicapped children without Down syndrome, both groups formed basic-level categories of objects in which function and shape of the objects were prominent features. Mervis argued that the formation of such categories could not be completely attributed to the mothers' labeling patterns. Mothers (particularly those of children with Down syndrome) did not consistently categorize objects for their children through their actions or words. In addition, the categories constructed by the children did not completely correspond with adult categories. Rather, children in both groups made overextension and underextension errors in their categorizations. Consequently, Mervis argues that "initial child-basic categories are formed on the basis of child cognitive structures rather than maternal labeling input."

The evolution of categories for both children with and without Down syndrome was also similar in the Mervis longitudinal study. The process of category change and redefinition was similar for both groups of children. For example, children with Down syndrome first constructed child-basic categories that did not coincide completely with the adult categories. However, the child-basic categories eventually became more differentiated as the poorest exemplars of a category eventually were included into other categories. When these changes occurred, the resultant categories appeared to approximate more closely those of adults. For both groups of children, the differentiation of concepts underlying categorization occurred slowly, with a period of overlap in which objects were simultaneously included in two categories at once. In addition, within both groups, categories could be modified by the emphasis of various features of the objects by adults.

Taken together, Mervis's findings suggest that children with Down syndrome and nonhandicapped children form similar concepts and categories of the world. The structure of the concepts and categories formed by each group seems to be similar, whereas the stages through which categories evolve are also similar. In both populations, children first form basic-level concepts that rely on the overall appearance and function of objects. However, through increased experience with the world and interactions with adults in which various features of objects are emphasized, the concepts that shape categories are modified and differentiated within each group.

Although the initial vocabulary and categories of children with and without Down syndrome may be similar, the rate of acquisition of vocabulary is not. Children with Down syndrome demonstrate the onset of language at the same MA, and same level of sensorimotor development as children without Down syndrome, but the rapidity with which their vocabularies increase at each stage differs. Mervis (in press) argues that this difference may be partially dependent on inherent difficulties that individuals with Down syndrome may have in the storage and retrieval of information from memory. Additionally, she argues that these difficulties are accentuated by the linguistic environment in which children with Down syndrome develop. Within the Mervis study, mothers of nonhandicapped children were more likely to (1) attend to their children's behaviors or the objects the children focused their attention on, and (2) focus their comments on the content of their children's actions than the mothers of children with Down syndrome. In contrast, mothers of children with Down syndrome tended to be more directive and less conversation eliciting and semantically contingent on their children's verbalizations. Correlational analyses indicated that the semantic contingency expressed by the mothers of the nonhandicapped children was related significantly to the number of words produced and comprehended by a child, whereas the directive style of the mothers of children with Down syndrome was not. Therefore, if vocabulary development is used as an index of categorization, conceptual development is affected by possible information-processing deficits in addition to maternal styles of interaction.

Early linguistic development

Results from the majority of studies focusing on the early language development of children with Down syndrome suggest that the sequence and structure of their language development is similar in many respects to that observed in normally developing children (see Fowler, in press; Miller, in press, for recent reviews). An examination of different domains within language (e.g., phonology, syntax, semantics, pragmatics) and relationships of language with cognition and social development also reveal striking similarities. There are also important differences. Perhaps the most striking difference is the dramatic delay in the expressive language development of children with Down syndrome (see Hodapp & Zigler, in press). Despite similarities in structure and sequence for most aspects of language, results of many studies document that individuals with Down syndrome show increasing linguistic deficits in relation to their nonverbal cognitive abilities with increasing chronological age (Miller, in press). For example, many individuals with Down syndrome do not progress beyond early stages of syntactic development (see Fowler, in press).

Studies of cognitive prerequisites for early language and the transition to first words in children with Down syndrome (e.g., Berger, in press; Dunst, in press; Mervis, in press) have documented that the onset of referential comprehension and production appears to be consistent with children's sensorimotor and cognitive attainments. That is, their first referential words (both in comprehension and production) occur in conjunction with the same levels of sensorimotor development (e.g., Piagetian stages 5–6 for object permanence and means–ends) and general cognitive development as measured by the Bayley Scale of Mental Development (1969) as those of nonhandicapped children (Mervis, in press). However, longitudinal studies of children at these very early language stages indicate that the rate of their early vocabulary development is significantly more delayed than that observed in normal children, even when level of cognitive development is considered (Mervis, in press).

Although much progress has been made in our understanding of language development in children with Down syndrome, our knowledge has been limited by the fact that much of this research has been based on small samples using cross-sectional designs. Beeghly and Cicchetti (1987) attempted to overcome this difficulty by assessing longitudinal changes in the early language of 41 children with Down syndrome over a 1-year period.

Forty-one children with Down syndrome (24 boys, 17 girls) and their mothers participated in this study. Dyads were observed interacting in various contexts during three laboratory visits spaced 6 months apart. All children were caucasian and reared in middle-class homes with their natural parents. At the first visit, children ranged in level of language development from prelinguistic to early multiword speech. Four children were prelinguistic (M CA = 24 months, range = 20–30 months); 7 children were at the single word stage (M CA = 40 months, range = 24–66 months); 19 children were beginning to combine words (early stage I; M CA = 44 months, range = 26–74 months); 8 children were in late stage I; M CA = 68 months, range = 60–82 months); and 3 were in stage 2 (M CA = 68 months, range = 61–76 months). Measures of children's productive and receptive language were coded from videotapes at each visit. Linguistic measures included mean length of utterance (MLU) in morphemes and in words, including MLU of the highest five utterances and upper bound, Lee's developmental sentence analysis (Lee, 1974), vocabulary diversity, proportion of lexicalized utterances, and proportion of unintelligible utterances. Pragmatic and communicative measures also were assessed (these are discussed in a later section).

Individual differences in age among children at each level of language development were marked, indicating that considerable heterogeneity in language development exists among children with Down syndrome. For most of the children in the Beeghly and Cicchetti (1987) sample, however, very minimal progress in language development was made over the course of the year. The majority of children (46%) remained at the same syntactic level for the entire year, whereas 37% progressed on substage or stage. Only 17% of the sample progressed through two language stages. This delay is especially notable in relation to the more rapid language growth of normal children (see Brown, 1973). In spite of the delayed development of Down syndrome children, an analysis of MLU distribution and Lee's developmental sentence structure indicated that the structure and course of their syntactic development was otherwise similar to that observed in nonhandicapped children. Although there was marked variation within sexes, girls tended to progress more rapidly than boys (e.g., 29% of girls but only 8% of boys progressed through two stages).

Vocabulary development was less delayed than syntactic development in children and appeared to be associated with children's age and cognitive maturity. Although children's vocabulary was significantly less diversified than that observed in nonhandicapped children matched to the children with Down syndrome on receptive vocabulary, older children with Down syndrome nonetheless tended to have larger productive vocabularies than younger children at any given language stage.

What can account for the inordinate language delay of these children? Partial answers may lie in both unique *child* characteristics (physical, neurophysiological, biochemical) and unspecified aspects of children's social and linguistic environments. For example, children with Down syndrome have a number of features that may serve to put these children at risk for expressive language problems (e.g., increased incidence of hearing and visual deficits; otitis media; structural anomalies in the speech apparatus; motor control problems affecting production; difficulties in verbal coding and decoding; memory deficits; and problems in arousal modulation, visuoproprioceptive feedback, dampened affect, and passivity; see Cicchetti & Beeghly, in press). These unique characteristics may in turn affect the quality of social interaction that children with Down syndrome experience, because social interaction patterns are reciprocal in nature (Bell & Harper, 1977). Many of the qualities listed here and other difficulties (e.g., decreased parental referencing during object play and social interaction, Berger, in press; Sorce, Emde, & Frank, 1982) may interfere with the establishment of turn taking and reciprocity during social interaction. These characteristics make it more difficult for adults to read, mark, and reward the behavior of Down syndrome children (Berger, in press).

Taken in tandem with the delayed developmental progress of Down syndrome children, these characteristics of Down syndrome children may also influence parents' beliefs and expectations for their children, which in turn could affect the type of input these children receive. Although the *structural* aspects of care giver speech to children with Down syndrome appear to be similar to care giver speech addressed to normally developing children at equivalent levels of language maturity (Buckhalt, Rutherford, & Goldberg, 1978; Buium, Rynders, & Turnur, 1974), other *functional* features of care giver input to children with Down syndrome (e.g., mother-directed interaction, semantic noncontingency) may be less than optimal for facilitating early language development (Mervis, in press).

Language and play

Piaget (1962) and other classical developmental theorists hypothesized that language and symbolic play were two aspects of an underlying emergent representational capacity – the semiotic function. From this viewpoint, one would expect to find close correspondence between language and symbolic play (as well as other types of symbolic functioning) in early development.

Partial support for a "neo-Piagetian" version of the cognitive (semiotic function) hypothesis comes from longitudinal studies of symbolic play, early language, and early gestural symbols. These studies have provided evidence for close correspondences in specific language and symbolic play abilities at several developmental points: first words, early word combinations, and emergence of syntax (Bates, Benigni, Bretherton, Camaioni, & Volterra, 1979). Other investigators have reported significant associations with more general aspects of language development and symbolic play maturity (e.g., Fein, 1979; Largo & Howard, 1979).

A stronger case for this hypothesis could be made with supporting evidence from children with delayed but heterogeneous linguistic and cognitive development, such as children with Down syndrome. In Beeghly and Cicchetti's studies of language and play, four parallels between symbolic play development and early language development were observed for children with Down syndrome (Beeghly & Cicchetti, 1987). These parallels are similar to those reported for normally developing children at similar stages of language and play development (e.g., McCune-Nicolich & Bruskin, 1982). Beeghly and Cicchetti observed the following correspondences. First, no prelinguistic child engaged in any symbolic play at any of the longitudinal visits. Second, children in the single-word stage of language development were observed to produce only single schemes during symbolic play. Third, children in early stage I of language development (initial word combinations) were observed to combine simple symbolic schemes during play (but did not combine words or schemes in a rule-governed or logical fashion). Finally, all children with more advanced language [i.e., in late stage I (MLU 1.50 to 1.99) or higher who showed evidence of rule-governed language] were observed to engage in planned hierarchically integrated symbolic play. At this stage, a marked increase in children's verbal and nonverbal symbolic fluency (productivity) was also noted. Considering the marked heterogeneity in CA of these children at each language level, these correspondences are striking.

Pragmatics and communicative skills

In the past several decades, increased attention has been given to pragmatic, or "social" aspects of language acquisition. Recently, investigators have emphasized the importance of both social experience and cognitive development for the acquisition of these social aspects of language, or "communicative competence" (see, for example, Bruner, 1983; Greenberg, 1983). Because children with Down syndrome typically show more advanced cognitive than linguistic development (Fowler, in press), it has been hypothesized that children with Down syndrome would be more communicatively competent during social interactions than nonhandicapped children at a similar level of syntactic development. That linguistic and pragmatic abilities can emerge asynchronously is supported by research with atypical populations of children (see Rosenberg, 1984, for a review). For example, the pragmatic skills of autistic children appear to lag behind their syntactic skills (see Schopler & Mesibov, 1985; Sigman & Mundy, 1987), whereas the reverse appears to be true for children with Down syndrome (Mundy, Sigman, Kasari, & Yirmiya, 1988).

Support for this hypothesis is provided by some (but not all) studies (see Miller, in press) of communicative competence in individuals with Down syndrome. Discrepancies in results are likely due at least in part to the wide variation in measures of discourse used in different studies. Several investigators have documented that adults with Down syndrome appear to be more advanced communicatively relative to their linguistic abilities, particularly when nonlinguistic aspects of communication (i.e., gestures, body movements) are also considered. Other investigators report that teenage subjects with Down syndrome showed more advanced communicative skills during peer interactions when observed in social contexts demanding higher levels of communicative competence (e.g., more questions asked, more topics introduced, use of longer utterances where appropriate). Even younger children with Down syndrome at very early stages of linguistic maturity show evidence of communicative competence. For example, Coggins and Stoel-Gammon (1982) found that 5 to 7-year-old children with Down syndrome in stage I of syntactic development (Brown,

1973; MLU 1.01–1.49) were able to respond appropriately to requests for clarification, as evidenced by repetitions or revisions of their utterances.

Beeghly and Cicchetti (1987) extended this research by comparing the communicative skills of a much larger group of children with Down syndrome and nonhandicapped children at a similar phase of syntactic development: early and late stage I (Brown, 1973). Stage I is an important phase of syntactic development because it marks children's transition from one-word to multiword speech. Changes in communicative and interactive skills of children with Down syndrome during early and late stage I of syntactic development were examined during two interactive situations varying in task demands for conversation maintenance. These skills were compared with those observed in two groups of nonhandicapped children individually matched to the children with Down syndrome for sex, demographics, and for either MLU in morphemes or for MA-equivalent scores.

Both normal children and children with Down syndrome in late stage I had significantly more mature communicative behavior than children in early stage I, with proportionally more lexicalized utterances, larger vocabularies, greater diversity of speech acts, longer chains of connected, conversationally relevant turns, and longer sequences of on-topic turns. Children in late stage I also differed in the content of their speech acts compared with children in early stage I, with more requests, statements, and description, and fewer conversational devices and turn fillers.

Results of group comparisons indicated that children with Down syndrome were more delayed linguistically than cognitively with respect to their vocabulary production and the lexicalization of their speech. In contrast, children with Down syndrome performed significantly better than their linguistically-matched controls (but not their MA-matched controls) when measures of communication and pragmatic development were considered, with longer sequences of on-topic turns and conversationally relevant turns, a greater diversity of speech acts, and more mature turn-taking skills. Children with Down syndrome also differed from their MLU controls (but not their MA matches) in the content of their speech acts, with fewer conversational devices and turn fillers, and more responses, descriptions, and statements. This pattern of results held true in both social contexts studied (structured picture book and free play).

These data reflect a marked asynchrony between syntactic and pragmatic development in children with Down syndrome (see Mundy et al., 1988, for similar findings). Although the communicative skills (and MAs) of all children increase significantly as MLU increased from early to late stage I, the children with Down syndrome had more mature communicative skills than their MLU matches. These results become less surprising when one considers the significant differences in children's MAs and CAs in the two groups. When one notes that the communicative performance of the children with Down syndrome did not differ from that of the MA-matched controls who were significantly older than the MLU controls and who had significantly longer MLUs and more elaborated vocabularies than the children with Down syndrome, the results become more striking. In sum, they highlight the significant role of both cognitive development and experience in the acquisition of social-communicative skills.

A notable difference in the communicative performance of the children with Down syndrome from that observed in their cognitively comparable controls was observed for one speech-act category. Although the children with Down syndrome did not differ from their MA controls in relative production of most speech-act categories studied, the children with Down syndrome nevertheless produced fewer requests than did their MA matches. Similar findings have been reported in other studies on initiating behavior of children with Down syndrome (Berger, in press). These results might also be explained by considering the characteristics of children with Down syndrome that may interfere with their tendency to take the initiative (e.g., problems in making eye contact). The results might also be partially accounted for by the fact that interactions with children with Down syndrome tend to be more mother-directed than those with non-handicapped children (Mervis, in press). When mothers are more directive, they provide fewer opportunities for their children to initiate social interaction. A directive style of interaction is a strategy commonly adopted when interacting with handicapped children, particularly more passive ones (Bell & Harper, 1977).

Conclusion

The organizational perspective holds that development occurs through the reorganization and restructuring of abilities into new behavioral or biological structures. Such restructuring is thought to be guided by the orthogenetic principle, which describes development as proceeding from simple undifferentiated forms to highly articulated structures and systems. A second, related line of research has focused on the extent to which the development and organization of behavioral systems differ from that of normally developing, nonhandicapped individuals. In this case, research has been directed toward the specific examination of the developmental sequences, stages and coherence of abilities important to development in various domains.

In most cases, the organizational perspective appears to be a useful framework for describing the development of abilities and characteristics of the Down syndrome population. Within the different domains examined, development seems to be guided by the orthogenetic principle. Although their pace of development is much slower than that of nonhandicapped, normally developing individuals, children with Down syndrome display increasingly more complex behaviors and thought structures as they mature and continue to interact with the world. Their responses to the world change as their representation of the world becomes more differentiated and abstract. Just as normally developing infants do, these individuals become less stimulus bound and more active in shaping and determining their interactions with the world. This developmental trend is apparent within the realms of socioemotional and intellectual development.

In terms of affective development, both normally developing children and children with Down syndrome demonstrate increasing differentiation in their expression of affect. For example, in terms of positive affect, Cicchetti and Sroufe (1976, 1978) have found that infants with Down syndrome first respond positively to intrusive, highly stimulating events. However, as they develop, they show appreciation for, and respond positively toward, more subtle, noninvasive social stimulation, whereas they decline in their positiveness toward intrusive stimulation. The expression of negative affect also changes with development, as infants with Down syndrome, just as nonhandicapped infants, do not initially show fear to stimuli such as the visual cliff and a looming object, but do so as they grow older. In both cases, the stages through which children progress reflect their changing cognitive abilities and the differentiation of affect. Moreover, the interaction between cognition and affect reflects coherence in the organization and structure of these developing systems.

Despite these similarities in development and organization, important qualitative differences also are apparent. The affect expressions of children with Down syndrome are significantly less intense relative to those of nonhandicapped children of similar developmental levels. Additional research has also shown that other behavioral differences emerge when the responsivity of children with Down syndrome is compared with that of normally developing children. Generally, duration of active engagement with toys, attention, and threshold of reactivity also have distinguished children with Down syndrome from nonhandicapped children.

These differences in responsivity to the world are reflected in the temperaments of children with Down syndrome. Although the Down syndrome population is very heterogeneous, these behavioral characteristics are often noted when group averages of temperament ratings or group observations are made. In part, these differences reflect lags in cognitive development, as suggested by the work of Cicchetti and Sroufe (1976, 1978). However, there is growing physiological evidence that such dampened reactivity may be related also to anomalies in the CNS that affect the development of forebrain inhibitory tracts and arousal systems. In the future, research that examines the interaction of physiological arousability and the expression of affect and cognition must be completed before conclusions can be drawn about organizations of Down syndrome children and their individual and joint impact on temperament.

Studies that have focused on attachment systems have also suggested that infants with Down syndrome develop similarly to nonhandicapped infants, although at a slower pace. In this case, Cicchetti and his colleagues (Cicchetti & Serafica, 1981; Serafica & Cicchetti, 1975; Thompson et al., 1985), studying infants and toddlers with Down syndrome in the strange situation, have found that reactions during separation from primary care givers are similar to those of nonhandicapped infants of the same MA. The responses of Down syndrome children reflect differentiated responses to people (i.e., stranger versus care givers) in addition to the coherent organization of various behavioral systems. In the latter case, the organization of attachment, affiliation, fear, and wariness interacts similarly to that of nonhandicapped infants.

This organization also appears to be tied to cognitive development and, again, to children's ability to evaluate their experiences. The most significant differences that emerge when MA comparisons are made lie in the intensity of reactions exhibited by children with Down syndrome. Generally, when separated from their caretakers, children with Down syndrome protest and search for their mothers, but do so more weakly and have longer latencies before responding than other infants. To date, however, studies that have examined the development of attachment systems longitudinally have not been conducted. Thus, although the attachment systems of children with Down syndrome are organized coherently and structured similarly to those of nonhandicapped children, and development seems to proceed to levels of increasing complexity, one cannot draw the same conclusions about the stages through which children with Down syndrome pass to arrive at such structures.

The development of self-perception also reflects development that proceeds from states of lack of differentiation to the differentiation of self and other. Children and infants with Down syndrome gradually acquire the ability to recognize their mirror images and to distinguish self from others. In mirror studies, toddlers with Down syndrome demonstrate visual self-recognition at the same developmental level that children without Down syndrome show self-recognition (Mans et al., 1978; Hill & Tomlin, 1981).

Beeghly and Cicchetti (1987) also have found that concepts of self and others become increasingly differentiated in play and in the child's expressive language. Such changes are reflected in the increasing abilities to decenter, integrate, and decontextualize play, and in the ability to represent one's self in hypothetical situations. Development in this area also appears to be tied to cognitive development, suggesting coherence in the organization of development. However, Beeghly and Cicchetti also note discordance between linguistic and symbolic abilities for children with Down syndrome, relative to normally developing children. Thus, unlike other domains of socioemotional development, the structuring of abilities may differ for these two groups of infants, with self-representation skills developing at a faster pace than linguistic skills.

In most of the studies of socioemotional development reviewed in this chapter, development seemed to be tied to information-processing skills and representational abilities. Children's ability to understand events and interactions in the world, coupled with the ability to represent these experiences symbolically, increasingly shape responses to the world. In many cases, the development of information-processing and representational skills in children with Down syndrome also parallels that of normally developing infants. Within these domains as well, individuals with Down syndrome move toward increasing differentiation and complexity in their capacities and seem to follow developmental pathways similar to those of nonhandicapped children.

Development in selective attention and information processing likewise reflects the orthogenetic principle. Infants and children with Down syndrome increasingly become attracted to and appear to appreciate configurations and stimuli of greater complexity as they mature. Presumably, their evaluations of stimuli become more sophisticated, based on an understanding of the more subtle aspects of configurations as well as past experiences and memory. These evaluations motivate the interest of children and drive their attention. Fantz and colleagues (1975) have shown that infants with Down syndrome demonstrate changes in their preference for visual stimuli similar to normally developing, nonhandicapped infants.

Research in other modalities has suggested that preference for various patterns, sounds, and shapes is correlated with developmental level for both groups of infants. In some cases, however, children with Down syndrome demonstrate preferences for cognitively complex tasks, such as intermodal matching, at a later developmental level than their normally developing peers. Such differences may reflect differences in motivation or interest, or possibly reflect different cognitive structures. Thus, taken together, these studies suggest that infants with Down syndrome and non-handicapped infants follow similar sequences and stages of development. However, the structure or coherence of systems that underlie information processing may differ. Future research should explore more closely specific phases of information processing to determine if the structure of evaluations is the same for both infants with and without Down syndrome (see Wagner et al., in press).

Sensorimotor development in this population reflects the movement from undifferentiated states to highly defined and developed abilities. Children with Down syndrome demonstrate increasingly complex behaviors with age (Cicchetti & Mans-Wagener, 1987; Dunst, in press). In addition, within the different domains of sensorimotor development, children with Down syndrome follow the same stage sequences as normally developing infants. However, within domains, children with Down syndrome may have more difficulty in moving from one stage of development to the next, and more difficulty in reorganizing their abilities into integrated, coherent structures as indicated by "false equilibriums" or "regressions." Nevertheless, both groups of children do demonstrate similar patterns of development, followed by periods of reorganization and consolidation. Consequently, children with Down syndrome, apart from developing at a slower pace, share many similarities in sensorimotor development.

Finally, the representational development of the child with Down syndrome also appears to adhere to the normal pattern. Studies that have examined the vocabulary development of children with Down syndrome have found that they attend to similar aspects of objects and organize concepts at the same level of abstractness as nonhandicapped, normally developing children (Mervis, in press). Furthermore, changes in concepts that arise from further interaction with objects are similar for both groups of children (Mervis, in press). Sensorimotor development (means–ends relationships and object concept) is also correlated with the onset of referential words for children with and without Down syndrome, indicating that sensorimotor skills, language, and conceptual skills interact, or that they reflect similar underlying thought structures (Mervis, in press).

In this regard, conceptual development in verbal children with Down syndrome and nonhandicapped children seems to follow the same sequence of development and structure of concepts. Differences emerge, however, in the child's rate of vocabulary acquisition. Such differences may be due to language difficulties rather than to differences in concept formation. Given findings of divergence between linguistic and representational skills, additional research that does not rely upon expressive language is needed.

In addition, future research should also focus on the organization of processes (i.e., coding, retrieval) by which children structure information and maintain concepts in memory.

Language development, which also reflects representational abilities, also demonstrates the usefulness of the orthogenetic principle in describing the development of individuals with Down syndrome. The language of children with Down syndrome becomes more complex in both content and structure. In terms of syntactic development, children with Down syndrome organize and develop skills similarly to normal children. Vocabulary development is less delayed than syntactic development and, likewise, is similar for both groups of children. In both cases, development seems to be tied to cognitive development. However, children with Down syndrome appear to be more delayed linguistically than cognitively.

In terms of pragmatic and communicative skills, development also seems to be related to developmental level. But in this case the discordance such as that observed between cognitive skills and syntactic and vocabulary development is not apparent. However, children with Down syndrome are more communicatively competent than linguistically competent. Consequently, there are asynchronies between syntactic and pragmatic development in children with Down syndrome that are not apparent in the normally developing population. Thus, similarities and differences exist between children with and without Down syndrome in the development of different aspects of language. Pragmatic development seems to be more similar to cognitive level than syntactic and vocabulary skills. However, although children with Down syndrome seem to undergo the same sequence of syntactic and vocabulary development as nonhandicapped children, their pace of development is slower than one would expect when comparisons are based on developmental level. Such asynchrony implies that although systems may be interrelated and coherent in their organization, the organization of these systems may differ from that of nonhandicapped normally developing children.

In terms of play, which also reflects their ability to symbolize, infants with Down syndrome progress from simple physical manipulation of toys to more sophisticated play schemes in which objects are combined, incorporated, and related in more complex ways, and as they acquire a greater appreciation of the functional qualities of each toy. In terms of the structure and density of play, children with Down syndrome are similar to normally developing children of the same MA. Likewise, although the rate of development of Down syndrome children is delayed, the sequence of appearance of new types of play for these children parallels that of normally developing children. However, although the play of children with Down syndrome becomes increasingly more abstract, it is still more concrete than the play of their normally developing peers of the same MA. Nevertheless, for both groups, such changes in the level of symbolic play are correlated significantly with MA.

Beeghly and Cicchetti (1987) also have illustrated that language and play seem to be interrelated. They note four parallels: (1) prerepresentational children did not engage in symbolic play, (2) children in the single-word stage of language development engaged in single scheme play, (3) children in the early stage of linguistic development combined only simply symbolic schemes in play, and (4) children who were most advanced in language development, demonstrating rule-governed language, also engaged in hierarchically structured symbolic play.

In summary, the development of individuals with Down syndrome across various domains follows a developmental course that is similar to that of nonhandicapped, normally developing persons. Although the pace of development is slower for children with Down syndrome, they demonstrate similar developmental trends, moving from states of low differentiation and simple interactions with the world, to the development of specific abilities, complex integrated thought, articulated concepts of the world, and a vast array of behaviors and schemes for interacting with the world. In this transition, the child ceases to be "stimulus bound," or simply a "reactor" to environmental events. Rather, children, through their increasing abilities to evaluate and mentally represent their experiences, start to shape their own reactions and actively manipulate their environment.

Additionally, when developmental level is taken into consideration, children with Down syndrome generally appear to progress through the same stages of development as normally developing children. Development occurs in an orderly fashion, with children from both populations acquiring increasingly more complex skills.

In terms of the structuring and integration of abilities, infants and children with Down syndrome demonstrate coherence in their development that in most cases parallels that of normally developing, nonhandicapped individuals. Underlying changes in the child's ability to evaluate and mentally represent the world are concomitantly reflected in affect, attachment, play, language, and self-systems. Such relationships suggest that development is highly organized and coherent.

However, despite the presence of these similarities, several differences are also apparent across different domains. First, the intensity of reactions emitted by the child with Down syndrome is weaker than that of normally developing children of the same CA or developmental level. Second, differences have been noted in the organization of linguistic skills, pragmatics, and cognitive development. In these cases, syntactic and vocabulary skills develop at a slower pace than pragmatic and cognitive skills. Thus, when children with Down syndrome are matched with nonhandicapped, normally developing children on the basis of developmental level, their syntax and vocabulary are significantly poorer than that of their normally developing peers.

This asynchrony may reflect the impact of interactions that arise between children with Down syndrome and their caretakers rather than significant differences in the organization of behavioral systems (Berger, in press; Mervis, in press). Because children with Down syndrome respond to their environment with dampened reactivity, or may seem to interact actively with their world less than normally developing children, caretakers may be more directive in their exchanges with their children. Indeed, directiveness is one parental strategy that appears to be negatively related to language development within this population. Mervis (in press) argues that this relationship is dependent on the low degree of contingency that characterizes directiveness. Thus, children with Down syndrome who experience such interactions do not learn as many words and their referents as children who experience a large amount of contingent exchanges with their parents. Berger (in press) has found that parental imitation of their children's responses brings attention to the child's abilities and fosters, in some children, increased responsivity and interactions. This research, therefore, underscores the importance of focusing on the child's abilities and showing sensitivity to the child's reactive capacities during interactions. In many regards, this task may be more difficult to carry out given the temperament qualities of many children with Down syndrome and the disappointment some parents experience when their children fail to meet developmental milestones early in infancy.

The organizational perspective, with its emphasis on the study of interacting behavioral and biological systems and on uncovering the relation between normal and atypical forms of development, provides an excellent theoretical framework for conceptualizing research on Down syndrome. Clearly, the organizational perspective has shed considerable light on the nature and course of development in infants and children with Down syndrome. Consequently, we believe that Zigler's position on the developmental–difference controversy in the field of mental retardation, when viewed from a broad developmental "world view" (Pepper, 1942), can also be generalized to organically retarded children. Even though children with Down syndrome do not function identically to MA-matched nonhandicapped youngsters, the application of a developmental approach reveals both the organization and coherence characteristic of their early development. We await the reporting of future multidisciplinary research on the developmental organization of older children and adults with Down syndrome. It is our belief that the results of this work will elucidate our understanding of normal and pathological ontogenesis.

References

Ainsworth, M.D.S., Blehar, M.C., Waters, E., & Wall, S. (1978). *Patterns of attachment: A psychological study of the strange situation.* Hillsdale, NJ: Erlbaum.

Bates, E. Benigni, L., Bretherton, I., Camaioni, L., & Volterra, V. (1979). *The emergence of symbols: Cognition and communication in infancy.* New York: Academic Press.

Bayley, N. (1969). *The Bayley scales of infant development.* New York: Psychological Corporation.

Becker, L., Armstrong, D., & Chan, F. (1986). Dendritic atrophy in children with Down's syndrome. *Annals of Neurology, 20* (4), 520–526.

Beeghly, M., & Cicchetti, D. (1987). An organizational approach to symbolic development in children with Down syndrome. *New Directions for Child Development, 36,* 5–29.

Beeghly, M., Weiss-Perry, B., & Cicchetti D. (1989). Affective and structural analysis of symbolic play in children with Down syndrome. *International Journal of Behavioral Development, 12,* 257–277.

Bell, R.Q., & Harper, L.V. (1977). *Child effects on adults.* Hillsdale, NJ: Erlbaum.

Belsky, J., & Most, R. (1981). From exploration to play: A cross-sectional study of infant free play behavior. *Developmental Psychology, 17,* 630–639.

Belsky, J., Rovine, M., & Taylor, D. (1984). The Pennsylvania Infant and Family Development Project: II: Origins of individual differences in infant–mother attachment: Maternal and infant contributions. *Child Development, 55,* 706–717.

Berger, J. (in press). Interactions between parents and their infants with Down syndrome. In D. Cicchetti and M. Beeghly (Eds.), *Children with Down syndrome: A developmental perspective.* New York: Cambridge University Press.

Berry, P., Gunn, P., & Andrews, R. (1980). Behavior of Down's syndrome infants in a strange situation. *American Journal of Mental Deficiency, 85,* 213–218.

Block, J.H., & Block, J. (1980). The role of ego-control and ego resiliency in the organization of behavior. In W.A. Collins (Ed.), *Minnesota Symposium on Child Psychology,* Vol. 13. Hillsdale, NJ: Erlbaum.

Bower, T.G.R., Broughton, J., & Moore, M.K. (1970). Infant responses to approaching objects. *Perception and Psychophysics, 9,* 193–196.

Bowlby, J. (1969/1982). *Attachment and loss* (Vol 1). New York: Basic Books.

Bretherton, I. (Ed.), (1984). *Symbolic play.* Orlando, FL: Academic Press.

Bretherton, I., & Ainsworth, M. (1974). Response of 1-year olds to a stranger in a strange situation. In M. Lewis & L. Rosenblum (Eds.), *The origins of fear.* New York: Wiley.

Bretherton, I., & Beeghly, M. (1982). Talking about internal states: The acquisition of an explicit theory of mind. *Developmental Psychology, 18,* 906–921.

Bridges, F., & Cicchetti, D. (1982). Mothers' ratings of temperament characteristics of Down syndrome infants. *Developmental Psychology, 18,* 238–244.

Bronfenbrenner, U. (1979). *The ecology of human development: Experiments by nature and design.* Cambridge, MA: Harvard University Press.

Brown, R. (1973). *A first language: The early stages.* Cambridge, MA: Harvard University Press.

Bruner, J. (1983). The acquisition of pragmatic commitments. In R. Golnikoff (Ed.), *The transition from prelinguistic to linguistic communication*. Hillsdale, NJ: Erlbaum.

Buckhalt, T.A., Rutherford, R.B., & Goldberg, K.E. (1978). Verbal and nonverbal interactions of mothers and their Down syndrome and nonretarded infants. *American Journal of Mental Deficiency, 72,* 337–343.

Buium, N., Rynders, J., & Turnur, J. (1974). Early maternal linguistic environment of normal and Down's syndrome language-learning children. *American Journal of Mental Deficiency, 79,* 52–58.

Campos, J., Hiatt, S., Ramsay, D., Henderson, C., & Svejda, M. (1978). The emergence of fear on the visual cliff. In M. Lewis & L. Rosenblum (Eds.), *The development of affect*. New York: Plenum.

Carey, W. (1973). Measurement of infant temperament in pediatric practice. In J.C. Westman (Ed.), *Individual differences in children* (pp. 298–304). New York: Wiley.

Casanova, M., Walker, L., Whitehouse, P., & Price, D. (1985). Abnormalities of the nucleus basalis in Down's syndrome. *Annals of Neurology, 18,* 310–313.

Cicchetti, D. (1984a). The emergence of developmental psychopathology. *Child Development, 55,* 1–7.

Cicchetti, D. (Ed.), (1984b). *Developmental psychopathology*. Chicago: University of Chicago Press.

Cicchetti, D., & Beeghly, M. (Eds.), (in press). *Children with Down syndrome: A developmental perspective*. New York: Cambridge University Press.

Cicchetti, D., & Hesse, P. (1983). Affect and intellect: Piaget's contributions to the study of infant emotional development. In R. Plutchik & H. Kellerman (Eds.), *Emotion: Theory, research and experience*, Vol. II. New York: Academic Press.

Cicchetti, D., & Mans-Wagener, L. (1987). Sequences, stages, and structures in the organization of cognitive development in infants with Down syndrome. In I. Uzgiris & J. McV. Hunt (Eds.), *Infant performance and experience: New findings with the ordinal scales* (pp. 281–310). Urbana: University of Illinois Press.

Cicchetti, D., & Pogge-Hesse, P. (1982). Possible contributions of the study of organically retarded persons to developmental theory. In E. Zigler & D. Balla (Eds.), *Mental retardation: The developmental–difference controversy*. Hillsdale, NJ: Erlbaum Associates.

Cicchetti, D., & Schneider-Rosen, K. (1986). An organizational approach to childhood depression. In M. Rutter, C. Izard, & P. Read (Eds.), *Depression in young people: Clinical and developmental perspectives*. New York: Guilford.

Cicchetti, D., & Serafica, F. (1981). The interplay among behavioral systems: Illustrations from the study of attachment, affiliation and manners in young Down syndrome children. *Developmental Psychology, 17,* 36–49.

Cicchetti, D., & Sroufe, L.A. (1978). An organizational view of affect: Illustration from the study of Down's syndrome infants. In M. Lewis & L. Rosenblum (Eds.), *The development of affect*. New York: Plenum.

Cicchetti, D., & Sroufe, L.A. (1976). The relationship between affective and cognitive development in Down syndrome infants. *Child Development, 47,* 920–929.

Coggins, T.E., & Stoel-Gammon, L. (1982). Clarification strategies used by four Down syndrome children for maintaining normal conversational interaction. *Education and Training of the Mentally Retarded, 17,* 65–67.

Cohen, L.B. (1981). Examination of habituation as a measure of aberrant infant development. In S.L. Friedman & M. Sigman (Eds.), *Preterm birth and psychological development* (pp. 241–253). New York: Academic Press.

Cohen, L.B., & Strauss, M.S. (1979). Concept acquisition in the human infant. *Child Development, 50,* 419–424.

Cowie, V. (1970). *A study of the early development of mongols*. Oxford: Pergamon Press.

Dunn, L.M., & Dunn, L. (1981). *The Peabody Picture Vocabulary Test – revised.* Circle Pines, MN: American Guidance Service.

Dunst, C.J. (1981). Social concomitants of cognitive mastery in Down syndrome infants. *Infant Mental Health Journal, 2,* 144–154.

Dunst, C. (in press). Sensorimotor development in infants with Down syndrome. In D. Cicchetti & M. Beeghly (Eds.), *Children with Down syndrome: A developmental perspective.* New York: Cambridge University Press.

Emde, R.N., & Brown, C. (1978). Adaptation to the birth of Down syndrome infants. *Journal of the American Academy of Child Psychiatry, 17,* 299–323.

Emde, R.N., Katz, E.L., & Thorpe, J.K. (1978). Emotional expression in infancy: II. Early deviations in Down syndrome. In M. Lewis and L.A. Rosenblum (Eds.), *The development of affect.* London: Plenum Press.

Fagan, J. (1976). Infant's recognition of invariant features of faces. *Child Development, 47,* 627–638.

Fantz, R.L., Fagan J.F., & Miranda, S.B. (1975). Early visual selectivity. In L.B. Cohen & P. Salapatek (Eds.), *Infant perception: From sensation to cognition, Vol. 1, Basic visual processes* (pp. 249–346). New York: Academic Press.

Fein, G. (1979). Echoes from the nursery: Piaget, Vygotsky and the relationship between language and play. In E. Winner & H. Gardner (Eds.), *Fact, fiction, and fantasy in childhood.* San Francisco: Jossey-Bass.

Fenson, L. (1984). Developmental trends for action and speech in pretend play. In I. Bretherton (Ed.), *Symbolic play.* New York: Academic.

Fowler, A. (in press). The development of language structure in children with Down syndrome. In D. Cicchetti & M. Beeghly (Eds.), *Children with Down syndrome: A developmental perspective.* New York: Cambridge University Press.

Fullard, W., McDevitt, S., & Carey, W. (1978). *Toddler Temperament Scale.* Philadelphia: Temple University Press.

Fullard, W., McDevitt, S., & Carey, W. (1984). Assessing temperament in one- to two-year old children. *Journal of Pediatric Psychology, 9,* 205–217.

Ganiban, J., Wagner, S., & Cicchetti, D. (in press). Temperament and Down syndrome. In D. Cicchetti & M. Beeghly (Eds.), *Children with Down syndrome; A developmental perspective.* New York: Cambridge University Press.

Gibson, D. (1978). *Down syndrome: The psychology of mongolism.* London: Cambridge University Press.

Gibson, E.J., & Walk, R. (1960). The "visual cliff." *Scientific American, 202,* 2–9.

Gillham, B. (1979). *The first worlds programme.* London: George Allen and Unwin.

Glenn, S.M., & Cunningham, C.C. (1983). What do babies listen to most? A developmental study of auditory preferences in nonhandicapped infants and infants with Down syndrome. *Developmental Psychology, 19* (3), 332–337.

Glenn, S.M., Cunningham, C.C., & Joyce, P.F. (1981). A study of auditory preferences in nonhandicapped infants and infants with Down's syndrome. *Child Development, 52,* 1303–1307.

Greenberg, M. (1983). Pragmatics and social interactions: The unrealized nexus. In L. Feagans, R. Golinkoff, & C. Garvey (Eds.), *The origins and growth of communication.* New York: Albex.

Gunn, P., & Andrews, P. (1985). The temperament of Down syndrome toddlers and their siblings. *Journal of Child Psychology and Psychiatry, 26,* 973–979.

Gunn, P., Berry, P., & Andrews, R. (1981). The temperament of Down syndrome infants: A research note. *Journal of Child Psychology and Psychiatry, 22,* 189–194.

Gunn, P., Berry, P., & Andrews, R. (1983). The temperament of Down syndrome toddlers: A research note. *Journal of Child Psychology and Psychiatry, 24,* 601–605.

Heffernan, L., Black, F., & Poche, P. (1982). Temperament patterns in young neurologically impaired children. *Journal of Pediatric Psychology*, *7*, 415–423.

Hesse, P., & Cicchetti, D. (1982). Perspectives on an integrated theory of emotional development. In D. Cicchetti & P. Hesse (Eds.), *New directions for child development*, *16*, 3–48.

Hill, P., & McCune-Nicolich, L. (1981). Pretend play and patterns of cognition in Down's syndrome infants. *Child Development*, *23*, 43–60.

Hills, S., & Tomlin, C. (1981). Self recognition in retarded children. *Child Development*, *52*, 145–150.

Hodapp, R., & Zigler, E. (in press). Applying the developmental perspective to individuals with Down syndrome. In D. Cicchetti and M. Beeghly (Eds)., *Children with Down syndrome: A developmental perspective*. New York: Cambridge University Press.

Inhelder, B. (1966). Cognitive development and its contribution to the diagnosis of some phenomena of mental deficiency. *Merrill-Palmer Quarterly*, *11*, 299–319.

Kagan, J. (1971). *Change and continuity in infancy*. New York: Wiley.

Kagan, J. (1981). *The second year*. Cambridge, MA: Harvard University Press.

Kaplan, B. (1966). The study of language in psychiatry: The comparative developmental approach and its application to symbolization and language in psychopathology. In S. Arieti (Ed.), *American Handbook of Psychiatry*. New York: Basic Books.

Kaplan, B. (1967). Meditations on genesis. *Human Development*, *10*, 65–87.

Kaplan, E. (1983). Process and achievement revisited. In S. Wapner & B. Kaplan (Eds.), *Toward a holistic developmental psychology*. Hillsdale, NJ: Erlbaum.

Keele, D., Richards, C., Brown, J., & Marshall, J. (1969). Catecholamine metabolism in Down's syndrome. *American Journal of Mental Deficiency*, *74*, 125–129.

Krakow, J.B., & Kopp, C. (1983). The effects of developmental delay on sustained attention in young children. *Child Development*, *54*, 1143–1155.

Lamb, M., Thompson, R., Gardner, W., Charnov, E., & Estes, D. (1984). Security of infantile attachment as assessed in the strange situation: Its study and biological interpretation. *Behavioral and Brain Sciences*, *7*, 124–147.

Largo, J., & Howard, J. (1979). Developmental progression in play behavior of children between nine and thirty months, II. *Developmental Medicine and Child Neurology*, *21*, 492–503.

Lee, L. (1974). *Developmental sentence analysis*. Evanston, IL: Northwestern University Press.

Lewis, M., & Brooks-Gunn, J. (1979). *Social cognition and the acquisition of self*. New York: Plenum Press.

Lewis, M., & Brooks-Gunn, J. (1984). Age and handicapped group differences in infants' visual attention. *Child Development*, *55*, 858–868.

Lewis, V., & Bryant, P.E. (1982). Touch and vision in normal and Down's syndrome babies. *Perception*, *11*, 691–701.

Lincoln, A., Courchesne, E., Kilman, B., & Galambos, R. (1985). Neurophysiological correlates of information processing by children with Down's syndrome. *American Journal of Mental Deficiency*, *89*, 403–414.

Loveland, K. (1987). Behavior of young children with Down syndrome before the mirror: Finding things reflected. *Child Development*, *58*, 928–936.

MacTurk, R., Vietze, P., McCarthy, M., McQuiston, S., & Yarrow, L. (1985). The organization of exploratory behavior in Down Syndrome and non-delayed infants. *Child Development*, *56*, 573–587.

Mahler, M., Pine, F., & Bergman, A. (1975). *The psychological birth of the human infant*. New York: Basic Books.

Mans, L., Cicchetti, D., & Sroufe, L.A. (1978). Mirror reactions of Down's syndrome infants and toddlers: Cognitive underpinnings of self-recognition. *Child Development*, *49*, 1247–1250.

Marcovitch, S., Goldberg, S., MacGregor, D., & Lojkasek, M. (1986). Patterns of temperament variation in three groups of developmentally delayed preschool children: Mother and father ratings. *Developmental and Behavioral Pediatrics, 7,* 247–252.

Matas, L., Arend, R., & Sroufe, L.A. (1978). Continuity in adaptation in the second year: The relationship between quality of attachment and later competence. *Child Development, 49,* 547–556.

McCune-Nicholich, L., & Bruskin, C. (1982). Combinatorial competency in symbolic play and language. In D. Pepler & K. Rubin (Eds.), *The play of children.* New York: Karger.

Mervis, C.B. (in press). Early conceptual development of children with Down syndrome. In D. Cicchetti & M. Beeghly (Eds.), *Children with Down syndrome: A developmental perspective.* New York: Cambridge University Press.

Mervis, C.B., & Cardoso-Martins, C. (1984). Transition from sensorimotor stage 5 to stage 6 by Down syndrome children: A response to Gibson. *American Journal of Mental Deficiency, 89,* 99–102.

Milgram, N. (1969). The rational and irrational in Zigler's motivational approach to mental retardation. *American Journal of Mental Deficiency, 73,* 527–535.

Milgram, N.A. (1973). Cognition and language in mental retardation: Distinctions and implications. In D.K. Routh (Ed.), *The experimental psychology of mental retardation.* Chicago: Aldine.

Miller, J.F. (in press). Language and communication characteristics of children with Down syndrome. In A. Crocker, S. Pueschel, J. Rynders, & C. Tingley (Eds.), *Down syndrome: State of the art.* Baltimore: Brooks.

Miranda, S.B., & Fantz, R.L. (1973). Visual preferences of Down syndrome and normal infants. *Child Development, 44,* 555–561.

Miranda, S.B., & Fantz, R.L. (1974). Recognition memory in Down syndrome and normal infants. *Child Development, 45,* 651–660.

Morss, J.R. (1983). Cognitive development in the Down's syndrome infant: Slow or different? *British Journal of Educational Psychology, 53,* 40–47.

Motti, F., Cicchetti, D., & Sroufe, L.A. (1983). From infant affect expression to symbolic play: The coherence of development in Down syndrome children. *Child Development, 54,* 1168–1175.

Mundy, P., Sigman, M., Kasari, C., & Yirmiya, N. (1988). Nonverbal communication skills in Down syndrome children. *Child Development, 59,* 235–249.

Nicholich, L. (1977). Beyond sensorimotor intelligence: Assessment of symbolic maturity through analysis of pretend play. *Merrill-Palmer Quarterly, 23,* 89–99.

Olson, G., & Sherman, T. (1983). Attention, learning, and memory in infants. In M.M. Haith & J. Campos (Eds.), *Infancy and developmental psychobiology* (pp. 1001–1080). (Vol. 2, P. Mussen, Ed., *Handbook of child psychology, 4th ed.*) New York: Wiley.

Pepper, S. (1942). *World hypotheses.* Berkeley: University of California Press.

Piaget, J. (1962). *Play, dreams, and imitation in childhood.* New York: Norton.

Purpura, D. (1975). Dendritic differentiation in human cerebral cortex: Normal and aberrant developmental patterns. In G. Kretzberg (Ed.), *Advances in neurology, Vol 12* (pp. 91–116). New York: Raven Press.

Reese, H., & Overton, W. (1970). Models of development and theories of development. In L.R. Goulet & P. Baltes (Eds.), *Life span developmental psychology: Research and theory.* New York: Academic Press.

Reznick, J.S., & Kagan, J. (1981). Category detection in infancy. Paper presented at the Biennial Meeting of the Society for Research in Child Development, Boston.

Rosch, E., & Mervis, C.B. (1975). Family resemblances: Studies in the internal structure of categories. *Cognitive Psychology, 7,* 573–605.

Rosenberg, S. (1984). Disorders of first-language development: Trends in research and theory. In E.S. Gollin (Ed.), *Malformations of development*. Orlando, FL: Academic Press.

Rothbart, M. (1981). Measurement of temperament in infancy. *Child Development, 52,* 569–578.

Rothbart, M., & Derryberry, D. (1981). The development of individual differences in temperament. In M. Lamb & A.L. Brown (Eds.), *Advances in developmental psychology, Vol. 1.* (pp. 37–86). Hillsdale, NJ: Erlbaum.

Rothbart, M., & Hanson, M. (1983). A care giver report comparison of temperament characteristics of Down syndrome and normal infants. *Developmental Psychology, 19,* 766–769.

Rubin, K., Fein, G., & Vandenberg, B. (1983). Play. In P. Mussen (Ed.), *Handbook of child psychology, Vol. 4: Socialization.* New York: Wiley.

Sackett, G., Sameroff, A., Cairns, R., & Suomi, S. (1981). Continuity in behavioral development: Theoretical and empirical issues. In K. Immelmann, G. Garlow, L. Petrinovich, & M. Main (Eds.), *Behavioral development.* Cambridge: Cambridge University Press.

Sameroff, A., & Chandler, M. (1975). Reproductive risk and the continuum of caretaking casualty. In F. Horowitz (Eds.), *Review of child development research* (Vol. 4). Chicago: University of Chicago Press.

Schneider-Rosen, K., & Cicchetti, D. (1984). The relationship between affect and cognition in maltreated infants: Quality of attachment and the development of visual self-recognition. *Child Development, 55,* 648–658.

Schopler, E., & Mesibov, G. (1985). *Communication problems in autism.* New York: Plenum.

Scott, B., Becker, L., & Petit, T. (1983). Neurobiology of Down's syndrome. *Progress in Neurobiology, 21,* 199–237.

Serafica, F.C., & Cicchetti, D. (1975). Down's syndrome children in a strange situation: Attachment and exploratory behaviors. *Merrill-Palmer Quarterly, 21,* 137–150.

Sigman, M., & Mundy, P. (1987). Symbolic processes in young autistic children. In D. Cicchetti and M. Beeghly (Eds.), *Atypical symbolic development.* San Francisco: Jossey-Bass.

Sorce, J., Emde, R., & Frank, M. (1982). Maternal referencing in normal and Down syndrome infants: A longitudinal analysis. In R. Emde and R. Harmon (Eds.), *The development of attachment and affilitative systems.* New York: Plenum.

Spiker, D., & Ricks, M. (1984). Visual self-recognition in autistic children: Deyelopmental relationships. *Child Development, 55,* 214–225.

Sroufe, L.A. (1979a). The coherence of individual development. *American Psychologist, 34,* 834–841.

Sroufe, L.A. (1979b). Socioemotional development. In J. Osofsky (Ed.), *Handbook of infant development.* New York: Wiley.

Sroufe, L.A., & Rutter, M. (1984). The domain of developmental psychopathology. *Child Development, 55,* 1184–1199.

Sroufe, L.A., & Waters, E. (1976). The ontogenesis of smiling and laughter: A perspective on the organization of development in infancy. *Psychological Reivew, 83,* 173–189.

Sroufe, L.S., & Wunsch, J. (1972). The development of laughter in the first year of life. *Child Development, 43,* 1326–1344.

Stanovitch, K. (1978). Information processing in mentally retarded individuals. *International Review of Research in Mental Retardation, 9,* 29–60.

Stern, D. (1985). *The interpersonal world of the infant: A view from psychoanalysis and developmental psychology.* New York: Basic Books.

Takashima, S., Becker, L., Armstrong, D., & Chan, F. (1981). Abnormal neuronal development in the visual cortex of the human fetus and infant with Down's syndrome: A quantitative and qualitative Golgi study. *Brain Research, 225,* 1–21.

Thompson, R., Cicchetti, D., Lamb, M., & Malkin C. (1985). The emotional responses of Down syndrome and normal infants in the strange situation: The organization of affective behavior in infants. *Developmental Psychology, 21,* 828–841.

Uzgiris, I., & Hunt, J. (1975). *Assessment in infancy.* Urbana, IL: University of Illinois Press.

Vietze, P., McCarthy, M., McQuiston, S., MacTurk, R., & Yarrow, L. (1983). Attention and exploratory behavior in infants with Down syndrome. In T. Field & A. Sostek (Eds.), *Infants born at risk: Perceptual and physical processes* (pp. 251–268). New York: Grune and Stratton.

Wagner, S., Ganiban, J.M., & Cicchetti, D. (in press). Attention, memory, and perception in infants with Down syndrome: A review and commentary. In D. Cicchetti & M. Beeghly (Eds.). *Children with Down syndrome: A developmental perspective.* New York: Cambridge University Press.

Watson, M., & Fischer, K. (1977). A developmental sequence of agent use in late infancy. *Child Development, 48,* 828–836.

Weinshilbaum, R., Thoa, N., Johnson, D., Kopin, I., & Axelrod, J. (1971). Proportional release of norepinephrine and dopamine-beta-hydroxylase from the sympathetic nerves, *Science, 174,* 1349–1351.

Weisz, J., & Yeates, K. (1981). Cognitive development in retarded and nonretarded persons: Piagetian tasks of the similar-structure hypothesis. *Psychological Bulletin, 90,* 153–178.

Weisz, J., & Zigler, E. (1979). Cognitive development in retarded and nonretarded persons: Piagetian tests of the similar-sequence hypothesis. *Psychological Bulletin, 86,* 831–851.

Werner, H. (1937). Process and achievement: A basic problem of education and developmental psychology. *Harvard Educational Review, 7,* 353–368.

Werner, H. (1948). *Comparative psychology of mental development.* Chicago: Follett.

Werner, H. (1957). The concept of development from a comparative and organismic point of view. In D. Harris (Ed.), *The concept of development.* Minneapolis: University of Minnesota Press.

Werner, H., & Kaplan, B. (1963). *Symbol formation: An organismic-developmental approach to language and the expression of thought.* New York: Wiley.

Wilson, R., & Matheny, A. (1986). Behavior-genetics research in infant temperament: The Louisville twin study. In R. Plomin & J. Dunn (Eds.), *The study of temperament: Continuities and challenges.* Hillsdale, NJ: Erlbaum.

Wing, L., Gould, J., Yeates, S., & Brierly, L. (1977). Symbolic play in severely mentally retarded and in autistic children. *Journal of Child Psychology and Psychiatry, 18,* 167–178.

Yates, C., Simpson, J., Maloney, A., Gorden, A., & Reid, A. (1980). Alzheimer-like cholinergic deficiency in Down's syndrome. *Lancet, 2,* 979.

Zahn-Waxler, C., & Radke-Yarrow, M. (1982). The development of altruism: Alternative research strategies. In N. Eisenberg (Ed.), *Development of social behavior.* New York: Academic Press.

Zigler, E. (1969). Developmental versus difference theories of mental retardation and the problem of motivation. *American Journal of Mental Deficiency, 73,* 536–556.

Zigler, E. (1973). The retarded child as a whole person. In D. Routh (Ed.), *The experimental study of mental retardation.* Chicago: Aldine.

Zigler, E., & Balla, D. (1977). Personality factors in the performance of the retarded: Implications for clinical assessment. *Journal of the American Academy of Child Psychiatry, 16,* 19–37.

Zigler, E., & Balla, D. (Eds.), (1982). *Mental retardation.* Hillsdale, NJ: Erlbaum.

9 Developmental issues in fragile X syndrome

Elisabeth Dykens and James Leckman

Fragile X syndrome is a recently identified X-linked disorder resulting in mental retardation and characteristic physical, cognitive, and behavioral features. Although data are now accumulating regarding the psychological functioning of fragile X males, previous research has focused almost exclusively on the genetic aspects and physical features of the disorder. As a result, the data are quite limited on the intellectual, adaptive, and behavioral functioning of boys and men with fragile X syndrome, and many questions remain about the development of fragile X males in virtually all areas of functioning.

In addition, the research reports on fragile X syndrome are found largely in the genetics literature, and less accessible to parents, educators, and health professionals who seek guidance with the daily management and education of these individuals. Given this need, and the relative newness of the disorder, this chapter will begin with a brief overview of fragile X syndrome, including its genetic features and enigmas and its physical phenotype. Data on the prevalence of fragile X syndrome, and the intellectual, adaptive, and behavioral functioning of fragile X males will then be presented. These findings will be discussed in relation to the two-group approach in mental retardation, the trajectory of intelligence, and the interplay between genetics and the environment.

Overview of fragile X syndrome

Genetic features

The chromosomal abnormality associated with fragile X syndrome was initially identified in 1969 by Lubs, who observed a pinched or constricted end on the X chromosomes of mentally retarded males in a large pedigree that followed an X-linked inheritance pattern. These chromosomal findings were not replicated until 1977, when Sutherland reported that in order to observe the abnormality on the X chromosome, tissue cells had to be grown in a culture deficient in folate. Even with these procedures, only a small percentage of the cells of affected males manifest the "fragile" site (15–40%), and it is not always consistently observed (Bregman, Dykens, Watson, Ort & Leckman, 1987). Recent advances in molecular genetic marking techniques are refining the accuracy of the fragile X diagnosis (Murphy, Kidd, Breg, Ruddle, & Kidd, 1985). Although there are many forms of X-linked retardation, the diagnosis of fragile X syndrome is generally reserved for cases in which the fragile site is identified through proper cytogenetic or molecular genetic procedures.

Fragile X syndrome is generally assumed to follow a Mendelian X-linked inheritance pattern. In this pattern, an unaffected female carrier has a 50% chance of transmitting the affected X chromosome to her daughters – who then become carriers – and a 50% chance of transmitting the affected X chromosome to her sons, who are affected with the disorder. Recent evidence, however, has pointed to considerable deviation from this pattern. Unlike other recessive X-linked disorders (e.g., color blindness, hemophilia), approximately one-third to one-half of the women carrying the fragile X marker are themselves mildly affected with the disorder, and may exhibit learning disabilities, a history of poor school performance, or mild to moderate mental retardation (Fishburn, Turner, Daniel, & Brookwell, 1983; Hagerman & Smith, 1983; Turner, Brookwell, Daniel, Selikowitz, & Zilibowitz, 1980). Recent estimates (Sherman et al., 1985) suggest that if the carrier female is affected herself, then 50% of her daughters will become carriers and all of her sons will inherit the disorder. If the carrier female is not clinically affected, then sons who inherit the affected X chromosome have a 75% of being clinically impaired, and daughters have a 30% chance of being affected.

In addition, segregation analyses suggest that as many as 20% of males who receive a fragile X chromosome by descent will fail to exhibit the fragile site cytogenetically and will be unaffected with the disorder (Sherman et al., 1985). The existence of these nonpenetrant carrier males has been confirmed using newer recombinant DNA techniques that allow investigators to follow the inheritance of segments of DNA from the affected region of the X chromosome. Although all of the daughters of these nonpenetrant, unaffected males will be carriers, they do not generally manifest clinical impairments. The sons of these males will not be affected with the disorder. Thus, fragile X syndrome presents several deviations from a recessive X-linked inheritance pattern that have important implications for the genetic counseling of families affected with this disorder.

Physical phenotype

Many mentally retarded males with fragile X syndrome exhibit characteristic physical features. Approximately 70% of these males have an
elongated face, a high forehead, and enlarged ears (see Bregman, Dykens,
Watson, Ort, & Leckman, 1987 for a review). Many of these features
become more pronounced after puberty. In addition, several investigators
have observed connective tissue dysplasia in some of their fragile X patients. These features include hyperextensible joints, a high arched palate,
and mitral valve prolapse (Hagerman, VanHousen, Smith, & McGauran,
1984). Macroorchidism, or enlarged testes, has also been consistently observed in fragile X males, particularly at postpubertal stages of development (see Bregman, Dykens, Watson, Ort, & Leckman, 1987 for a
review). The increased frequency of macroorchidism in fragile X syndrome, although not necessarily unique to this form of retardation, has led
many investigators to explore the neuroendocrine functioning of fragile
X males. These studies do not generally point to abnormal neuroendocrine
functioning, although some affected males may exhibit gonadal dysfunction and slight abnormalities in the hypothalamic–pituitary regulation of
the thyroid.

Prevalence of fragile X syndrome

Recent estimates of the prevalence of fragile X syndrome in the population
(0.73–0.92 per 1,000 males) suggest that it is second only to Down syndrome in terms of a known chromosomal cause of retardation (Herbst &
Miller, 1980; Webb, Bundey, Thake, & Todd, 1986). As Down syndrome
is rarely transmitted as a genetic disorder from Down syndrome parent to
Down syndrome child, fragile X syndrome is thought to be the most common heritable cause of mental retardation. Surveys of retarded populations indicate that fragile X syndrome may account for 2–7% of all cases
of retardation among males (Webb, Bundey, Thake, & Todd, 1986). Thus,
fragile X syndrome is estimated to be quite prevalent among mentally
retarded males. As discussed next, both the prevalence of the disorder and
the patterns of its genetic transmission (e.g., affected carrier females) have
important implications for the classification of retarded individuals, specifically for the two-group approach.

Fragile X syndrome and the "two-group" approach

In contrast to defect or difference theorists, developmental theorists have
generally relied on the "two-group" approach to differentiate among

mentally retarded individuals (Zigler, 1967; 1969). Within this approach, approximately 25% of mentally retarded individuals are assumed to have organic etiologies, and 75% to have nonorganic, or familial retardation (Zigler & Hodapp, 1986). A review of large-scale population studies, however, has identified a 50-50 split between organic and familial retardation (Zigler & Hodapp, 1986). Recently, Zigler and Hodapp (1986) revised this two-group approach, extending the two groups into four groups, and calling for further differentiation of those individuals with organic and nonorganic impairments.

In the expanded classification system of Zigler and Hodapp (1986), 25% of retarded individuals are assumed to have organic impairments with known etiologies, 35% to have familial retardation, 35% are classified as polygenic isolates, and less than 5% are construed as experiencing severe environmental deprivation. The authors acknowledge that these percentages are estimates and are subject to change, and the recent discovery of fragile X syndrome, including its prevalence and pattern of genetic transmission, certainly provides several important sources of change for the percentages noted. For example, Zigler and Hodapp (1986) assert that an "undisputed fact" about nonorganic retardation is "that it tends to run in immediate families" (p. 51). In addition, familial–cultural retardation is defined as existing in those cases in which at least one parent has an IQ below 70, and in which the range of retardation in the affected members is mild to moderate. Fragile X syndrome certainly runs in both immediate and distant family members, and the mean IQ of affected males is in the moderate range (Chudley, 1984).

Approximately 33% of carrier females, including mothers, exhibit learning difficulties or mild to moderate retardation. Thus, it appears that many cases of fragile X syndrome fit the typical description of familial mental retardation. This overlap in clinical description, as well as the estimated prevalence and frequency of fragile X, makes it quite likely that fragile X syndrome will result in a decrease of cases classified as familial–cultural and an increase in cases classified as organic.

Although Zigler and Hodapp's (1986) revised classification system has refined the description of nonorganic retarded individuals, it has not attempted to refine the classification of individuals with organic retardation. Recently, Burack, Hodapp, and Zigler (1988) emphasized the need for further differentiation among organically impaired individuals. These authors note that the predominant tendency in MR research is to classify groups according to level of impairment, not by etiology. Yet, as Burack, Hodapp, and Zigler (1988) demonstrate, classifying groups solely by level of impairment may obscure important differences between various etiological groups. These group differences may be manifest in both psychological and behavioral functioning, including intellectual and adaptive strengths and weaknesses, the trajectories of intelligence throughout development, and patterns of maladaptive behavior. Recent data pertaining to the psychological and behavioral functioning of boys and men with fragile X syndrome provide considerable support for the classification of research groups based on etiology, as opposed to level of impairment. These data are presented next, and are also disscussed in relation to an underlying area of weakness that appears to permeate various domains of functioning in fragile X males.

Intellectual functioning

Although fragile X males display the full range of intellectual impairments from borderline to profound, most are moderately affected, with IQs in the 35–40 range (Chudley, 1984). Affected fragile X males with average or near average IQs have also been reported (Daker, Chidiac, Fear, & Berry, 1981). Several investigators (Chudley, 1984; Herbst, Dunn, Dill, Kalousek, & Krywaniuk, 1981) have reported that fragile X males perform lower on certain subtests of the Wechsler Intelligence Scale for Children-Revised (WISC-R) (e.g., information, digit span, arithmetic) and higher on others (e.g., picture completion, similarities). The implication of these findings, however, remains unclear, as the authors did not advance hypotheses regarding the underlying cognitive processing of their subjects.

Recently, Dykens, Hodapp, and Leckman (1987) systematically examined the intellectual functioning of fragile X males by identifying their strengths and weaknesses and relating them to putative styles of cognitive processing. These authors aimed to measure "two types of mental functioning that have been identified independently by cerebral specialization researchers ... Luria and his followers ... and cognitive psychologists" (Kaufman & Kaufman, 1983, p. 2). The two types of mental functioning are *sequential processing*, or solving problems bit by bit in serial or temporal order, and *simultaneous processing*, or integrating stimuli in a holistic, frequently spatial manner. These processing domains have proven useful in formulating educational strategies that capitalize on individual processing strengths and minimize processing weaknesses.

Utilizing the Kaufman Assessment Battery for Children (K-ABC; Kaufman & Kaufman, 1983), these authors reported that fragile X males exhibited consistent and significant difficulties with sequential-processing tasks. Deficits in sequential processing have also been observed by Kemper,

Hagerman, and Altshul-Stark (1987). This difficulty in sequential processing indicates significant weaknesses in auditory, visual, and motoric short-term memory. Achievement in mathematics also emerged as an area of significant weakness in these males (Dykens, Hodapp, & Leckman, 1987) and is consistent with the association between poor sequential-processing skills and problems in the retention of math facts (Kaufman, Kaufman, & Goldsmith, 1984).

In contrast to their findings of relative weaknesses in sequential processing, Dykens, Hodapp, and Leckman (1987) found significant strengths for fragile X males in simultaneous processing. This strength in simultaneous processing was particularly noteworthy in subjects' abilities to make perceptual inferences, and to complete tasks that required perceptual closure, flexibility and organization. This distinct pattern of relative strengths in simultaneous processing and weaknesses in sequential processing, was evident for all fragile X males in this study.

Although the intellectual profiles identified by Dykens, Hodapp, and Leckman (1987) may be unique to males with fragile X syndrome, additional data are necessary to confirm this hypothesis. Utilizing the K-ABC with Down syndrome subjects, Pueschel, Gallagher, Zartler, and Puezzullo (1987) have reported no particular strengths or weaknesses in the sequential and simultaneous-processing abilities of these children. A significant strength emerged, however, in a sequential task assessing visual–motoric short-term memory. This task emerged as the lowest subtest score for all of the fragile X subjects in the Dykens, Hodapp, and Leckman (1987) study. Thus, what appears to be a significant strength in Down syndrome children is a significant weakness in fragile X boys. Still, the uniqueness of these profiles remains unclear, and more systematic comparisons between Down syndrome, fragile X, and other etiological groups are necessary to address this issue.

Even without clarifying data, however, the identification of specific strengths and weaknesses in the fragile X and Down syndrome samples conflicts with previous analyses of educable and trainable mentally retarded children. Silverstein, Goldberg, Kasner, and Solomon (1984), for example, found no significant strengths or weaknesses in the intellectual functioning of educable mentally retarded children. Similarily, Kaufman and Kaufman (1983) reported no significant difference between sequential and simultaneous processing, and little variability in achievement tests, in groups of educable and trainable mentally retarded children. In these studies, the etiology of the children's retardation was not considered in data analysis. This classification of retarded individuals according to their level of functioning may obscure potential differences in the cognitive profiles of various etiological groups (Burack, Hodapp, & Zigler, 1988). The identification of specific cognitive profiles in fragile X syndrome, and in other groups such as Down syndrome, confirms the importance of classifying groups on the basis of etiology rather than overall level of impairment. Further refinement of classification, and of intervention approaches with individuals with organic retardation, requires that workers in the field of mental retardation begin to adopt this perspective in their research methodologies.

In addition to confirming the importance of research groups based upon etiology, it may be that the specific pattern of cognitive strengths and weaknesses in fragile X males affects their functioning and development in other domains. Specifically, compromised sequential processing and relative strengths in simultaneous processing may be evident in areas other than intellectual functioning. Indeed, recent evidence suggests that sequential-processing difficulties and strengths in simultaneous processing in fragile X males are found in their linguistic functioning and in their patterns of maladaptive behavior. Sequential-processing deficits may also be apparent in the adaptive behavior skills of these males. The linguistic and adaptive functioning and the maladaptive behavior of fragile X males are presented next, and are discussed in relation to this apparently pervasive sequential-processing defect.

Linguistic functioning

The linguistic functioning of fragile X males has been characterized as disabled, with distinctive problems in auditory memory, reception, and articulation (Howard-Peebles, Stoddard, & Mims, 1979). It has also been described as jocular, abrupt, and repetitive, with rhythmic, litany-like phrasing, echolalia and palilalia, and dysfluent and dyspraxic traits (Jacobs et al., 1980; Paul, Cohen, Breg, Watson, & Herman, 1984; Turner, Brookwell, Daniel, Selikowitz, & Zilibowitz, 1980).

It remains unclear if these language characteristics are unique to fragile X syndrome or shared with other etiological groups. In a comparison of institutionalized fragile X and nonfragile X retarded men, Paul, Dykens, Leckman, Watson, Breg, and Cohen (1987) found no patterns of strength or weakness, or distinctive group differences, in receptive or expressive language functioning.

Areas of significant strength and weakness have been found, however, in studies of noninstitutionalized fragile X boys and young men. Marans, Paul, and Leckman (1987) have reported significant strengths in both expressive and receptive vocabulary of noninstitutionalized fragile X subjects, and relative strengths in vocabulary have also been observed by Sudhalter (1987). In contrast, fragile X males have been found to have significant weaknesses in sentence imitation tasks and in the mean length of utterance (MLU) (Marans, Paul, & Leckman, 1987). Both sentence imitation and longer MLUs require auditory short-term memory and the ability to organize and express words in an orderly, step-by-step, linear manner. As such, they tap many processes inherent in sequential processing. Thus, it appears that the underlying cognitive deficit in sequential processing also manifests itself in the linguistic functioning of many fragile X males. In addition, their linguistic strengths in receptive and expressive vocabulary may be related to their cognitive strengths in simultaneous processing; strengths in both of these domains reflect the ability to understand and label the overall meaning or goal of a task.

Maladaptive behavior and psychopathology

Although many fragile X males have been described as cooperative, cheerful, and pleasant (Chudley, 1984; Herbst, Dunn, Dill, Kalousek, & Krywaniuk, 1980), males with this syndrome have been shown to exhibit significant levels of maladaptive behavior (Dykens, Hodapp, & Leckman, 1989), as well as specific patterns of behavioral difficulties (Bregman, Leckman, & Ort, in press). In particular, problems with aggressive outbursts, hyperactivity, gaze aversion, attention deficits, stereotypy, and self-injurious behavior have been frequently observed (Bregman, Dykens, Watson, Ort, & Leckman, 1987; Fryns, Jacobs, Kleczkowska, & Van den Berghe, 1984; Jacobs et al., 1980; Lejune, 1982; Mattei, Mattei, Aumeras, Auger, & Giraud, 1981).

Many of these maladaptive behaviors may be related to the presence of certain psychiatric disorders in the fragile X population. For example, given the stereotypical behaviors and communication problems in some fragile X boys, several investigators have explored the relationship between fragile X syndrome and infantile autism. Reports of the prevalence of autism in fragile X males are quite variable, with estimates ranging from 7% (Bregman, Leckman, & Ort, in press) to 14% (Fryns, Jacobs, Kleczkowska, & Van den Berghs, 1984) to 47% (Hagerman, Jackson, Levitas, Rimland & Braden, 1986). Numerous investigators have also screened their autistic samples, testing for the fragile X marker in boys already diagnosed with autism. The frequency of fragile X among males with autism is also quite variable, ranging from 15% to none (see Bregman, Dykens, Watson, Ort, & Leckman, 1987 for a review). Thus, there may be a modest degree of overlap in the two syndromes, and it is quite likely that some of the variability in the literature may be attributable to discrepancies among investigators in their diagnostic procedures and subject samples. These discrepancies make it difficult to ascertain a precise estimate of the degree of overlap between the disorders at present.

Unlike the controversy over the diagnosis of infantile autism, there appears to be a consensus in the literature that many boys and young men with fragile X syndrome exhibit significant problems with attention, hyperactivity, and impulsivity (e.g., Hagerman, Murphy, & Wittenberger, 1987). Indeed, Bregman, Leckman, and Ort (in press) determined that 93% of their noninstitutionalized fragile X sample met the Diagnostic and Statistical Manual of Mental Disorders (DSM-III; American Psychiatric Association, 1980) criteria for Attention Deficit Disorder with Hyperactivity. In addition, these authors found that approximately 29% of their sample met DSM-III criteria for Anxiety Disorder. Anxiety problems were noted to be particularly problematic in interpersonal situations and in the social arena. It appears that these anxiety and attentional problems may characterize both young, noninstitutionalized boys and older institutionalized fragile X men (Dykens, Hodapp, & Leckman, 1989).

It may also be the case that attentional problems may change depending upon the age of the fragile X males. Although additional longitudinal data are needed, it seems that the hyperactive, impulsive, and aggressive symptoms that frequently accompany attentional deficits are less problematic among older fragile X subjects (Dykens, Hodapp, & Leckman, 1989). Thus, attention deficits in fragile X boys have been consistently observed by several investigators, and they may persist in many adults as well, but without the motoric involvement often noted in younger subjects.

It may be that the anxiety disorders noted in some fragile X males contribute to their difficulties in sustaining appropriate levels of attention and concentration. It is also quite likely that these attention deficits are related to the underlying deficit in sequential processing that characterizes many fragile X males. Adequate sequential processing requires some competency in short-term memory functioning; short-term memory is generally impaired when the ability to attend and concentrate is compromised. Although the relationship between these two problematic areas remains unclear, it is hypothesized that they are interdependent in that one deficit may serve to exacerbate the other.

Adaptive functioning

The ability to adapt socially – or to perform "daily activities required for personal and social sufficiency" (Sparrow, Balla, & Cicchetti, 1984, p. 6) –

is essential for the success of retarded persons living in a variety of settings. For example, social adaptation has been identified as more important than IQ for the ultimate life success of retarded individuals living in the community (Baller, Charles, & Miller, 1967; Windle, 1962). In addition, adaptive behavior is critical in determining the success or failure of individuals in group homes (Hill & Bruininks, 1984; Landesman-Dwyer & Sulzbacher, 1981) and in the large institutional setting (King, Raynes, & Tizard, 1971).

In assessing the importance of social adaptation, however, most studies have relied on data from mixed etiological groups. As such, data remain limited regarding the adaptive functioning of specific etiological groups such as fragile X syndrome.

Herbst (1980) noted that there may be a relationship between "social adaptability" and IQ in fragile X males, but did not specify how, or if, social adaptation was measured. Utilizing the Vineland Adaptive Behavior Scales (Sparrow, Balla, & Cicchetti, 1984), which assess communication, daily living, and socializations skills, Dykens, Leckman, Paul, and Watson (1987) compared older fragile X individuals to other residents of a large institution. These authors found that fragile X males exhibited significantly higher domestic daily living skills than their nonspecific retarded and autistic counterparts, and were apt to demonstrate adaptive skills that exceeded mental age (MA) expectations. Further examination of both institutionalized and noninstitutionalized fragile X males (Dykens, Hodapp, & Leckman, 1989) pointed to significant relative strengths in both groups in their daily living skills compared with communication and socialization abilities. Within the daily living skills domain, personal skills (e.g., toileting, grooming) and domestic skills (e.g., cleaning, cooking) were better developed than community skills (e.g., managing money, using a phone).

Although the institutional sample in this study demonstrated particular deficits in expressive and written communication compared with the noninstitutionalized group, the overall pattern of adaptive functioning identified by these authors persisted across samples that varied widely in their residential status, age, and degree of impairment. In addition, Wolff, Gardner, Lappen, Paccia, and Schnell (1987) have also recently reported strengths in domestic and personal daily living skills in a sample of fragile X children and adults. Although these authors did not relate the living status or functioning level of their subjects, it appears that strengths in daily living skills apply to many fragile X males regardless of their age, IQ, and residential status.

This profile of adaptive behavior may be consistent with sequential-processing deficits, and with the apparent strength of these males in tasks requiring vocabulary and factual knowledge. Achievement tasks tapping skills in vocabulary and general environmental knowledge are similar to daily living skills in that both areas often involve tasks that are susceptible to repeated training (see Baker, 1984). Given the weakness in sequential processing and short-term memory, fragile X males may be particularly adept at performing behaviors that are typically overtrained and that do not necessarily rely upon short-term memory. Thus, although fragile X males exhibit levels of adaptive behavior that are generally commensurate with their levels of cognitive ability (Dykens, Leckman, Paul, & Watson, 1987), their adaptive skills may exceed MA expectations in tasks that are repeatedly taught and that deemphasize sequential processing.

As presented here, the hypothesis of sequential-processing deficits in many males with fragile X syndrome has received support from their profiles of strength and weakness in cognitive, linguistic, and adaptive functioning, as well as from their patterns of maladaptive behavior. This underlying sequential-processing deficit thus appears to pervade many aspects of functioning in these males and should be an important consideration in the development of appropriate intervention strategies for this group. The strengths of many fragile X males in simultaneous processing and in tasks requiring vocabulary and environmental knowledge provide additional guidelines for the development of effective educational tactics and intervention strategies.

Individuals with strengths in simultaneous processing solve problems best by mentally processing many parallel pieces of information at the same time. Simultaneous processing may be particularly important in recognizing the shape and appearance of numbers and letters, understanding the overall meaning of a story or situation, interpreting the overall meaning of visual stimuli such as pictures, charts, diagrams and maps, and visualizing solutions to problems in their entirety (Kaufman, Kaufman, & Goldsmith, 1984). As such, many fragile X males who demonstrate a relative strength in simultaneous processing may respond well to a teaching strategy that emphasizes the overall meaning of a task, or groups of details or images, before breaking down the task or grouping into its component parts. This teaching style might include helping fragile X males to visualize what is to be learned, offering a sense of the whole by appealing to their visual–spatial orientation, and making tasks concrete whenever possible with manipulative materials such as graphs, models, pictures, maps, and diagrams.

Many individuals with relative strengths in simultaneous processing and relative weaknesses in sequential processing exhibit difficulty with word attack skills, decoding and phonetics, the rules of grammar, breaking down arithmetic problems into their component parts, remembering specific sequences or details of a story, and understanding and following oral instructions or a sequence of steps or rules (Kaufman, Kaufman, & Goldsmith, 1984). As such, fragile X males who exhibit this profile may not respond well to teaching strategies that appeal to their verbal–temporal functioning, that emphasize verbal cues and auditory memory, or that present materials in a step-by-step manner that gradually leads up to the presentation of the entire concept.

The deficits in sequential processing shown by many fragile X males may be exacerbated by overactivity, impulsivity, and poor concentration and attention, particularly in younger boys. In many fragile X youngsters, including those with diagnoses of attention deficit hyperactivity disorder, these behaviors contribute to considerable management problems in both their classroom and home environments. In situations where traditional behavioral modification programs aimed at reducing impulsivity and increasing on-task behavior fail, families and physicians may consider a trial of stimulant medication. In particular, methylphenidate has been noted to improve the attention span of some fragile X boys (Hagerman, Murphy, & Wittenberger, 1987), and clonidine has been reported as effective in other youngsters (Leckman, 1987).

Trajectory of intelligence

The specific profiles of strength and weakness in fragile X syndrome and in other etiological groups offer guidelines as to *how* one may best intervene with these individuals. Of equal importance, however, is *when* one should intervene. It is generally assumed that intervention programs may meet with more success if they are implemented at specific times in an individual's course of development (e.g., early intervention programs), and considerable attention has focused on the timing of programs that optimize cognitive functioning (e.g., Zigler & Seitz, 1982).

The timing of interventions aimed at cognitive functioning have generally been based upon data pertaining to the trajectory of intelligence in normal individuals and in mentally retarded individuals of mixed etiologies. However, proponents of the developmental approach to mental retardation suggest that trajectories of intelligence may differ across various etiological groups (Burack, Hodapp, & Zigler, 1988). For example, Hodapp and Zigler (in press) have reviewed longitudinal studies of Down syndrome children that showed decelerating rates of intellectual development from infancy throughout adolescence. This pattern contrasts with studies of retarded cerebral palsy subjects in which fairly stable IQ's over time were noted, with some indications of slight increases in IQ over time (e.g., Cruickshank, Hallahan, & Bice, 1976).

These findings contrast with the long-term IQ stability noted in educable children of mixed etiologies over a 4-year span (Silverstein, 1982), and in mildly retarded adults, also of mixed etiology, when followed for a period of 35 years (Ross, Begab, Dondis, Giampiccolo, & Meyers, 1985). Thus, whereas data pertaining to mixed etiological groups point to long-term IQ stability, specific etiological groups may manifest markedly different trajectories of intellectual development. Additional data on the trajectories of IQ in specific etiological groups such as fragile X syndrome could help clarify the issue of IQ stability versus change in retarded populations.

Some reports have noted that the intellectual functioning of many younger boys with fragile X syndrome lies in the borderline or mildly retarded range, whereas adult males are more often severely or profoundly retarded (Hagerman, Kemper, & Hudson, 1985; Opitz, 1984). Thus, there may be a deceleration of IQ in fragile X males that is related to CA (Borghgraef, Fryns, Dielkens, Pyck, & Van den Berghe, 1987). Lachiewicz, Gullion, Spiridigliozzi, and Aylsworth (1987) report that this IQ decline begins in early childhood. In contrast, Dykens, Hodapp, Ort, Finucane, Shapiro, and Leckman (1989) have reported that IQ declines and MA plateaus in the late childhood or early adolescent years (ages 10–15 years). An additional report (Hagerman, Schreiner, Kemper, Wittenberger, Zahn, & Habicht, submitted) indicates that the greatest drop in IQ in their sample occurred between the ages of 8 and 12 years, spanning the age ranges in the two studies noted. Thus, although there is agreement that IQs eventually decline in many fragile X males, the exact point at which this is likely to occur remains unclear. Additional longitudinal and cross-sectional studies with large numbers of fragile X males are needed to precisely delineate the parameters of the age range in which IQ declines and MA plateaus.

The question of why IQ remains relatively stable at early ages but declines in the early teen years remains problematic. Some researchers have speculated that this premature decline in IQ may be related to regulatory factors responsible for the initiation of puberty in that the earliest signs of cognitive plateauing in these males appear to coincide with the earliest signs of their pubertal development (Dykens, Hodapp, Ort, Finucane, Shapiro, & Leckman, 1989). Other researchers, however, have hypothesized that the drop in IQ occurs because the abstract reasoning and symbolic language skills that are stressed in the intellectual assessments of later childhood may be problematic for many fragile X males (Hagerman, Schreiner, Kemper, Wittenberger, Zahn, & Habicht, submitted). These hypotheses raise the question of whether IQ changes are due to changes in the "developmental tasks" facing the child or to changes in the development of the neurological system. This issue of task versus maturation has been discussed in relation to Down syndrome children (Hodapp & Zigler, in press; see chapter 12) and the development of normal children (McCall, Eichorn, & Hogarty, 1977). Additional longitudinal research should examine the contribution that these or other hypotheses make in explaining the IQ changes observed in fragile X males.

Implications for intervention

Studies of IQ trajectory confirm the importance of classifying research groups by etiology in that identifying differences between IQ trajectories of various groups will ultimately allow for more fine-tuned intervention efforts. Although it is too early to conclude that declines in IQ are an inevitable consequence of fragile X syndrome, findings from these studies may help in planning the timing and intensity of educational and vocational efforts with fragile X males; indeed these findings provide renewed impetus for the "earlier the better" focus of many intervention programs. Parents and teachers should be counseled that these findings do not necessarily signal a deterioration or loss of acquired cognitive skills. Rather, they should be informed about the possibility that in contrast to non-retarded children, whose cognitive development plateaus from 16 to 18 years of age, fragile X boys may plateau at an earlier period, somewhere between the ages of 10 to 15 years. Thus, fragile X children doing comparatively well in their earlier years may ultimately perform lower on IQ tests than previously thought. In addition, parents and educators should be counseled that this decline in IQ may not be apparent in the child's adaptive behavior, and that the relationship between IQ decline and the adaptive functioning of fragile X males remains unknown at present.

The family environment and fragile X syndrome

Although developmental theorists and researchers have traditionally focused on changes and processes within the child alone, there has been an increasing emphasis on the role played by the child's external environment at various points in both normal and atypical development (e.g., Sameroff, chapter 5, this volume). A considerable amount of this work in developmental psychology has been devoted to the child's immediate, interpersonal environment – primarily the family and mother–child interactions.

Fragile X syndrome provides several unique opportunities to examine environmental issues of concern to developmentalists – such as the child's family environment and mother–child interaction – that are not readily afforded in other retardation syndromes or in families with atypical members.

As previously discussed, approximately one-third to one-half of the females who carry the fragile X marker are themselves affected with the syndrome. These women may manifest mild to moderate mental retardation, or learning problems and disabilities that may be similar to the profiles of cognitive weaknesses manifest by affected males, such as poor attention span, difficulty with numerical reasoning, and auditory short-term memory (e.g., Kemper, Hagerman, Ahmad, & Mariner, 1986). Thus, some boys with fragile X syndrome reside in families in which their mothers and/or female siblings exhibit retardation or learning problems, others may have similarly affected male siblings, and still others may have families in which their mothers, sisters, and/or brothers are not at all affected with the syndrome. These variations in family constellation provide opportunities for researchers to compare mother–child interactions, sibling–child interactions, and so on in families with or without an affected mother or sibling, and to relate the findings to the affected males' intellectual, adaptive, and behavioral functioning. In short, the variable pattern of expression seen in fragile X syndrome provides a unique opportunity to tease apart the effects of the retardation syndrome from surrounding environmental stimulation.

In addition, recent research has suggested that many carrier females exhibit psychological and emotional difficulties such as anxiety (Hagerman & Smith, 1983), psychotic problems and shyness (Fyrns, 1986), and autistic behavior (Hagerman, Chudley, Knoll, Jackson, Kemper, & Ahmad, 1986). Most recently, Reiss, Hagerman, Vinogradov, Abrams, and King (1988) have reported an increase of schizophrenia spectrum disorders and a history of chronic affective disorders in a sample of 35 carrier mothers compared with a matched control group of mothers of developmentally delayed and behaviorally dysfunctional youngsters. Research on mother–child interactions in depressed and schizophrenic mothers in general points to considerable problems in maternal responsiveness to the needs of their children (Tronick & Field, 1986), as well as to deviant maternal communication patterns (Bateson, Jackson, Haley, & Weakland, 1956; Massie, 1982). As no studies have yet been reported that describe mother–child interactions of fragile X females who exhibit psychiatric or cognitive impairments, it is difficult to describe the impact that these maternal problems may have in the development of their sons and daughters affected with fragile X syndrome. It may be hypothesized, however, that the offspring of carrier females with multiple psychiatric and cognitive difficulties are at increased risk compared with fragile X boys with "normal" mothers. Until research that explores this hypothesis is available, the present findings of increased vulnerability to psychiatric and learning disabilities among some carrier females suggest that intervention efforts need to be carefully tailored to the needs of each individual family. For example, some families may require extra support and involvement from school officials, mental health agencies, outreach programs, and parent aid/education programs, and others will require less intensive or minimal efforts.

Directions for future research

Although data are fast accumulating on the genetic, behavioral, cognitive, adaptive, and maladaptive features of males with fragile X syndrome, many questions remain about their development in all areas of functioning. In addition, there are considerable gaps in our knowledge of carrier females, their profiles of cognitive and behavioral strengths and weaknesses, and the impact that affected mothers and siblings may have on family functioning.

Of particular interest to those concerned with the developmental approach to mental retardation are questions regarding the specificity of the cognitive, adaptive, linguistic, and behavioral profiles previously described, as well as the specificity of the IQ trajectory in fragile X syndrome. Further research is necessary to identify the extent to which these profiles and trajectories are shared by other etiological groups, and to describe how these findings confirm or contradict the extension of the two-group approach in organic retardation. In addition, the implication of the pervasive sequential-processing deficit observed in this syndrome for defect versus developmental theory needs to be described.

Many questions also remain that may have more immediate applicability to educators, parents, and health professionals who intervene on a daily basis with fragile X boys and men. For example, the relationship between the decline in IQ and the adaptive functioning of these males remains unclear, as does the age at which this decline is most apt to occur. The reasons why all boys with fragile X syndrome do not manifest this IQ decline also remain to be elucidated. In addition, there is a need to systematically evaluate the effectiveness of educational efforts and vocational strategies that capitalize on potential strengths in simultaneous processing and minimize the pervasive sequential-processing deficits often observed in these males. Finally, if future research identifies similarities in the cognitive and behavioral profiles of carrier females, nonpenetrant males, and affected males, then effective intervention strategies that optimize the functioning of all affected family members will have to be developed.

This recommendation for future research will be particularly helpful if it also describes the impact that carrier females with and without psychiatric and cognitive disabilities may have upon family functioning, mother–child interactions, and the development of their offspring affected with fragile X syndrome. Given the nature of these questions, future work in fragile X syndrome will necessarily require collaboration between many fields, including genetics, developmental and clinical psychology, child psychiatry, and special education.

References

American Psychiatic Association (1980). *Diagnostic and statistical manual of mental disorders* (3rd ed.). Washington, DC: American Psychiatric Association.

Baker, B. (1984). Intervention with families with young, severely handicapped children. In J. Blacher (Ed.), *Severely handicapped young children and their families*. New York: Academic Press.

Baller, W., Charles, P., & Miller, E. (1967). Mid-life attainment of the mentally retarded: A longitudinal study. *Genetic Psychology, 75*, 235–239.

Bateson, G., Jackson, D., Haley, J., & Weakland, J. (1956). Toward a theory of schizophrenia. *Science, 1*, 251–264.

Borghraef, M., Fryns, J., Dielkens, A., Pyck, K., & Van den Berghe J. (1987). Fragile X syndrome: A study of the psychological profile of 23 patients. *Clinical Genetics, 32*, 179–186.

Bregman, J., Dykens, E., Watson, M., Ort, S., & Leckman, J. (1987). Fragile X syndrome: Variability in phenotypic expression. *Journal of the American Academy of Child and Adolescent Psychiatry, 26*, 463–471.

Bregman, J., Leckman, J., & Ort, S. (in press). Fragile X syndrome: A model of genetic predisposition to psychopathology. *Journal of Autism and Developmental Disorders*.

Burack, J., Hodapp, R., & Zigler, E. (1988). Issues in the classification of mental retardation: Differentiating among organic etiologies. *Journal of Child Psychology and Psychiatry, 29*(6), 765–779.

Chudley, A. (1984). Behavioral phenotype. In J. Opitz & G. Sutherland (Eds.), Conference report: International workshop on the fragile X and X-linked mental retardation. *American Journal of Medical Genetics, 17*, 45–50.

Cruickshank, W., Hallahan, P., & Bice, H. (1976). The evaluation of intelligence. In W. Cruickshank (Ed.), *Cerebral palsy: A developmental disability* (3rd ed.). Syracuse, NY: Syracuse University Press.

Daker, M., Chidiac, P., Fear, L., & Berry, A. (1981). Fragile X in a normal male: A cautionary note. *Lancet, 1*, 780.

Dykens, E., Hodapp, R., & Leckman, J. (1987). Strengths and weaknesses in the intellectual functioning of males with fragile X syndrome. *American Journal of Mental Deficiency, 92*, 234–236.

Dykens, E., Hodapp, R., & Leckman, J. (1989). Adaptive and maladaptive functioning of institutionalized and noninstitutionalized fragile X males. *Journal of the American Academy of Child and Adolescent Psychiatry, 28*(3), 427–430.

Dykens, E., Hodapp, R., Ort, S., Finucane, B., Shapiro, L, & Leckman, J. (1989). The trajectory of cognitive development in males with fragile X syndrome. *Journal of the American Academy of Child and Adolescent Psychiatry, 28*(3), 422–428.

Dykens, E., Leckman, J., Paul, R., & Watson, M. (1987). The cognitive, behavioral, and adaptive functioning of fragile X and non-fragile X retarded men. *Journal of Autism and Developmental Disorders, 18*, 41–52.

Fishburn, J., Turner, G., Daniel, A., & Brookwell, R. (1983). The diagnosis and frequency of X-linked conditions in a cohort of moderately retarded males with affected brothers. *American Journal of Medical Genetics, 14*, 713–724.

Fryns, J. (1986). The female and the fragile X. *American Journal of Medical Genetics, 23*, 157–170.

Fyrns, J., Jacobs, P., Kleczkowska, A., & Van den Berghe, H. (1984). The psychological profile of the fragile X syndrome. *Clinical Genetics, 25*, 131–134.

Hagerman, R., Chudley, A., Knoll, J., Jackson, A., Kemper, M., & Ahmed, R. (1986). Autism in fragile X females. *American Journal of Medical Genetics, 23*, 375–380.

Hagerman, R., Jackson, A., Levitas, A., Rimland, B., & Braden, M. (1986). An analysis of autism in 50 males with fragile X syndrome. *American Journal of Medical Genetics, 23*, 359–374.

Hagerman, R., Kemper, M., & Hudson, M. (1985). Learning disabilities and attentional problems in boys with fragile X syndrome. *American Journal of Diseases in Children, 139*, 674–678.

Hagerman, R., Murphy, M., & Wittenberger, M. (1987, December). *A controlled trial of stimulant medication in children with the fragile X syndrome.* Paper presented to the First National Fragile X Conference, Denver, CO.

Hagerman, R., Schreiner, R., Kemper, M., Wittenberger, M., Zahn, B., & Habicht, K. *Longitudinal IQ changes in fragile X males.* Manuscript submitted for publication.

Hagerman, F., & Smith, A. (1983). The heterozygous female. In R. Hagerman & P. McBogg (Eds.), *The fragile X syndrome: Diagnosis, biochemistry, and intervention.* Dillon, CO: Spectra Publishing.

Hagerman, R., VanHousen, K., Smith, A., & McGauran, L. (1984). Consideration of connective tissue dysfunction in the fragile X syndrome. *American Journal of Medical Genetics, 17*, 111–121.

Herbst, D. (1980). Nonspecific X-linked mental retardation I: A review with information from 24 families. *American Journal of Medical Genetics, 7*, 443–460.

Herbst, D., Dunn, H., Dill, F., Kalousek, D., & Krywaniuk, L. (1981). Further delineation of X-linked mental retardation. *Human Genetics, 58*, 366–371.

Herbst, D., & Miller, J. (1980). Nonspecific X-linked mental retardation II: The frequency in British Columbia. *American Journal of Medical Genetics, 7*, 461–470.

Hill, B., & Bruininks, R. (1984). Maladaptive behavior of mentally retarded individuals in residential facilities. *American Journal of Mental Deficiency, 88*, 380–387.

Hodapp, R., & Zigler, E. (in press). Applying the developmental perspective to individuals with Down syndrome. In D. Cicchetti & M. Beeghly (Eds.), *Children with Down syndrome: A developmental perspective.* New York Cambridge University Press.

Howard-Peebles, O., Stoddard, G., & Mims, M. (1979). Familial X-linked mental retardation, verbal disability, and marker X chromosomes. *American Journal of Medical Genetics, 31*, 214–222.

Jacobs, P., Glover, T., Magner, M., Fox, P., Gerrard, J., Dunn, H., & Herbst, D. (1980). X-linked mental retardation: A study of 7 families. *American Journal of Medical Genetics, 7*, 471–489.

Kaufman, A., & Kaufman, N. (1983). *Kaufman assessment battery for children.* Circle Pines, MN: American Guidance Service.

Kaufman, A., Kaufman, N., & Goldsmith, B. (1984). *Kaufman sequential or simultaneous (K-SOS): A leaders guide.* Circle Pines, MN: American Guidance Service.

Kemper, M., Hagerman, R., Ahmad, R., & Mariner, R. (1986). Cognitive profiles and the spectrum of clinical manifestations in heterozygous fra (X) females. *American Journal of Medical Genetics, 23,* 139–156.

Kemper, M., Hagerman, R., & Altshul-Stark, D. (1987, December). *Cognitive profiles of boys with the fragile X syndrome.* Paper presented to the First National Fragile X Conference, Denver, CO.

King, R., Raynes, N., & Tizard, J. (1971). *Patterns for residential care: Sociological studies in institutions for handicapped children.* London: Routledge & Kegan Paul.

Lachiewicz, A., Gullion, C., Spiridigliozzi, G., & Aylsworth, A. (1987). Declining IQs of males with fragile X syndrome. *American Journal of Mental Retardation, 92,* 272–278.

Landesman-Dwyer, S., & Sulzbacher, F. (1981). Residential placement and adaptation of severely and profoundly retarded individuals. In R. Bruininks, C. Meyers, C. Stiedard, & K. Lakin (Eds.), *Deinstitutionalization and community adjustment of mentally retarded people.* Washington, DC: American Association on Mental Deficiency.

Leckman, J. (1987, December). *Cognitive and neuropsychological features of the fragile X syndrome.* Paper presented to the First National Fragile X Conference, Denver, CO.

Lejune, J. (1982). Is the fragile X syndrome amenable to treatment? *Lancet, 1,* 273–274.

Lubs, H. (1969). A marker-X chromosome. *American Journal of Medical Genetics, 21,* 231–244.

Marans, W., Paul, R., & Leckman, J. (1987, November). *Speech and language profiles in males with fragile X syndrome.* Paper presented to the American Speech and Hearing Association Annual Convention, New Orleans, LA.

Massie, H.N. (1982). Affective development and the organization of mother-infant behavior from the perspective of psychopathology. In E.Z. Tronick (Ed.), *Social interchange in infancy: Affect, cognition, and communication.* Baltimore: University Park Press.

Mattei, J., Mattei, M., Aumeras, C., Auger, M., & Giraud, F. (1981). X-linked mental retardation with the fragile X: A study of 15 families. *Human Genetics, 59,* 281–289.

McCall, R.B., Eichorn, D., & Hogarty, P. (1977). Transitions in early mental development. *Monographs of the Society for Research in Child Development, 42.*

Mundy, P., & Kasari, C. (this volume). The similar structure hypothesis and differential rate of development in mental retardation. Chapter 4.

Murphy, P., Kidd, J., Breg, R., Ruddle, F., & Kidd, K. (1985). An anonymous single copy X-chromosome clone, DX 579, from Xq26–Xq28, identifies a moderately frequent RFLP [HGM 8 provisional no. DX 579]. *Nucleic Acids Research, 13,* 3015.

Opitz, J. (1984). History, nosology, and bibliography of X-linked retardation. In J. Opitz & G. Sutherland (Eds.), Conference report: International workshop on the fragile X and X-linked retardation. *American Journal of Medical Genetics, 17,* 19–33.

Paul, R., Cohen, D., Breg, R., Watson, M., & Herman, S. (1984). Fragile X syndrome: Its relation to speech and language disorders. *Journal of Speech and Hearing Disorders, 49,* 328–332.

Paul, R., Dykens, E., Leckman, J., Watson, M., Breg, R., & Cohen D. (1987). A comparison of language characteristics of mentally retarded adults with fragile X syndrome and those with nonspecific retardation and autism. *Journal of Autism and Developmental Disorders, 17,* 457–468.

Pueschel, S., Gallagher, P., Zartler, A., & Puezzullo, J. (1987). Cognitive and learning processes in children with Down syndrome. *Research in Developmental Disabilities, 8,* 21–37.

Reiss, A., Hagerman, R., Vinogradov, S., Abrams, M., & King, R. (1988). Psychiatric disability in female carriers of the fragile X chromosome. *Archives of General Psychiatry, 45,* 25–30.

Ross, R., Begab, M., Dondis, E. Giampiccolo, J., & Meyers, C. (1985). *Lives of the mentally retarded: A forty year follow-up study*. Stanford: Stanford University Press.

Samaroff, A. (1990). The role of the environment in developmental theory. In R. Hodapp, J. Burack, & E. Zigler (Eds.), *Issues in the developmental approach to mental retardation*. New York: Cambridge University Press.

Sherman, S.L., Jacobs, P.A., Morton, N., Froster-Iskenivs, V., Howard-Peebles, P.N., Nelson, K.B., Partington, M.W., Sutherland, G.R., Turner, G., & Water M. (1985). Further segregation analysis of the fragile X syndrome with special reference to transmitting males. *Human Genetics, 69*, 289–299.

Silverstein, A. (1982). A note on the constancy of IQ. *American Journal of Mental Deficiency, 87*, 227–228.

Silverstein, A., Goldberg, C., Kasner, A., & Solomon, B. (1984). An attempt to determine the intellectual strengths and weaknesses of EMR children. *American Journal of Mental Deficiency, 88*, 435–437.

Sparrow, S., Balla, D., & Cicchetti, D. (1984). *Vineland scales of adaptive behavior*. Circle Pines, MN: American Guidance Service.

Sudhalter, V., (1987, December). Speech and language characteristics and intervention strategies with fragile X patients. Paper presented to the First National Fragile X Conference, Denver, CO.

Sutherland, G. (1977). Fragile sites on human chromosomes: Demonstration of their dependence on the type of culture medium. *Science, 17*, 119–123.

Tronick, E., & Field, T. (1986). Maternal depression and infant disturbance. In E. Tronick & T. Field (Eds.), *New directions for child development, No. 34*. San Francisco: Jossey-Bass.

Turner, G., Brookwell, R., Daniel, A., Selikowitz, M., & Zilibowitz, M. (1980). Heterozygous expression of X-linked mental retardation and X-chromosome marker fra(X) (q27). *New England Journal of Medicine, 303*, 662–664.

Webb, T., Bundey, S., Thake, A., & Todd, J. (1986). Population incidence and segregation ratios in the Martin-Bell syndrome. *American Journal of Medical Genetics, 23*, 573–580.

Windle, C. (1962). Prognosis of mental subnormals. *American Journal of Mental Deficiency, 66* (Monograph Supplement to No. 5).

Wolff, P., Gardner, J., Lappen, J., Paccia, J., & Schnell, R. (1987, December). *Social adaptation and behavior in males with the fragile X syndrome*. Paper presented to the First National Fragile X Conference, Denver, CO.

Zigler, E. (1967). Familial mental retardation: A continuing dilemma. *Science, 155*, 292–298.

Zigler, E. (1969). Developmental versus difference theories of mental retardation and the problem of motivation. *American Journal of Mental Deficiency, 73*, 536–556.

Zigler, E., & Hodapp, R. (1986). *Understanding mental retardation*. New York: Cambridge University Press.

Zigler, E., & Seitz, V. (1982). Future research on socialization and personality development. In E. Zigler, I. Child, & M. Lamb (Eds.), *Socialization and personality development* (2nd ed.). New York: Oxford Univerity Press.

10   Deviance and developmental approaches in the study of autism

Fred R. Volkmar, Jacob A. Burack, and Donald J. Cohen

Deviance and developmental approaches

The study of atypical development and behavior, particularly of the most deviant kind, is valuable in understanding the universality of the human "blueprint" for development. It has been argued that certain aspects of psychological growth are common to all persons and that even the most atypical behaviors and developmental patterns must be viewed within the context of normal developmental processes (see chapter 3). The study of children with autism provides a particularly cogent test of this hypothesis. The disorder is characterized by an early onset of extreme impairments in social, communicative, and cognitive development, and an extremely poor outcome. The pattern of social-communicative deviance observed in autism is unusual; as Rutter and Garmezy (1983) have pointed out, autism is "in some respects the clearest example of a disease entity in child psychiatry" (p. 794). Given the distinctiveness and severity of the condition, any observation of commonalities of development between autistic and less severely handicapped and nonhandicapped individuals would support the notion of developmental "universals"; similarly, the great variability of developmental functioning within autistic individuals, and the heterogeneity of syndrome expression of the disorder, provides potentially important insights into the limits of behavioral organization in the developing individual. Conversely, the utilization of developmental theory may provide a framework within which certain aspects of behavior and developmental functioning in autistic persons can be understood.

Dr. Burack is now at the Hebrew University in Jerusalem, Israel. This work was supported in part by the William T. Grant Foundation, MHCRC Grant 30929, CCRC Grant RR00125, NICHD Grant HD-03008, NIMH Grant MH00418, the John Merck Fund, and Mr. Leonard Berger.

246

Important effects of developmental level in relation to syndrome expression of autism have been recognized; yet, traditional developmental frameworks do not seem to adequately explain the clinical features of autism. Early studies suggested that the development of autistic children was erratic and characterized by lags and spurts (Fish, Shapiro, Halpern, & Wile, 1965; NSAC, 1978; Ritvo, 1976), was uneven (DeMyer, Hintgen, & Jackson, 1981; Loveland & Kelley, 1988; Snow, Hertzig, & Shapiro, 1987; Treffert, 1988; Volkmar, Sparrow, Goudreau, Cicchetti, Paul, & Cohen, 1987), and was sometimes characterized by unusual patterns of developmental regression (Harper & Williams, 1975; Hoshino, Kancko, Yashima, Kumashiro, Volkmar, & Cohen, 1987). Such notions are not compatible with usual concepts of developmental orderliness and invariance, and suggest major limitations in the application of usual developmental models in the study of autistic individuals.

This view has recently been questioned by studies of atypical populations (see chapter 1) and by attempts to view development in autism within usual developmental frameworks (e.g., Morgan, 1986). The observations that many autistic individuals are also mentally retarded and that many severely retarded individuals show increased levels of autistic-like behavior (Freeman, Schroth, Ritvo, Guttue, & Wake 1980; Wing & Gould, 1979) have emphasized the importance of viewing developmental characteristics of autistic individuals within the context of general developmental delay. It has become increasingly evident that neither deviance nor developmental approaches alone can provide a comprehensive framework for the study of autism. On the one hand, the deviance model ignores the importance of developmental level and change observed. On the other hand, the developmental model alone cannot explain many of the bizarre and deviant characteristics of the disorder. The study of autism offers an important opportunity to integrate both developmental and deviance approaches in the attempt to derive a truly developmental psychopathology of the condition – that is, one that encompasses developmental factors and behavioral deviance.

Autism as a diagnostic concept

The reluctance to study autism from a developmental perspective can best be understood within a historical framework. This framework provides a context for initial and subsequent views on the validity and definition of the disorder. Such a framework illustrates the importance of explicit and implicit assumptions that guide research in developmental psychopathology.

Historical background

In 1943, Leo Kanner described 11 children with an unusual – and previously unrecognized – syndrome characterized by profound social disinterest and insistence on sameness, as well as unusual language development, unusual sensitivities to aspects of the inanimate environment, and highly unusual motor and other behaviors. Kanner coined the term early infantile autism to suggest the apparent congenital nature of the condition and the withdrawn, inner-directed quality of these children. He carefully framed his observations of social deviance within a developmental context and emphasized the markedly deviant social disinterest of these cases. Although his phenomenological description has proven remarkably robust, some of the early speculations of Kanner and others suggested false leads for research.

Kanner's concept aroused considerable controversy, particularly because it questioned existing assumptions about psychopathology. For example, many investigators assumed that some fundamental continuity must exist between psychiatric disorders in adults and those observed in children. This assumption was reflected in the presumption that autism was a type of psychosis much like adult psychoses, particularly schizophrenia. This view minimized the role of developmental aspects of reality testing (Piaget, 1955) and the difficulties inherent in employing such concepts in children with marked communication problems. The notion that autism must represent the earliest manifestation of schizophrenia similarly reflected an assumption of continuity based on (1) severity, (2) broad concepts of schizophrenic illness, and (3) the unintended point of confusion introduced by Kanner's use of the term "autism."

Another source of controversy arose in regard to Kanner's observation that the parents of his cases were unusually successful people who interacted in rather unusual ways with their children. Although Kanner's initial description emphasized the apparent congenital nature of the condition, this mention of deviant parenting style suggested a potential role of early experience in syndrome pathogenesis (e.g., Bettleheim, 1967; Desperet, 1956). Early psychodynamic views minimized the influence of the child on mediating parent–child interaction, and often seemed to blame parents for the child's disorder. Kanner also suggested that the disorder was not associated with other medical conditions, nor with mental retardation. Accordingly, for many years, children who exhibited an autistic-like condition in association with some obvious medical condition or organic insult were thought to exhibit secondary autism, and deficits in intellectual skills observed during administration of IQ tests were attributed to poor testability or negativism.

Validity of the diagnostic concept

These controversies were resolved over the course of several decades as various lines of evidence that supported the validity of autism as a meaningful diagnostic concept became available. Studies of series of cases of childhood "psychosis" (Kolvin, 1971; Volkmar, Cohen, Hoshino, Rende, & Paul, 1988) revealed that autistic children differed from children with more classic schizophrenia in many ways – including clinical features, age of onset, family history, course, IQ, and associated organic problems. They differed from nonautistic retarded children and children with severe language disorders in terms of the pattern of their social, communicative, and cognitive development (Rutter, 1978). Longitudinal and other data suggested that some aspects of Kanner's description and speculations had to be modified. For example, it became clear that autism was often associated with other medical conditions (e.g., seizures) and with other disorders (e.g., congenital rubella); that autistic children typically functioned within the mentally retarded range when appropriate tests were employed; and that the IQ was relatively stable and predictive of adult outcome (Alpern, 1962; DeMyer, Hintgen, & Jackson, 1981). Similarly, it became apparent that whereas the disorder was fairly uncommon (Zahner & Pauls, 1987), it could be found in all social classes (Wing, 1980), and that neither specific deficits in parenting nor parental psychopathology could account for the condition (Cantwell, Rutter, & Baker, 1978; Cox, Rutter, Newman, & Partak, 1975).

It should also be noted that investigators have tended to assume that various aspects of the syndrome were, in some sense, primary. Speculation centered, for example, around such varied notions as disturbances in perception (Ornitz & Ritvo, 1968), arousal (Tinbergen & Tinbergen, 1972), cognition (Prior, 1979), and language (Rutter, Bartak, & Newman, 1981). Cairns (1979) has described an implicit cognitive primacy hypothesis – that children's cognitions are the predominant determinants of behavior – that has contributed to a relative neglect of certain aspects of development in autism, particularly those relating to social development.

Organic factors

There is now considerable evidence suggesting the importance of organic factors in the pathogenesis of autism. Signs of CNS dysfunction include the persistence of primitive reflexes and various abnormalities on neurological examination, an increased incidence of seizure disorders, and abnormalities on EEG, CT, and MRI examination, etc. (Courchesne, Yeung-Courchesne, Press, & Jernigal, 1988; Golden, 1987). Seizure disorders are common among autistic individuals, and the pattern of seizure onset, usually in adolescence, is unusual (Deykin & McMahon, 1979; Rutter 1970). It is also now clear that autism can be observed in association with a wide variety of medical conditions – for example, congenital infections (e.g., congenital rubella), metabolic disorders (e.g., PKU), chromosome abnormalities (e.g., fragile X syndrome). However, no single disorder or laboratory finding has been invariably associated with autism, and it remains unclear why some individuals with certain specific conditions are autistic whereas others are not.

Along with other lines of evidence, the observation of associations of autism with various conditions has given rise to various attempts to identify potential neuropathological models for the disorder (Ornitz, 1987). Defects have been hypothesized at various anatomic sites and in various neurobiological systems; at present, there is little evidence to support any precise hypothesis. Neuropathological and neuroanatomic studies have provided conflicting results (e.g., Williams, Hauser, Purpura, Delong, & Swisher, 1980; Courchesne, Yeung-Courchesne, Press & Jernigan, 1988). Neurochemical studies have consistently revealed an increased peripheral level of the neurotransmitter serotonin in about 40% of cases (Anderson & Hoshino, 1987). The relevance of this finding is unclear because elevated serotonin levels are found in other disorders including mental retardation, serotonin levels are not related to aspects of syndrome expression, and the relationship of peripheral levels of serotonin to CNS functioning remains unclear.

The possibility that genetic mechanisms may play a role in the pathogenesis of the disorder is supported by the observation that the incidence of the condition increased in siblings, particularly in monozygotic twins (see Pauls, 1987 for a review). Higher rates of autism are also noted among siblings of autistic children, and nonautistic siblings are more likely to exhibit some cognitive impairment (August, Stewart, & Tsai, 1981).

Although precise mechanisms accounting for syndrome pathogenesis remain to be clearly established, overt evidence of organicity is associated with greater degrees of intellectual impairment and worse outcomes. Autistic individuals with IQs of less than 50, for example, are more likely to develop seizure disorders. Autistic individuals with higher levels of organic involvement, as evidenced by greater frequency of physical anomalies, have been noted to have lower IQ scores (Links, Stockwell, Abichandani, & Simeon, 1980). Volkmar et al. (1988) assessed the degree of apparent organic involvement in relation to intellectual functioning in 142 clinically autistic individuals. Cases were grouped into three categories – idiopathic (no evidence of organic pathology), stigmatic (some evidence

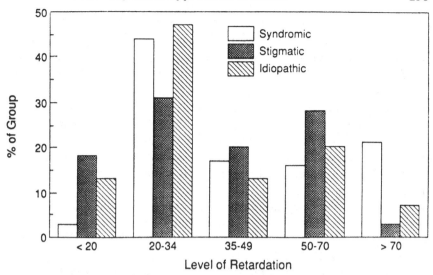

Figure 10.1. Degree of organic involvement in a series of 122 autistic individuals in relation to level of mental retardation. Adapted from Volkmar et al., 1988.

of organic pathology not diagnostic of a specific syndrome or seizure disorder), and syndromic (clear association with a specific syndrome or seizure disorder). Nearly 50% of this autistic sample showed some evidence of overt organicity (see Figure 10.1). The degree of organicity was inversely related to IQ – autistic children with lower IQ scores had the highest proportion of organic pathology.

Diagnosis and definition

As the validity of the autistic syndrome was recognized, attempts were made to refine the diagnostic concept using both categorical and dimensional approaches. The task of arriving at truly operational, reliable, and valid definitions of the disorder is complicated by the need to address both issues of development change and behavioral deviance (Zigler, 1969).

Categorical approaches

Categorical approaches to diagnosis of autism reflected the consensus on the validity of the diagnostic concept and the advent of new diagnostic approaches such as multiaxial classification (Rutter, Shaffer, & Shepherd, 1975) and diagnostic criteria (Spitzer, Endicott, & Robins, 1978). Rutter's (1978) synthesis of Kanner's original description and subsequent research was particularly influential. He proposed features essential for the diagnosis: (1) onset before 30 months, (2) impaired social and communicative development of a distinctive type (not simply the result of intellectual level), and (3) a variety of unusual behaviors subsumed under the general category of insistence on sameness (e.g., resistance to change, unusual preoccupation, and abnormal play patterns). The National Society for Autistic Children (1978) definition also emphasized the importance of social and communicative deviance, and additionally included disturbances in rates and sequencs of development and disturbed responses to sensory stimuli. Although neither of these proposed definitions specified explicit, operational diagnostic criteria (i.e., how impaired must social development be and in what specific ways), the availability of these definitions, particularly that of Rutter (1978), significantly facilitated subsequent research. Rutter's definition was in large part the basis of the definition of autism included in DSM III (APA, 1980).

Autism's inclusion as an "official" psychiatric diagnosis for the first time in DSM III (APA, 1980) reflected substantial agreement on the validity, distinctive course, and clinical features of the disorder. In DSM III, infantile autism was included in a new diagnostic class, the pervasive developmental disorders. Diagnostic criteria for autism emphasized the early onset (before 30 months) of pervasive social unresponsiveness, unusual patterns of communication, and of environmental responsivity, and the absence of signs and symptoms more typical of schizophrenia. Advantages and disadvantages of this scheme were apparent (see Cohen, Paul, & Volkmar, 1987 for a review). Problems included a general overemphasis on the infantile aspect of autism (i.e., criteria proposed were most applicable to younger children) (Volkmar, Cohen, & Paul, 1986). The implicit notion that autistic individuals grew out of autism was suggested by the inclusion of a residual autism category. This view was not supported by evidence that suggested persistence of significant difficulties into adult life (DeMyer et al., 1981). An attempt was made to deal with these problems in DSM III-R (APA, 1987), the revision of DSM III.

The DSM III-R criteria for autistic disorder are more elaborate than in DSM III, and were greatly influenced by the work of Lorna Wing and her collaborators, which suggested the need for a somewhat broader view of the disorder (Wing & Gould, 1979) than that of Rutter (1978). This broadened concept was meant to include both low functioning (Wing & Gould, 1979) and very high functioning (Wing, 1981) individuals. Criteria proposed for autistic disorder were more developmentally oriented in an attempt to encompass the entire range of syndrome expression over various ages and developmental levels. The infantile aspects of the disorder were deemphasized, and criteria were explicitly framed with a developmental context. Although many of these changes appeared to be justified, recent work (Volkmar et al., in press) suggests that the concept has been significantly broadened. A general problem with this and other categorical diagnostic approaches has been the importance of framing observations of social and communicative behavior within a developmental context without explicit methods for doing so. Dimensional approaches to diagnosis offer important alternative ways of defining the disorder that can take developmental factors into account.

Dimensional approaches

Various instruments have been developed for diagnosis, assessment, and behavioral characterization of autism (Parks, 1983). These instruments differ from categorical approaches in important ways, although many such instruments also provide for a categorical diagnosis. The development and use of these instruments is complicated by several factors (Volkmar & Cohen, 1988a). Given the communicative problems of affected persons, parental or teacher reports are sometimes unreliable. Observational instruments suffer from other problems – for example, symptoms may vary in response to differences in the environment (Volkmar, Hoder, & Cohen, 1985), and some important but low-frequency behaviors (e.g., self-abuse) may be difficult to incorporate within observational schemes. Typically, a deviance model as opposed to a developmental model (Zigler, 1969) is employed because deviant behaviors are sampled or rated, and issues of standardization are particularly problematic.

The developmental approach to assessment is also represented in the use of well standardized, normative assessment instruments for cognitive and communicative functioning (Cohen et al., 1987). Volkmar et al., (1987) have recently extended this approach to operational definitions of social dysfunction as well.

Subtypes of autism

Various attempts to categorize autistic individuals into subgroups have been made over the years, and reflect an awareness of the tremendous range in syndrome expression (Volkmar & Cohen, 1988a). Early attempts to develop subgroups were based on the absence or presence of associated medical conditions (i.e., "primary" vs. "secondary" autism). Similar attempts have been made around various features such as biological findings (e.g., hyperserotonemia), age of onset and severity (e.g., as in DSM III), early perinatal and prenatal factors, and so on. Wing has recently proposed (Wing & Atwood, 1987) a subtyping system related to social characteristics of affected individuals. Probably the most commonly proposed subtyping system has revolved around IQ (see Volkmar, 1987b). Lower IQ (<55) individuals have a worse prognosis, are more likely to exhibit seizures, and so on. The prepotence of IQ as a predictor of outcome is, of course, not limited to autism, and serves as a reminder of the importance of developmental level for ultimate adjustment.

Syndrome expression: Developmental and deviance aspects

As issues of syndrome validity and definition were gradually clarified, it became possible to examine specific aspects of development in autistic individuals. These studies have helped to suggest which aspects of syndrome expression are best understood within a developmental framework as opposed to those features that represent truly deviant patterns of development. For example, the recognition that autism was typically observed in association with mental retardation suggested that one could examine important potential contributions of developmental level (e.g., MA) per se to aspects of syndrome expression. Studies have revealed areas both of developmental continuity and discontinuity between individuals with autism and those with other developmental disabilities. The delineation of areas in which development is truly deviant has important implications for our understanding of autism and for developmental psychopathology in general.

Onset

In his use of the words "early" and "infantile" in his initial term for autism, Kanner (1943) noted an important and distinctive feature of the disorder – its very early onset. Initially, Kanner thought that the disorder was truly congenital – that is, present from birth – although he and others subsequently noted that autism occasionally appeared after a relatively short period of apparently normal development. Subsequent research (e.g., Kolvin, 1971) has confirmed the importance of this observation. Most definitions of the disorder emphasize this early onset by indicating that the disorder either must be present by 30 or 36 months of age (e.g., APA, 1980; Rutter, 1978) or that this usually is so (APA, 1987).

Volkmar, Stier, and Cohen (1985) ascertained apparent age of onset (or, as it might more properly be termed, age of recognition) of autism in 103

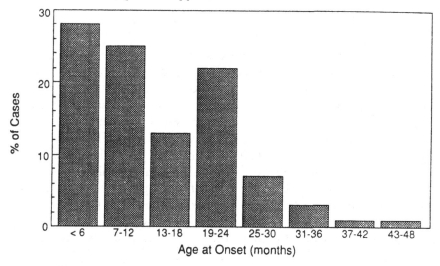

Figure 10.2. Age of onset (recognition) of autism. Adapted from Volkmar, Stier, and Cohen, 1985.

autistic individuals. Data from this study are presented in Figure 10.2. The vast majority of cases were identified in the first 2 years of life. Moreover, the rare case with an onset after age 3 years was often observed in association with some medical condition that appeared to affect the CNS. Given the centrality of marked social dysfunction as a diagnostic hallmark of the syndrome, and the usual sociability of infants, the observation that cases are identified early in life may not seem surprising. It does, however, suggest an important difference from other disorders.

In mental retardation not associated with autism, typically only the most severely retarded individuals are identified early in life, with milder degrees of retardation identified later in childhood (Tarjan, Wright, Eyman, & Keeran, 1973). In autism, however, almost all cases are identified by age 3 years, and most by age 2 years. Although it might be argued that the degree of retardation is the salient factor for recognition – that the early recognition reflects the severity of the associated retardation – this does not seem to be the case for several reasons. Nonretarded autistic individuals are also typically detected early in life. Although Volkmar et al. (1985) noted that onset was not significantly related to IQ, Short and Schopler (1988) noted that severity of autism could be related to onset, and that 94% of cases were recognized by age 3 years. Thus, in terms of apparent onset of the condition, autism appears to differ from mental retardation per se. This difference appears to be based on the early social-communicative deviance as originally described by Kanner.

Cognitive development

Although early investigators tended to invoke notions like "untestability" (Alpern, 1962) or "negativism" (Cowan, Hoddinott, & Wright, 1965) to account for poor performance on standard assessment instruments, a considerable body of research has subsequently shown autism to be related to basic cognitive deficits that involve impairments in symbolic, sequencing, abstracting, and coding skills (DeMyer et al., 1981; Prior, 1979; Rutter & Garmezy, 1983). The pattern of intellectual skills in autism is often marked by unusual scatter and "splinter" skills unlike that typically observed in mental retardation not associated with autism (Zigler & Hodapp, 1986). Autistic individuals tend in general to perform better on tasks involving memory or visual–spatial skills compared with tasks that require verbal encoding or sequencing of information or imitation. Some autistic individuals exhibit remarkable – and isolated – skills. These can include great feats of memory, calculation (e.g., the ability to correctly predict days of the weeks for dates years in advance), or drawing (e.g., Selfe, 1977; Treffert, 1988).

This pattern of performance differs from that typically observed in mental retardation and may to some extent have accounted for early impressions of normal intellectual level. However, it is clear that a majority of autistic individuals function in the mentally retarded range, with many being severely and profoundly retarded (DeMyer et al., 1974; Volkmar & Cohen, 1988a, b). Full scale IQ data from a series of 229 cases evaluated at the Child Study Center at Yale University are presented in Figure 10.3. In this series, over half the cases had full-scale IQ scores of 50 or less. This result is consistent with other studies, which suggest that between 50% and 75% of autistic children have IQs below 50 (DeMyer et al., 1974; Rutter & Lockyer, 1967), and with other reports of distribution of levels of retardation in persons with organic retardation (Zigler & Hodapp, 1986). Individuals with IQs of 50 or less have the worst long-term prognosis, are more likely to be mute and to exhibit seizures, and so on. (Rutter & Garmezy, 1983).

Although the distribution of scores over levels of mental retardation has varied somewhat between samples (Volkmar & Cohen, 1988a, b), presumably reflecting differences in diagnostic practices and criteria, it seems reasonably clear that autistic individuals are even more impaired than nonautistic mentally retarded individuals with the same intellectual level, reflecting in part the associated problems in communication and social interaction. Follow-up studies of autistic individuals with normal levels of intelligence have noted the persistence of marked abnormalities in

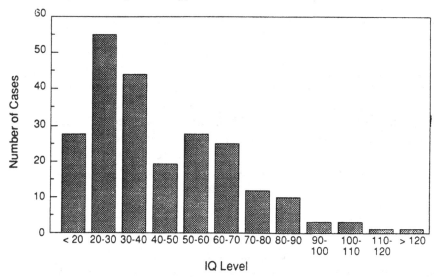

Figure 10.3. Distribution of full-scale IQ scores in a sample of 229 autistic individuals.

social relationship and adjustment in adulthood (Volkmar & Cohen, 1985; Rumsey, Rapoport, & Scerry, 1985).

Relationships between autism and level of intelligence are of great theoretical importance. To the extent that autistic individuals also suffer from associated mental retardation, it becomes critically important to identify which aspects of the syndrome may, most parsimoniously, be viewed as a reflection of IQ. The observation that "autistic-like" behaviors are more common among severely retarded individuals raises an important – and complicated – issue (Freeman et al., 1980; Wing & Gould, 1979). Variations in diagnostic practices are greatest at either end of the IQ distribution. Some investigators (e.g., Wing & Gould, 1979) advocate a broad concept of autism that may include many severely retarded persons; the utility of this broader concept remains to be clearly established (Rutter & Garmezy, 1987). Conversely, the examination of autistic individuals functioning within the normal range of intelligence may suggest which aspects of the syndrome are least related to developmental level per se.

To address potential confoundings with developmental level, behavioral and developmental features must be examined in relationship to other groups of mentally retarded persons at similar MA and IQ levels. Such comparisons are particularly important for assessment of developmental notions of similar developmental sequence (see chapter 3) and structure (see chapter 4); these comparisons help to identify specific developmental features or behaviors that are not simply a reflection of developmental level.

The notion that autism increases dramatically as IQ declines has been taken to suggest the primacy of cognitive factors in syndrome pathogenesis. In this view, impaired cognitive processes leading to problems in communication and social relationships are fundamental to the disorder, and behavioral and emotional problems are viewed as secondary aspects of the condition. However, the occurrence of autism in persons with IQs in the normal range suggests that autism cannot be totally accounted for by developmental delay unless, of course, it is assumed that the condition is fundamentally different in such individuals.

Social development

The social dysfunction observed in autism is unique in several respects. It is not like that observed even in normal infants; it differs from that usually observed in retarded, nonautistic, individuals; and it cannot be accounted for simply by general developmental level (Cohen et al., 1987). Unlike normally developing infants who are profoundly social creatures (Stern, 1985), young autistic children show little interest in social interaction (see Volkmar, 1987a, for a review). For example, the human face appears to be of little interest to these children, who fail to engage in the early social-communicative dialogues of infancy and who fail to form specific attachments to care givers unlike children with Down syndrome (Berry, Gunn, & Andrews, 1980). Although the social deficits in autism are most profound among the youngest and most severely affected individuals, even the highest functioning autistic adults exhibit marked deficits in social interaction (Volkmar & Cohen, 1985).

Despite the fact that investigators have emphasized the importance of social deficits, surprisingly little research has been done on social aspects of autism (Volkmar, 1987a). This has reflected both the operation of an implicit "cognitive primacy hypothesis" (Cairns, 1979) and the awareness that some rudimentary capacities for social interaction often develop as the child grows older. This lack of research is surprising because social deficits are consistently regarded as being central for purposes of syndrome definition, and some diagnostic schemes (e.g., Rutter, 1978) emphasize the deviance of social developmental level relative to general developmental level. Although a few attempts have been made to provide greater description and operational definitions of social dysfunction (Parks, 1983; Volkmar et al., 1987), this aspect of the disorder remains poorly characterized and understood. An understanding of the pathogenesis of social dysfunction and its relationship to other aspects of development may be particularly important for understanding the limits of developmental organization in autistic individuals.

Language and communication

Language and communication skills are particular areas of deficit in autistic persons that apparently cannot be simply explained by developmental delay (Paul, 1987), suggesting some limitations of the developmental approach and similar-sequence hypothesis in communicative development. Early in life, autistic children show deficits in play and in the usual social-communicative transactions of infancy that are considered to be important precursors to the development of language and communication skills (Bartak, Rutter, & Cox, 1975; Sigman & Ungerer, 1981). Paul (1987) has noted the marked preverbal limitations typically apparent in autism, especially those that require joint attention and social reference. Similarly, language often fails to develop at all, and as many as 50% of autistic individuals remain mute throughout their lives. Ultimate outcome depends on both the acquisition of communicative speech by age 5 years (Eisenberg & Kanner, 1956) and on cognitive skills. When language does develop, it is typically very deviant, and is characterized by echolalia, pronoun reversal, marked abnormalities in intonation, and by quite limited use within social contexts. The language and communication deficits observed in autism differ from those observed both in mental retardation and developmental language disorders (Paul, 1987).

At the same time, developmental perspectives do clarify at least some aspects of those communication skills that do develop. Echolalia, for example, was often viewed as an attempt to avoid social interaction. Recent work (e.g., Prizant & Schuler, 1987) has noted that echoed utterances may serve various adaptive functions, and echolalia is also seen in normal development (Weir, 1962; Paul, 1987). There is some evidence to suggest that when language skills are attained, they are done so in a similar manner to that observed in the general population (Burack et al., 1988).

Behavioral features and developmental level

The association of autism and mental retardation presents important problems and opportunities for research studies. It is clear that developmental level must be considered in examining aspects of behavioral and developmental functioning in autistic individuals (Yule, 1978). Some deficits, apparently specific to autism, appear on closer examination to be more primarily a function of MA. For example, Lovaas and colleagues (e.g., Lovaas, Schreibman, Koegel, & Rehm, 1971) suggested that autistic children are overselective in their responses to multiple sources of stimulation – that is, they respond to only part of a relevant cue or to minor or irrelevant features – and this apparent stimulus overselectivity was suggested to account for many characteristics of autism. Subsequent research, however, suggested that overselectivity may more parsimoniously be accounted for as a function of low MA (Schover & Newson, 1976; Yule, 1979), and is also observed in nonautistic mentally retarded children (Anderson & Rincover, 1982; Litrownik, McInnis, Wetzel-Pritchard, & Filipelli, 1978). Although there is some evidence to suggest that autistic persons may be more overselective than nonautistic mentally retarded individuals even when IQ and MA are taken into account (Frankel, Simmons, Fichter, & Freeman, 1984), this concept can no longer be viewed as unique to autism.

Similarly, deficits in self-recognition and self-perception were commonly considered to be characteristic of autistic persons (e.g., Bettleheim, 1967). However, empirical studies have generally revealed that capacities for self-recognition reflect developmental level (Ferrari & Matthews, 1983; Spiker & Ricks, 1984). Dawson and McKissick (1984) reported that 2 of 15 young autistic children lacked self-recognition, and these two children had commensurate deficits in object permanence. Similar issues have been noted in the study of perception (Hermelin & O'Connor, 1970) and cognitive abilities (Sigman & Ungerer, 1981; Hobson, 1984). These findings suggest that behavioral characteristics must be viewed in light of developmental level. In addition, the findings suggest that for at least some purposes, the study of nonretarded autistic children may be particularly helpful.

An additional complication is posed by the observation that some aspects of autism change over the course of development. This observation poses a particular problem for the development of assessment and diagnostic instruments as well as for research studies (Parks, 1983; Volkmar & Cohen, 1988a). One solution to this problem is to focus only on either very young children or on the early development of older children and adults. This has the disadvantage of ignoring potentially interesting aspects of developmental change in syndrome expression, and introduces the problems attendant to parental retrospection (Robbins, 1963).

Typically, social-communicative deficits are most profound in younger autistic children. By the time the child reaches school age, some selective attachments to parents and greater communicative skills often develop (Sigman & Ungerer, 1984). Behavior problems, such as stereotyped and self-stimulatory behaviors, may become more marked over the course of development, and significant changes in adjustment can be observed in adolescence. Although even the highest functioning autistic adults typically exhibit significant degrees of disturbance, our understanding of developmental changes in syndrome expression remains quite limited and is an important topic for future research.

The similar-sequence hypothesis and autism

The notion of orderly and invariant sequences of development (see chapters 1 and 3) has been emphasized in most developmental theories (e.g., Kohlberg, 1969; Piaget, 1955), which suggest that specific developmental sequences should be the same for all children regardless of culture, level of intellectual functioning, and type of impairment. Most studies of retarded populations have noted that stages of development appear in the same order as in nonretarded populations, regardless of the etiology of the retardation (see Weisz & Zigler, 1969, and chapter 3). Autism provides a cogent test of this hypothesis, particularly because some definitions (e.g., NSAC, 1978) have emphasized unusual development patterns as characteristics of the disorder.

Burack et al. (1988) examined sequences of development in motor, receptive, and communication skills in autistic and nonautistic but developmentally disordered individuals. A series of analyses revealed that whereas both groups were delayed in acquisition of certain milestones, usual sequences of development were observed. Similarly, Wenar, Ruttenberg, Kalish-Weiss, & Wolf (1986) compared the scores of preschool autistic children with the series of a large group of normally developing young children; they found that less-disturbed autistic children progressed, albeit at a slower rate, through the same developmental sequence as did normal 2- and 3-year olds. They also noted, however, that many autistic children, particularly the more impaired ones, exhibited marked degrees of deviant and maladaptive behavior that would not be considered normal at any stage of development. Similar concerns have been raised regarding sequences in the language development of autistic persons. As a practical matter, it should be noted that assumptions about similar sequences are extensively used in developing intervention programs.

Rate of development

Unusual and unique developmental rates have been attributed to autistic individuals. For example, Fish et al. (1965) suggested that early development in autistic children is unpredictable and is often characterized by both significant lags and abrupt spurts of skill acquisition. This notion was included in some diagnostic classifications – for example, NSAC, 1978. Although many investigators and clinicians have accepted the lag-spurt hypothesis, however, empirical studies have not consistently supported the concept. Ornitz, Guthrie, and Farley (1977) found that the development of autistic children, based on parental reports, was significantly delayed but stable. Snow et al. (1987) reported relatively high levels of stability in various developmental areas over a period of 9 months in preschool autistic children. Lotter (1978) also noted developmental stability in older autistic children.

Available research suggests that *within* a given domain of functioning, rates of development are relatively stable for those skills that do develop. This does not, however, mean that relationships *between* domains of functioning are stable, as discussed later (also see chapters 4 and 12). As noted previously, many autistic individuals, for example, never speak, and some important developmental landmarks may never be achieved. An additional problem in attribution of developmental irregularities as specific to autism is raised by the observation that some discontinuities and bursts of development are noted in normally developing children (Fischer, Pipp, & Bullock, 1984).

Developmental regressions

Although the lag–spurt hypothesis has not generally received extensive empirical support, several studies have suggested that autistic children are more likely to exhibit episodes of marked developmental regression (Harper & Williams, 1975; Hoshino et al. 1987; Lotter, 1966). For example, a child who was able to speak in sentences may markedly deteriorate and lose this skill altogether. Hoshino et al. (1987) noted that such regressions were reported in lexical and gestural communication and in imitation, attachment, and self-care skills, with nearly half the sample exhibiting such regressions. Estimates of the prevalence of autistic persons who show such behavioral regressions range from 21% (Rutter, 1985) to 67% (Koizumi & Usada, 1980).

Behavioral regressions have also been observed in childen with mental retardation and other developmental disabilities, although less commonly than is observed in autism (Hoshino, Watanabe, & Yokoyama, 1986). Burack et al. (1988) similarly noted that autistic children were more likely than other developmentally disabled children to lose previously acquired communicative skills. Very rarely, children appear to develop normally for a period of several years prior to the onset of a marked and profound developmental regression. Although such children exhibit many behavioral features of autism, they have an even worse prognosis, and some classification systems include a specific diagnostic category (disintegrative disorder or disintegrative psychosis) to account for these children (Volkmar & Cohen, in press). The observation of more frequent episodes of developmental and behavioral regressions in autistic individuals suggests an important exception to the similar-sequence hypothesis, which otherwise is observed within a given developmental domain.

The similar-structure hypothesis and autism

Development is organized in such a manner that functioning across domains generally is integrated and interdependent (Cicchetti & Pogge-Hesse, 1982). For example, the relationship between social skills and impaired cognitive functioning has been investigated in a variety of cognitively impaired populations. The study of autistic individuals provides important information about the organization of behavior across domains of functioning. Although there is considerable controversy on the question of whether or not all groups of mentally retarded persons show atypical structures (Zigler & Hodapp, 1986; Weisz, Yeates, & Zigler, 1982; chapters 4 and 7) it is clear that autistic individuals display unusual patterns of behavior, unusual patterns of performance on IQ tests, and unusual discrepancies between certain developmental skills (DeMyer et al., 1981; Loveland & Kelley, 1988; Snow et al., 1987; Volkmar et al., 1987).

Concerning the similar-structure hypothesis in familial retarded individuals, Zigler (1967, 1969) has argued that these persons should not differ from nonretarded persons of the same MA in any specific area of functioning. In a more expanded developmental approach, the similar-structure hypothesis can even be extended to persons with mental retardation from organic etiologies, and can provide a theoretical framework through which profiles of the cognitive and behavioral functioning of these groups can be assessed (Hodapp & Zigler, in press). Models of developmental structure can be particularly informed by the extent that marked differences between areas of developmental functioning are observed in atypical populations. The observation of marked dysynchronies between aspects of developmental functioning may suggest important relationships between developmental skills.

Although overall performance on standard IQ tests is considerably below average, autistic children show significant variation among domains of functioning on a variety of standard psychometric assessment instruments, including the WISC-R (Tymchuk, Simmons, & Neafsey, 1977), the

Gesell Developmental Scales (Snow et al., 1987), and the revised Vineland Adaptive Behavior Scales (Loveland & Kelley, 1988; Volkmar et al., 1987). In general, autistic children do better on nonverbal tasks such as block design and objects assembly and worse on verbal tasks that require abstract reasoning (DeMyer et al., 1974). Tymchuk et al. (1977) found that autistic adolescents scored highest on the digit span and block design subtests of the WISC and lowest on the comprehension, coding, and picture arrangement subtests. Snow et al. (1987) reported that autistic children did significantly better on motor and perceptual performance than on language and personal-social tasks.

Volkmar et al. (1987) examined patterns of performance on the revised Vineland Adaptive Behavior Scales (Sparrow et al., 1984) in the areas of communication, daily living, and socialization in a series of 57 consecutive cases (22 autistic and 35 nonautistic) seen in a clinic for individuals with developmental disabilities. The autistic and nonautistic groups were roughly comparable in age, IQ, and MA. Significant group differences in Vineland age-equivalent scores were observed for receptive communication and all three socialization areas (interpersonal relationships, play and leisure time, and coping skills). The ratio of adaptive behavior age-equivalent scores to MA provided a direct test of the hypothesis that social and communicative development in autism is abnormal even when MA is taken into account. The results of this series of comparisons are presented graphically in Figure 10.4.

In some areas (particularly daily living skills), the performance of the autistic group was similar to that predicted by MA, whereas socialization and communication skills were markedly delayed relative to other skills and to MA. Loveland and Kelley (1988) noted that the functioning of autistic children in socialization and communication was less advanced than that of nonhandicapped persons of similar nonverbal MA, but comparable to that of nonhandicapped persons of similar verbal MA. This observation suggests the high degree of interdependence of communicative and social skills.

In the study by Volkmar et al. (1987), a series of pairwise comparisons between Vineland subdomain age-equivalent scores revealed that the autistic cases exhibited significantly greater discrepancy between Vineland subdomains even when a conservative statistical approach was employed. This result was confirmed in another sample by Burack et al. (1988). The observation suggests a limitation in the application of the similar-structure hypothesis. Although it might be argued that the unusual degree of developmental unevenness observed in autism reflects the presence of "organicity," it should be noted that unusual patterns of performance across

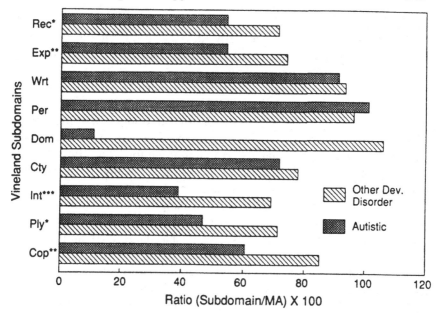

Figure 10.4. Ratios of Vineland Subdomain scores to MA (× 100) in autistic (*n* = 35) and nonautistic, developmentally disordered (*n* = 22) individuals. Rec = receptive, Exp = expressive, Wrt = written, Per = personal, Dom = domestic, Cty = community, Int = interpersonal relationships, Ply = play and leisure time, Cop = coping skills. Mann-Whitney U tests: $^*p \leq .05$, $^{**}p \leq .01$, $^{***}p \leq .001$. Adapted from Volkmar et al., 1987.

domains of functioning are also observed in individuals who function within the normal range of intelligence and who do not exhibit overt evidence of organicity.

Future directions

The study of individuals with autism provides an important opportunity to test basic tenets of developmental theory in the effort to derive a psychopathological model that encompasses both the important deviance and developmental aspects of the syndrome. On the one hand, aspects of syndrome expression are related to developmental level and the developmental model continues to guide rehabilitation. On the other hand, certain aspects of autism do not correspond to existing developmental models. To some extent this is not surprising – that is, autism is typically defined on the basis of marked social-communicative deviance and delay not attributable to developmental level. Discrepancies between areas of developmental functioning have repeatedly been noted in autistic individuals. Similarly, the early onset of social-communicative deviance in autism is distinctive, as is the developmental course of affected individuals. Several areas will be important topics for future research.

Given the nature of social deficits and deviance for definition and expression of the syndrome, it is remarkable that so little is known about the pathogenesis of the syndrome. As with other developmental disorders in which organic factors are implicated, the more precise explication of the nature of the underlying organicity is an important topic for future research (see chapter 2). Similarly, the role of social-communicative deviance in the expression of deviant patterns of development in other areas remains essentially unexplored. It is possible, for example, that the study of autism may suggest important ways in which various lines of development are interdependent – for example, it is possible that the study of autistic social dysfunction may illuminate ways in which social development serves an important regulatory and integrative function. Future studies may profitably focus on selected samples of autistic individuals – for example, of very high functioning adults or very young children – to help explicate important effects of developmental level and developmental changes in syndrome expression. Similarly, the debate about the prevalence of the disorder among very low functioning persons may illuminate aspects of syndrome continuity/discontinuity. Such research should facilitate our understanding both of the disorder and developmental factors in other forms of psychopathology.

References

Alpern, G.D. (1962). Measurement of "untestable" autistic children. *Journal of Abnormal Psychology, 72,* 478–496.

American Psychiatric Association. (1980). *Diagnostic and Statistical Manual,* 3rd ed., Washington, DC.

American Psychiatric Association. (1987). *Diagnostic and Statistical Manual* 3rd rev. ed., Washington, DC.

Anderson, G.M., & Hoshino, Y. (1987). Neurochemical studies of autism. In D. Cohen & A. Donnellan (Eds.), *Handbook of autism and pervasive developmental disorders.* New York: Wiley.

Anderson, N.B., & Rincover, A. (1982). The generality of overselectivity in developmentally disabled children. *Journal of Experimental Child Psychology, 34,* 217–230.

August, G.J., Stewart, M.A., & Tsai, L. (1981). The incidence of cognitive disabilities in the siblings of autistic children. *British Journal of Psychiatry, 138,* 416–422.

Bartak, L., Rutter, M., & Cox, A. (1975). A comparative study of infantile autism and specific developmental receptive language disorder: I. The children. *British Journal of Psychiatry, 126,* 127–145.

Berry, P, Gunn, P., & Andrews, R. (1980). Behavior of Down's syndrome infants in a strange situation. *American Journal of Mental Deficiency, 85,* 213–218.

Bettelheim, B. (1967). *The empty fortress: Infantile autism and the birth of the self.* New York: Free Press.

Burack, J.A., Malik, N., & Volkmar, F.R. (1988). *Sequences and structure of development in autistic and nonautistic, developmentally disabled children.* Under editorial consideration.

Cairns, R.B. (1979). *Social development: the origins and plasticity of interchanges.* San Francisco: Freeman.

Cantwell, D., Rutter, M., & Baker, L. (1978). Family factors. In M. Rutter & E. Schopler (Eds.), *Autism: A reappraisal of concepts and treatment.* New York: Plenum.

Cicchetti, D., & Pogge-Hesse, P. (1982). Possible contributions of the study of organically retarded persons to developmental theory. In E. Zigler & D. Balla (Eds.). *Mental retardation: The developmental–difference controversy.* Hillsdale, NJ: Erlbaum.

Cohen, D.J., Paul, R., & Volkmar, F.R. (1987). Issues in the classification of pervasive developmental disorders and associated conditions. In D. Cohen & A. Donnellan (Eds.), *Handbook of autism and pervasive developmental disorders,* New York: Wiley.

Courchesne, E., Yeung-Courchesne, R., Press, G.A., & Jernigal, T.L. (1988). Hypoplasia of cerebellar vermal lobules VI and VII in autism. *New England Journal of Medicine, 318,* 1349–1354.

Cowan, P.A., Hoddinott, B.A., & Wright, B.A. (1965). Compliance and resistance in the conditioning of autistic children. *Child Development, 36,* 913–923.

Cox, A., Rutter, M., Newman, S., & Partak, L.A. (1975). A comparative study of infantile autism and specific developmental receptive language disorder: I. Parental characteristics. *British Journal of Psychiatry, 126,* 146–159.

Dawson, G., & McKissick, F.C. (1984). Self-recognition in autistic children. *Journal of Autism and Developmental Disorders, 14,* 383–394.

DeMyer, M.K., Barton, S., Alpern, G., Kimberlin, C., Allen, J., Yang, E., & Steele, R. (1974). The measured intelligence of autistic children. *Journal of Autism and Childhood Schizophrenia, 4,* 42–60.

DeMyer M.L., Hintgen J.N., & Jackson, R.K. (1981). Infantile autism reviewed: A decade of research. *Schizophrenia Bulletin, 7,* 388–451.

Desperet, J. (1956). Some considerations relating to the genesis of autistic behavior in children. *American Journal of Orthopsychiatry, 20,* 335–350.

Deykin, E.Y., & McMahon B. (1979). The incidence of seizures among children with autistic symptoms. *American Journal of Psychiatry, 136,* 1310–1312.

Eisenberg, L., & Kanner, L. (1956). Early infantile autism 1943–1955. *American Journal of Psychiatry, 112,* 556–566.

Ferrari, M., & Matthews, W.S. (1983). Self-recognition deficits in autism: Syndrome-specific or general developmental delay? *Journal of Autism and Developmental Disorders, 13,* 317–324,

Fischer, K.W., Pipp, S.L., & Bullock, D. (1984). *Continuities and discontinuities in development.* New York: Plenum.

Fish, B., Shapiro, T., Halpern, F., & Wile, R. (1965). The prediction of schizophrenia in infancy. *American Journal of Psychiatry, 121,* 768–775.

Frankel, F., Simmons, J.Q., Fichter, M., & Freeman, B.J. (1984). Stimulus overselectivity in autistic and mentally retarded children: A research note. *Journal of Child Psychology and Psychiatry, 25,* 147–155.

Freeman, B.J., Schroth, P., Ritvo, E., Guthrie, D., & Wake, L. (1980). The behavior observation scale for autism (BOS): Initial results of factor analyses. *Journal of Autism and Developmental Disorders, 10,* 343–346.

Golden, G.S. (1987). Neurological functioning. In D. Cohen & A. Donnellan (Eds.), *Handbook of autism and pervasive developmental disorders.* New York: Wiley.

Harper, J., & Williams S. (1975). Age and type of onset as critical variables in early infantile autism. *Journal of Autism and Childhood Schizophrenia, 5*, 25–35.

Hermelin, B., & O'Connor, N. (1970). *Psychological experiments with autistic children.* Oxford: Pergamon.

Hobson, R.P. (1984). Early childhood autism and the question of egocentrism. *Journal of Autism and Developmental Disorders, 14*, 85–104.

Hodapp, R.M., and Zigler, E. (in Press). Applying the developmental perspective to individuals with Down syndrome. In D. Cicchetti & M. Beeghly (Eds.), *Children with Down syndrome: A developmental perspective.* New York: Cambridge University Press.

Hoshino, Y., Kancko, M., Yashima, Y., Kumashiro, H., Volkmar, F.R., & Cohen, D.J. (1987). Clinical features of autistic children with setback course in their infancy. *Japanese Journal of Psychiatry and Neurology, 41*, 237–246.

Hoshino, Y., Watanabe, K., & Yokoyama, F. (1986). The clinical features of autistic children who show setback course. *Seishin Igaku, 28*, 629–640.

Kanner, L. (1943). Autistic disturbances of affective contact. *Nervous Child, 2*, 217–250.

Kohlberg, L. (1969). Stage and sequence: The cognitive-developmental approach to socialization. In D. Goslin (Ed.), *Handbook of socialization theory and research.* Chicago: Rand McNally.

Koizumi, T., & Usada, S. (1980). The developmental and biological factors of autistic children and speech retarded children in infancy. *Japanese Journal of Child and Adolescent Psychiatry, 21*, 178–185.

Kolvin, I. (1971). Studies in childhood psychoses. I. Diagnostic criteria and classification. *British Journal of Psychiatry, 118*, 381–384.

Links, P.S., Stockwell, M., Abichandani, F., & Simeon, J. (1980). Minor physical anomalies in childhood autism. Part I: Their relationship to pre- and perinatal complications. *Journal of Autism and Developmental Disorders, 10*, 273–285.

Litrownik, A.J., McInnis, E.T., Wetzel-Pritchard, A.M., & Filipelli, D.L. (1978). Restricted stimulus and inferred attentional deficits in autistic and retarded child. *Journal of Abnormal Psychology, 87*, 554–562.

Lotter, V. (1966). Epidemiology of autistic conditions in young children. *Social Psychiatry, 1*, 124.

Lotter, V. (1978). Follow-up studies. In M. Rutter & E. Schopler (Eds.), *Autism: A reappraisal of concepts and treatment.* New York: Plenum.

Lovaas, O.I., Schreibman, L., Loegel, R., Rehm, R. (1971). Selective responding by autistic children to multiple sensory input. *Journal of Abnormal Psychology, 77*, 211–222.

Loveland, K.L., & Kelley, M.L. (1988). Development of adaptive behavior in adolescents and young adults with autism and Down syndrome. *American Journal of Mental Deficiency, 93*, 84–92.

Morgan, S.B. (1986). Autism and Piaget's theory: Are the two compatible? *Journal of Autism and Developmental Disorders, 16*, 441–457.

National Society for Autistic Children (NSAC) (1978). National Society for Autistic Children definition of the syndrome of autism. *Journal of Autism and Developmental Disorders, 8*, 162–167.

Ornitz, E.M. (1987). Neurophysiologic studies of infantile autism. In D. Cohen & A. Donnellan (Eds.), *Handbook of autism and pervasive developmental disorders.* New York: Wiley.

Ornitz, E.M., Guthrie, D., & Farley, A. J. (1977). Early development of autistic children. *Journal of Autism and Childhood Schizophrenia, 7*, 207–229.

Ornitz, E.M., & Ritvo, E.R. (1968). Perceptual inconstancy in early infantile autism. *Archives of General Psychiatry, 18*, 76–98.

Parks, S.L. (1983). The assessment of autistic children: A selective review of available instruments. *Journal of Autism and Developmental Disorders, 13*, 255–267.

Paul, R. (1987). Communication in autism. In D. Cohen & A. Donnellan (Eds.), *Handbook of autism and pervasive developmental disorders*. New York: Wiley.

Pauls. D. (1987). The familiarity of autism and related disorders: A review of the evidence. In D. Cohen & A. Donnellan (Eds.), *Handbook of autism and pervasive developmental disorders*. New York: Wiley.

Piaget, J. (1955). The construction of reality in the child. London: Routledge & Kegan Paul.

Prior, M.R. (1979). Cognitive abilities and disabilities in infantile autism: A review. *Journal of Abnormal Child Psychology, 7*, 357–380.

Prizant, B., & Schuler, A. (1987). Facilitating communication: Theoretical foundations. In D. Cohen & A. Donnellan (Eds.), *Handbook of autism and pervasive developmental disorders*. New York: Wiley.

Ritvo, E.R. (Ed.). (1976). *Autism: Diagnosis, current research and management*. New York: Spectrum.

Robbins L.C. (1963). The accuracy of parental recall of aspects of child development and child rearing practices. *Journal of Abnormal and Social Psychology, 6*, 261–270.

Rumsey, J.A., Rapoport, J.L., & Scerry, W.R. (1985). Autistic children as adults: psychiatric, social, behavioral outcomes. *Journal of the American Academy of Child Psychiatry, 24*, 465–473.

Rutter, M. (1970). Autistic children: Infancy to adulthood. *Seminars in Psychiatry, 2*, 435–450.

Rutter, M. (1978). Diagnosis and definition. In M. Rutter & E. Schopler (Eds.), *Autism: A reappraisal of concepts and treatment*. New York: Plenum.

Rutter, M. (1985). Infantile autism and other pervasive developmental disorders. In M. Rutter & L. Hersov (Eds.), *Child and adolescent psychiatry*. London: Blackwell Scientific Publications.

Rutter, M., Bartak, K., & Newman, S. (1971). Autism – A central disorder of cognition and language. In M. Rutter (Ed.), *Infantile autism: Concepts, characteristics, and treatment*. London: Churchill Livingstone.

Rutter, M., & Garmezy, N. (1983). Developmental psychopathology. In E.M. Hetherington (Ed.), *Handbook of child psychology, Vol. 4.*, New York: Wiley.

Rutter, M., & Lockyer, L. (1967). A five to fifteen-year follow-up study of infantile psychosis. *British Journal of Psychiatry, 113*, 1169.

Rutter, M., Shaffer, D., & Shepherd, M. (1975). *A multiaxial classification of child psychiatric disorders*. Geneva: World Health Organization.

Schover, L.W., & Newson, C.D. (1976). Overselectivity, developmental level, and overtraining in autistic and normal children. *Journal of Abnormal Child Psychology, 4*, 289–298.

Selfe, L. (1977). *Nadia: A case of extraordinary drawing ability in an autistic child*. London: Academic Press.

Short, A.B., & Schopler, E. (1988). Factors relating to age of onset in autism. *Journal of Autism and Developmental Disorders, 18*, 207–216.

Sigman, M., & Ungerer, J. (1981). Sensorimotor skills and language comprehension and autistic children. *Journal of Abnormal Child Psychology, 9*, 149–165.

Sigman, M., & Ungerer, J. (1984). Attachment behaviors in autistic children. *Journal of Autism and Developmental Disorders, 14*, 231–244.

Snow, M.E., Hertzig, M.E., & Shapiro, T. (1987). Rate of development in young autistic children. *Journal of the American Academy of Child Psychiatry, 26*, 834–835.

Sparrow, S., Balla, D., & Cicchetti, D. (1984). *Vineland Adaptive Behavior Scales*. Circle Pines, MN: American Guidance Service.

Spiker, D., & Ricks, M. (1984). Visual self-recognition in autistic children: Developmental relationships. *Child Development, 55*, 214–225.

Spitzer, R.L., Endicott, J.E., & Robins, E. (1978). Research diagnostic criteria. *Archives of General Psychiatry, 35*, 773–782.

Stern, D. (1985). *The interpersonal world of the human infant*. New York: Basic Books.

Tarjan, G., Wright, S.W., Eyman, R.K., Keeran, C.V. (1973). Natural history of mental retardation: Some aspects of epidemiology. *American Journal of Mental Deficiency, 77*, 369–373.

Tinbergen, E.A., & Tinbergen, N. (1972). Early childhood autism: An ethological approach. *Advances in Ethology, Journal of Comparative Ethology*, Supplement No. 10. Berlin: Paul Perry.

Treffert D.A. (1988). The idiot savant: A review of the syndrome. *American Journal of Psychiatry, 145*, 563–572.

Tymchuk, A.J., Simmons, J.A., & Neafsey, S. (1977). Intellectual characteristics of adolescent childhood psychotics with high verbal ability. *Journal of Mental Deficiency Research, 21*, 133–138.

Volkmar, F.R. (1987a). Social development. In D.J. Cohen & A. Donnellan (Eds.), *Handbook of autism and pervasive developmental disorders*. New York: Wiley.

Volkmar, F.R. (1987b). Annotation: Diagnostic issues in the pervasive developmental disorders. *Journal of Child Psychology and Psychiatry, 28*, 365–369.

Volkmar, F.R., Bregman, J., Cohen D.J., & Cicchetti, D.V. (in press). DSM III vs. III-R diagnoses of autism. *American Journal of Psychiatry*.

Volkmar F.R., & Cohen D.J. (1985). The experience of infantile autism: A first person account by Tony W. *Journal of Autism and Developmental Disorders, 15*, 47–54.

Volkmar, F.R., & Cohen, D.J. (1988a). Classification and diagnosis of childhood autism. In E. Schopler & G.B. Mesibov (Eds.), *Diagnosis and assessment in autism*. New York: Plenum.

Volkmar, F.R., & Cohen, D.J. (1988b). Issues in the diagnosis and classification of infantile autism. In B. Lakey & A. Kazdin (Eds.), *Advances in clinical child psychology*. New York: Plenum.

Volkmar, F.R., & Cohen, D.J. (in press). Disintegrative psychosis or "late onset" autism? *Journal of Child Psychology and Psychiatry*.

Volkmar, F.R., Cohen, D.J., Hoshino, Y., Rende, R., & Paul, R. (1988). Phenomenology and classification of the childhood psychoses. *Psychological Medicine, 18*, 191–201.

Volkmar, F., Cohen, D.J., & Paul. R. (1986). An evaluation of DSM-III criteria for infantile autism. *Journal of the American Academy of Child Psychiatry, 25*, 190–197.

Volkmar, F.R., Hoder, E.L., & Cohen, D.J. (1985). Compliance, "negativism" and the effects of treatment structure in autism: A naturalistic, behavioral study. *Journal of Child Psychology and Psychiatry, 26*, 865–877.

Volkmar, F.R., Sparrow, S.A., Goudreau, D., Cicchetti D.V., Paul, R., & Cohen, D.J. (1987). Social deficits in autism: An operational approach using the Vineland Adaptive Behavior Scales. *Journal of the American Academy of Child and Adolescent Psychiatry, 26*, 156–161.

Volkmar, F.R., Stier, D.M., Cohen, D.J. (1985). Age of recognition of pervasive developmental disorder. *American Journal of Psychiatry, 142*, 1450–1452.

Weir, R. (1962). *Language in the crib*. The Hague: Mouton.

Weisz, J., Yeates, J., & Zigler, E. (1982). Piagetian evidence and the developmental-difference controversy. In E. Zigler & D. Balla (Eds.). *Mental retardation: The developmental-difference controversy*. Hillsdale, NJ: Erlbaum.

Weisz, J., & Zigler, E. (1979). Cognitive development in retarded and nonretarded persons: Piagetian tests of the similar-sequence hypothesis. *Psychological Bulletin, 86*, 831–851.

Wenar, C., Ruttenberg, B.A., Kalish-Weiss, B., & Wolt, E.G. (1986). The development of normal and autistic children: A comparative study. *Journal of Autism and Development Disorders, 16,* 317-333.

Williams, R.S., Hauser, S.L., Purpura, D., Delong, R., & Swisher, C.N. (1980). Autism and mental retardation: Neuropathological studies performed on four retarded persons with autistic behavior. *Archives of Neurology, 37,* 749-753.

Wing, L. (1980). Childhood autism and social class: A question of selection? *British Journal of Psychiatry, 137,* 410-417.

Wing, L. (1981). Asperger's syndrome: A clinical account. *Psychological Medicine, 11,* 115-129.

Wing, L., & Atwood, A. (1987). Syndromes of autism and atypical development. In D.J. Cohen & A. Donnellan (Eds.), *Handbook of autism and pervasive developmental disorders.* New York: Wiley.

Wing, L., & Gould, J. (1979). Severe impairments of social interaction and associated abnormalities in children: Epidemiology and classification. *Journal of Autism and Developmental Disorders, 9,* 11-30.

Yule, W. (1978). Research methodology: What are the "correct controls?" In M. Rutter & E. Schopler (Eds.), *Autism: A reappraisal of concepts and treatment.* New York: Plenum.

Zahner, G.E.P., & Pauls, D.L. (1987). Epidemiological surveys of infantile autism. In D. Cohen & A. Donnellan (Eds.), *Handbook of autism and pervasive developmental disorders.* New York: Wiley.

Zigler, E. (1967). Familial mental retardation: A continuing dilemma. *Science, 155,* 292-298.

Zigler, E. (1969). Developmental versus difference theories of mental retardation and the problem of motivation. *American Journal of Mental Deficiency, 73,* 536-549.

Zigler, E., & Hodapp, R.M. (1986). *Understanding mental retardation.* New York: Cambridge University Press.

11 The issues of multiple pathways in the development of handicapped children

Claire B. Kopp and Susan L. Recchia

Multiple pathways, a term found in the developmental literature, suggests that major end-points in development (e.g., sensorimotor period, preschool years) as well as particular attainments (e.g., object permanence, problem solving, conservation) can be reached without necessarily invoking specific systems or processes for information intake and encoding. Although some might have reservations about this premise (Gesell, 1948; Piaget, 1970), recent research provides partial support. The perception of form can be obtained by visual or manual exploration, or both (e.g., see Spelke, 1987). Similarly, the functional fine tuning of learning and retrieval may occur by using auditory rehearsal strategies, reliance on visual clues, or invention of acronyms (e.g., see Brown, Bransford, Ferrara, & Campione, 1983).

The concept of multiple (or alternative) pathways has been used to account for the developmental attainments of handicapped children (e.g., Kopp & Shaperman, 1973). However, systematic, comprehensive studies that test models of multiple pathways have yet to be made, although Millar's (1988) programmatic research with the congenitally blind is an important beginning. Millar has focused on spatial abilities, and argues on the basis of data that vision is neither necessary nor sufficient for coding spatial information. She does state that sense modalities are often specialized, but systems do interconnect such that there is the possibility of overlapping inputs. Millar further states that "... sensory information is normally convergent and complementary, and can be sampled at any point during processing" (p. 71). In Millar's view, the acquisition of spatial information depends on the source and form of input, one's prior knowledge base, and how the current inputs are encoded. She also notes

Preparation of this chapter was supported in part by NSF grant BNS 87-10028 and DOE grant GOO 86 35232 to CBK. Appreciation is extended to Claire Hamilton for her perceptive comments.

272

that when particular systems are typically specialized for certain kinds of knowledge (e.g., vision for spatial information), impairments of the system can be associated with more difficult acquisition of knowledge than might otherwise occur.

Millar's research has been methodical and her conclusions have been drawn carefully. It is reasonable to invoke the concept of multiple pathways with respect to the blind and their potential for spatial understanding. However, basic questions remain. How far does the concept extend in the development of handicapped children? Does it apply to performance in all domains – perception, cognition, social interaction, emotional development, communication? Can we expect that with the provision of seemingly appropriate experiences, blind children will invariably understand the nuances of emotional signals even though salient visual cues are not seen, that deaf children will learn rules for family life even though admonishments and vocal inflections are not heard, and that children with major arm impairments will discern the operating systems of mechanical toys even though motor explorations are impossible?

Our aim in this chapter is to explore issues similar to these. We focus on development in the early years, with a primary interest on children who are blind, deaf, or have motor impairments, who have intact central nervous systems, whose handicap began early, and whose condition is major. Further, we examine capability in relation to several domains of functioning – cognition, language, social interactions – but we emphasize communication and social abilities. We describe relevant theory and research rather than present an inclusive review of the literature.

Background

In this section, we discuss two perspectives that influence our approach to multiple pathways. The first relates to the *origins* of behavior (biological, experiential, both) and how these can be linked to views about alternative pathways. We propose that an analysis of origins forces consideration of the meaning of a behavior for an individual's survival, growth, and development. We argue that behaviors with biological underpinnings are likely to pertain to organism survival and basic adaptations, and therefore may be most likely to involve multiple processes as a form of insurance. However, if survival is not at stake, evidence suggests guarantees are unlikely, particularly for learned and complex behaviors.

The second perspective turns on the issue of definition of behavioral performance. In the final analysis, the criterion of performance is used to infer that multiple pathways operate. We submit that the most rudimentary forms of behavior are the least credible exemplars of performance; rather, a more viable case can be made for mature forms of behaviors. Equally important is consideration of the quality of behaviors that are shown.

Both of these issues have bearing on how one determines if multiple pathways have the potential to be activated. This in turn has ramifications for the interventions provided to handicapped children.

The origins of behavior

The 1970s marked a turning point in views about biological influences on early development; increasingly, biological underpinnings of behavior were accepted and their implications described (Flavell, 1972; Gould, 1977; Kagan, 1971; Scarr-Salapatek, 1976). Influenced by Piaget, this thinking also stemmed from advances made in the study of genetics and biology, the growing importance of ethological perspectives, and detailed studies of comparative development.

Since the 1970s, more refined conceptualizations have appeared. Two that have particular relevance for early behavior have been articulated by Horowitz (1987) and Black and Greenough (1986). Horowitz proposes categories of universal and nonuniversal behaviors with implications for each. Universals I are hard-wired, extremely probable behaviors that quickly emerge in the infant repertoire. Early sensory and perceptual abilities such as contrast discriminations, habituation, and awareness of movement are examples. Universals II require environmental stimulus feedback for shaping and influencing level of attainment. These behaviors include species-specific behaviors such as Piagetian sensorimotor intelligence. Nonuniversals are behaviors that result from specific learning experiences. Numerous and extensive, these behaviors include various kinds of knowledge and skills (e.g., historical facts, arithmetic principles, moral conventions, cultural information, family rules, sports, problem-solving approaches, and dress codes).

Horowitz's categories suggest that more elaborate conceptualizations of behavioral underpinnings can be helpful in thinking about the probabilities that certain behaviors will appear in the repertoire, and what is needed to further development. Black and Greenough's (1986) model moves us closer to this challenge.[1] They provide a conceptual framework for understanding and studying ". . . when and how environmental input and genetic constraints interact during development" (p. 2). These authors use the terms "maturation," "maintenance," "facilitation," and "induction"

---

[1] This model is itself adapted from the writings of Richard Aslin and Gilbert Gottlieb. The work of these authors is discussed in Black and Greenough (1986).

Table 11.1. *Biology and experience in early development: An epigenetic model*

I. Foundation processes (genotype-driven)

Themes: Can have complex neural systems
Experience is not necessary to "carve out" neural structures
Experience may be useful

Process	Example	Developmental implications
Maturation		
Behaviors that occur without experiential input	Sucking, looking, rooting	Species and individual survival and adaptation
Maintenance		
Fully emerged behaviors whose continued expression depends on adequate and/or appropriate experience	Babbling, phonemes, speech of a cultural group	May be particularly relevant for culturally prescribed communication patterns – "tool" use
Facilitation		
Behaviors that can develop without specific experience, but mature more rapidly with experiential input	Walking, reach and grasp, depth perception (?)	Experience may also "refine" skills

II. Induction processes (experience-driven)

Themes: Experiences may provide general information to all members of a species
Idiosyncratic experiences may be necessary for adaptation to a particular environment
Quality of the environment is important
"Structure" of experience is incorporated into brain structure (neural modifications)

Process	Examples	Developmental implication
Induction		
Behaviors that will not fully emerge unless appropriate experience is provided	Social rules, book knowledge, cultural information, games – domain-specific knowledge	One induction process may set the stage for another

Source: Adapted from Black & Greenough (1986).

to characterize processes and to differentiate influences of biology and the environment. Table 11.1 is a slightly revised version of their model, and provides definitions and examples.

In Black and Greenough's view, there is no doubt about the pervasive importance of environmental experiences for induction processes for learning about one's milieu. However, it is also clear that fundamental behaviors appear in the repertoire of the young human with very little experiential influence. Maturation processes function on their own, whereas facilitation processes use experience to advance development but can operate without stimulation from the environment. As an example, Dennis (1940) documented that infants reared primarily on cradle boards walked about when expected. Maintenance is more complicated because this process uses experience to build a new behavior from the basics of a wired-in behavior. Reach and grasp are intrinsic to humans, but the use of pencils, forks, hammers, and computers is not. Experiences help humans construct skills for tools.

Using Black and Greenough's model as a point of departure, it is possible to generate ideas about how and when multiple pathways can be called into play. Consider first the needs of most species. At a most basic level, immature members of a species need to be able to survive if the species itself is to survive. Extending this line of reasoning, inferences can be made about the behaviors needed to survive. These include the ability (1) to discriminate touch early in life, (2) to be aware of pain or danger, and (3) to recognize sounds and scents of familiar others. Beyond providing systems of behaviors, evolutionary thrusts could ensure survival by guaranteeing redundancy in information intake. That is, if one system became inoperable, another could take over. If vision were impaired, the perception of surface and texture could be discerned by touch. Thus, multiple pathways should be available to ensure the emergence of behaviors that are intrinsic to species survival and early adaptations.

Evidence for dual-system activation in human infancy comes from findings reported by Spelke (1987, 1988), among others, who have shown that young infants have the capacity for some forms of intermodal perception. Each sensory modality provides a means of discriminating the surrounding environment. Equally important, one modality can provide information to another. A 5-month-old infant can touch a covered object and identify it on the basis of past visual experience with it. Recent evidence demonstrates that intermodal functioning is quite extensive. For example, infant auditory perception is in part influenced by input from the visual system (Kuhl, 1987), and kinesthesis and vision are linked at least by the fifth month (Bahrick & Watson, 1985).

Turning to induction processes – behaviors that develop because of experience – the case for multiple pathways is more complicated. Some knowledge and skills evolve only from a single type of experience; therefore, the issue of multiple pathways is irrelevant. Phonemic development demands exposure and responsivity to a certain linguistic environment. In order to pronounce words correctly according to the standards of a culture, one has to hear the sounds that are emphasized in conversational speech by members of that culture. Similarly, a sports ability is acquired only by action – by using a tennis racket, hitting a baseball, or throwing a basketball. The skill can be sharpened by meditation, imagery exercises, or reading, but the specific activity itself is basic.

Alternatively, other skills develop because of inputs from a broad array of experiences. In these instances, multiple pathways have the potential to be activated. The development of arithmetic skills is an example – the principles of numeration can be learned by using one's fingers, manipulating objects, visualizing groups of objects, or counting. Similarly, communication skills involve elements of vocal production, touch, vision, and hearing. Most of us utilize all four modalities, but Helen Keller used touch almost exclusively, and Beethoven relied extensively on vision and touch.

In sum, consideration of the origins of behaviors is a first step in analyzing the probabilities that multiple pathways exist. An additional step requires the evaluation of performance on specified tasks. Here, judgments about the functional quality of behaviors become important; this is the focus of the next section.

Behavioral competencies

Our second background point turns on the definition of performance, particularly as it pertains to handicapped children. We argue that rudimentary levels of behaviors (e.g., being able to count to two) or those that are inappropriately manifested (e.g., noncontingent smiles or use of words irrelevant to the context) ought not to be used as an index of knowledge or skill.

Judgments about the adequacy of child performance should include evaluation of (1) the nature of a behavior's expression (e.g., is a social smile dampened, is a behavior ambiguous?); (2) *functional* appropriateness to the context (e.g., smiling is evidenced by a child, but rarely in interaction with care givers): and (3) behavioral generalization to multiple situations (e.g., recognizing that safety rules about parking lots applies to all parking lots, not just the one at the neighborhood supermarket). More precise descriptions of child ability will lead to more precise inferences about the influence or operation of multiple pathways.

In the rest of this chapter, we draw on these background perspectives in our examination of research. The first section focuses on infancy. Discussion begins with current views of infancy, and moves to the implications of these views for the development of handicapped infants. We cite evidence that suggests that the basic sensorimotor repertoire is achieved by handicapped infants, implicating the processes of multiple pathways. In contrast, we highlight some of the difficulties experienced by handicapped infants in developing reciprocal social interactions, and suggest limitations with the concept of multiple pathways.

The second section focuses on preschoolers and the capabilities they need to make the successful transition to childhood. We emphasize language because of its importance, and specifically examine the language of handicapped children in the context of social interactions. We conclude that language dysfunctions impede the passage to social competence.

In the concluding section, we offer suggestions for interventions. Our premise is that alternative paths exist for communicative competencies, whereas alternatives are few for effective social interactions. Interventions may benefit by helping care givers and handicapped children develop to the fullest extent possible those competencies that involve multiple pathways. This may make it easier to facilitate the development of skills that evolve from restricted pathways.

Infancy

Developmentalists have come to appreciate that human infancy is a special period in the course of the life span. Scarr-Salapatek (1976) persuasively argued that infant intelligence represents "... a dynamic interplay of genetic preadaptations and developmental adaptations to features of the caretaking environment" (p. 166). Infant intelligence is less variable than later intelligent behavior because of its evolutionary background, and individual differences in infant behavior are restricted by genetic preadaptations (canalization). These constraints, according to Scarr-Salapatek, permit the emergence of key infant behaviors irrespective of relative variations in rearing environments. The environment does influence the rate at which development proceeds but not the essential form or characteristics of behavior. Almost all infants develop object permanence, but when this behavior emerges and the range of contexts within which it is elicited vary with particular infant experience.

Within the realm of early social interactions and attachments, many of the same arguments apply. For example, Bowlby (1969) described preadaptations for social interactions and attachments, and noted the different types of behaviors that facilitate the infant's earliest interaction with others (e.g., looking, clinging, crying). Others such as Gould (1977) have suggested evolutionary-based physical adaptations that bring adults close to the young. These include the appealing facial and body attributes of the immature (e.g., large head on a small body, wide forehead, large eyes).

Thus, evolution and biology have provided mechanisms that will bring infant and care giver together and, equally, will allow the infant to respond to the tactual, kinesthetic, visual, and auditory inputs provided by others. This interaction and mutual responsivity has the potential to occur for infants and care givers irrespective of rearing milieu (Kagan, 1984).

Implications for handicapped infants

What conclusions can be drawn from these facts about infant development? First, the basic sensorimotor and social repertoires and other behaviors in the Universal I and II domains, or those influenced by maturation or facilitation processes, can be expected to appear in handicapped infants. These behaviors include the ability to discriminate between different sensations, produce vocalizations, and habituate to simple stimuli. How these behaviors are used (i.e., their functional quality and appropriateness) depends on the nature of the child's handicapping condition.

Second, the specific inputs (e.g., direct teaching, opportunities for observation) that are required in order for older infants and toddlers to learn (1) the language of their culture, (2) the expectations that care givers have for behavior, and (3) social norms, *are also required for the handicapped child.* However, whether these behaviors are learned and how the child will use them will be a function of three factors: (1) the system that is impaired, (2) the ability of care givers to provide experiences that are singularly relevant to the task to be learned, and (3) the infant's ability to understand and integrate the information that is being offered.

Pretend play provides an example of a behavior that requires environmental interactions. This kind of play develops toward the end of the second year of life, and involves (1) prior cognitive attainments (e.g., representation – assigning a word (cat) to an object (a four-legged animal that says "meow") and (2) numerous experiences that involve exploring and playing with objects.

Pretend play should be possible for a blind child if the following occurs: Sequences of play that focus on behavioral episodes (e.g., using a toy spoon to stir make-believe food in a bowl) are modeled for the child in a meaningful way; the child has the potential to recognize the functional characteristics of real objects that the toys are meant to simulate; the child is aware that children themselves can initiate a play activity of the kind modeled for her.

Research with handicapped infants

Several lines of research converge to show unequivocally that blind, deaf, and motorically impaired infants develop Piagetian sensorimotor skills and basic reciprocal social interactions. In a landmark study of Thalidomide infants, Decarie (1969) demonstrated the development of object permanence and attachment behaviors. Kopp and Shaperman (1973) found evidence for competency in numerous components of sensorimotor intelligence (e.g., object permanence, spatial knowledge, problem-solving, and discrimination of means–ends relationships) with a totally limbless boy (non-Thalidomide). Granted, the usual ways of interacting with objects differed for these children from those observed with motorically intact infants. The limbless boy rolled toward objects, and if they were small enough, he held them between his head and shoulders. In formal tests of sensorimotor skills, head turning, direction of looking, and vocal responses were used as measurement indexes.

Fraiberg (1977) and colleagues documented numerous social and cognitive abilities demonstrated by blind infants (e.g., object permanence, attachment, functional play); these results have been replicated by Rogers and Puchalski (1988). The appearance of many of these behaviors is delayed, sometimes by as much as a year; indeed, Fewell (1983) notes that most aspects of sensorimotor development appear late in blind infants within Piagetian stages 3 through 6. She notes failures as well, including the inability (1) to understand the cause of object activation, (2) to determine the relationships between actions and solution, and (3) to categorize objects by salient features. Fewell's description suggests that understanding of causality may be one of the more difficult sensorimotor achievements for the blind infant. There are seemingly few ways to demonstrate cause-and-effect object relationships with preverbal children who cannot see object and event sequences. These data nicely complement Millar's comments about late-appearing behaviors when systems have specialization for information intake.

Overall, the findings from the studies mentioned suggest that the basic sensorimotor repertoire is present, and largely functional, in blind, motorically impaired, and deaf infants (Mogford, 1977).

Turning to research in which other behaviors were examined provides a mixed view of capabilities and problems. Consider the social smile. Its biological underpinnings are apparent in that it appears in blind infants at about the same time as in sighted infants. But its functional use has significant limitations in that it is irregular in appearance, and often dampened when it does appear (Fraiberg, 1971).

What about more advanced, learned social behaviors? Here we refer to abilities such as reciprocity and turn-taking in interactions, joint attention, drawing a care giver into play, using care givers as a resource when help is needed, or even teasing care givers both to test knowledge of the world and to determine limits (e.g., Bretherton & Bates, 1979; Kopp, in press; Uzgiris, 1967). These and other social skills develop out of and build upon basic social abilities that are probably biologically driven (Black & Greenough, 1986). What evolves are social interactions that become finely tuned, and expectancies about the other's behaviors (e.g., Brazelton, Koslowski, & Main, 1974; Kaye & Fogel, 1980; Stern, 1985; Tronick, Cohn, & Shea, 1986).

At all levels, social interactions require contingent verbal or nonverbal communication patterns that are engaged in by both infant/toddler and care giver. Communication here refers to care givers' use of verbalizations, emotional expressions, gestures, or touch, and to infants' use of sounds, affective displays, interest, or motor responsivity.

Research suggests that the more advanced social interactions and related communication exchanges of nonhandicapped infants differ from those experienced by many handicapped infants/toddlers.[2] Turn-taking, for instance, appears to be infrequent for the latter. Part of the problem stems from difficulties experienced by each partner in reading and interpreting cues. Oftentimes, there is not a great deal of consistency found in signal production; thus, each interaction, which ordinarily would depend on past experiences, has to be treated as a novel event. One morning, a blind infant lowers its head and becomes still in order to discriminate clues that signal mother is approaching. Another morning, the infant becomes more animated as she approaches. Both kinds of behavior actually represent infant interest, but if mother cannot detect a discernible pattern, she does not know how to respond. If infant and mother can decode the others' signals, successful mutual engagement will occur. If decoding is unsuccessful, the interaction will be confused.

Social interaction-communication problems are not unique to blind infants. Hearing-impaired infants and their care givers have difficulties establishing reciprocity (e.g., Schlesinger & Meadow, 1972), attributed to

---

[2] It is important to recognize that not all handicapped infants and young children have problems with communication and social competencies.

problems that arise in working out appropriate contingencies (Wood, Wood, Griffiths, & Howarth, 1986).

We see in our own research the marked sensitivities care givers need to have in order to let toddlers discover their worlds without unduly inhibiting them. Praise for solitary play, highly affective interchanges in mutual engagements, explanations about forbidden activities, and time-outs for noncompliance all demand both attentiveness from partners and responses that are related to the previous activities. Touch, vision, and hearing are involved.

In contrast, consider what may occur with the dyad of a 15-month-old deaf girl and her hearing care giver. Mother wants to teach the child to stay seated in her highchair while eating, that she use her spoon instead of fingers, and that she *ask* for more food instead of banging her tray. All the while, mother attempts to maintain a pleasant mealtime interaction and to provide clear signals. In turn, the child has to stay visually attentive in order to receive the messages; this can be difficult for toddlers. The child may understand the entire sequence of expectations or she may miss important cues. In any event, the mother has to assess as best she can how much the child encodes the mealtime message. Errors in evaluation may lead to nonappropriate reinforcements.

Given these challenges, it is not surprising that care-giver inputs to hearing-impaired and blind infants are more directive and constrained than those provided to sighted infants (e.g. Fraiberg, 1977). Mutual exchanges are often not achieved because the dyad is not coordinated in terms of signals. Interestingly, the same pattern occurs with motorically impaired infants and toddlers (e.g., Seidman, Allen, & Wasserman, 1986). Impatience about slow movements may partially account for this.

These distortions in communication and social interactions often have ripple effects. For example, the sense of *agency* and the notion of *identity* that typically develop during the second year may show dysfunction and may provoke additional problems with communication.

Implications for multiple pathways

Multiple-pathway processes potentially apply to communicative effectiveness. As noted, early communication is multifaceted, and includes visual, auditory, and tactual means to give and to receive messages. All are potentially useful communication modes. However, if communication between care giver and infant/toddler is ineffective, it is almost certain that more advanced social interactions will be ineffective. It seems unlikely that multiple pathways play a role because the infant's and toddler's *learned* social interactive skills are intertwined with communication; there is no substitute, no alternative, for communicative competence.

Conclusions

In general, the concept of multiple pathways may be particularly applicable to some aspects of infancy because of behavioral underpinnings and species requirements. The biological underpinnings of many of the young infant's behaviors allow for considerable redundancy in input. The concept of multiple pathways may not be as applicable to infant and toddler skills that develop because of specialized environmental inputs. One has to consider the competency that is being acquired, the nature of the handicap, and the ability of the partners to give and receive information.

The preschool years

In the last section we focused on general communication skills of handicapped infants, and discussed the implications of impairments in this ability for social interactions. In this section, we turn to communication that involves words and symbols. We examine language problems with handicapped preschoolers and note their implications for social skills. And we again explore handicaps vis-a-vis restricted and alternative pathways to competence. To set the stage, we begin with current views of preschool capabilities.

The abilities of preschoolers

Our culture has distinct expectations for preschool-aged children. They are expected to become knowledgeable about their society, care givers, siblings, and peers. They must learn to communicate effectively, organize their thinking, recognize others' needs, become a partner in play, understand rules for behavior, and control their own emotions.

These challenges would be difficult to meet even if preschoolers were fully prepared. However, recent studies reveal the marked degree of imbalance that characterize their capabilities. Most apparent in thought, imbalances are actually evident in almost every domain of functioning.

Cognitively, preschoolers are at once sensitive to others' perspectives, understand some principles, know about categories, and show some planning and strategic behavior. But they are also unable to generate rules for the way the physical world operates, perceptual transformations mystify them, and they have difficulty organizing information, accessing their knowledge, and monitoring their own actions (e.g., Borke, 1975; Brown, Bransford, Ferrara, & Campione, 1983; Flavell, 1985; Gelman & Gallistel, 1978; Seigler, 1978; Wellman, 1985).

Socially, preschoolers recognize themes in play, the social requirements of interactions, and the need to continuously negotiate daily peer exchanges, but they rarely evaluate their actions (e.g., Corsaro, 1979, 1985; Garvey, 1974). Emotionally, they shift from affirmations of self-assurance and maturity to displays of fear, rivalry, and negativism (Goodenough, 1931; Jones & Burks, 1936; Murphy, 1956; Wenar, 1982).

By the end of the preschool years, children no longer appear to be in an imbalanced state. The transition to more advanced behaviors takes place on two fronts. Care givers increase their demands and expectations (Rogoff, Sellers, Pirrotta, Fox, & White, 1975) and expose children to additional explanations, rules, and admonitions. The children themselves show motivation to grow and to understand themselves and others.

As children grow, the use of language takes on greater significance in communication with others and also as an aid to their own learning. Children become more proficient in understanding symbols, and employ language for self-instruction, to resolve uncertainties and fears, to facilitate attention to task demands, to move toward self-monitoring, and to explore roles in fantasy play (e.g., Corsaro, 1985; Dunn, Bretherton, & Munn, 1987; Gottman & Parker, 1987). Further, language enriches the development of categories so that information can be systematically organized and remembered about one's social and object world (e.g., social roles, normative conventions) (Fischer, Hand, Watson, van Parys, & Tucker, 1986).

Language used with peers and care givers has coherence, shows adaptations to the partner, and has many features of conversational sophistication (Schaffer, 1984). Moreover, Schaffer notes that during this age, children's language becomes more contingent and relevant, and the range of interpersonal uses increases. "Conversations thus become lengthier, more explicit, and more cohesive ..." (p. 151). In short, language serves the young child as a particularly important channel to additional achievements. The richer the language, the more opportunity to try out words in a variety of settings.

Language skills within specific handicaps

Children with specific handicaps such as blindness, deafness, and physical disability are at particular risk for impaired development of language competence (Fraser, 1986; Seidman, Allen, & Wasserman, 1986). The progression of language development may be slowed appreciably or the language repertoire may be impoverished.

Research in the development of communication competence in children with nonorganic language impairments is sparse, and is referred to only briefly in this section. Some difficulties have been noted in structure and lexicality, rate of syntactic development, and use of productive vocabularies (Seidman et al., 1986). Confounds related to home-rearing conditions and lengthy hospitalizations have not been fully explored.

Recent research indicates salient differences in the quality and complexity of blind children's language (Andersen, Dunlea, & Kekelis, 1984). Examining language in context (as opposed to simply defining content), findings revealed that totally blind children often acquire largely unanalyzed labels rather than true word meanings. Further, pragmatic development is deviant (Kekelis & Andersen, 1984). The authors cite the example of a blind child using the word "more" to ask for another cookie in a specific context, but not in general to indicate an additional quantity. From a functional standpoint, the verbal communication system has significant limitations.

Studies of deaf children reveal widespread problems related to their inability to encode age-relevant language-mediated messages. The deaf also have a high rate of illiteracy (Liben, 1978; Meadow, 1980; Wood et al., 1986). Until recently, the 90% of deaf children born to hearing parents typically had only primitive systems of communication available to them throughout their early childhood (Liben, 1978).

Both blind and deaf children tend to give confusing signals to others. This occurs even when sign language is used by young deaf children. Although deaf children produce gestures that have linguistic and communicative properties (i.e., gestures used to refer to objects or to indicate an action) (Goldin-Meadow & Mylander, 1983, 1984), they also produce idiosyncratic gestures and use a single gesture to convey several meanings. This process, called overextension, is akin to that found in the one-word-period of young hearing children (see Clark, 1983). It is far more difficult for care givers to interpret overextensions when gestures are used alone than when they are combined with sounds and words.

Although young blind children have often learned words and phrases, their language is frequently combined with idiosyncratic gestures, facial expressions, and body language. All provide conflicting signals. Further, the children's limited experiences may help produce verbal communications that have obscure meanings. Consider the following example. A preschool-aged blind child repeatedly says "face" while exploring a plastic ball that has several cutout holes. What can this verbal activity mean to the care giver or peer who does not know that the child recently learned the word "face" in connection with touching and exploring the configuration of the human face?

In sum, within the realm of verbal communication, the handicapping conditions of deafness and blindness impede the growth of language. Children, in part, find it difficult to make sense of the information given, they give ambiguous messages to others, and the feedback they receive from others is not always appropriate. Perhaps most important, the conversational skills that evolve with nonhandicapped preschoolers are severely constrained.

Implications

Alternative pathways. Research with the deaf shows that an alternative path to symbolic knowledge using a sign system does, in time, appreciably facilitate child functioning. Harris (1978) found better impulse control in deaf children of deaf parents than in deaf children of hearing parents. The former were exposed to sign language early in life. Data suggest that the introduction of symbolic language allowed children to learn specifically what was expected of them. Results from this study clearly indicate that manual language is an alternative path to communication when others are knowledgeable about signs.

Other evidence supports the existence of sign language as an alternative pathway for deaf children's language development. Petitto (1987) notes discontinuities in the deaf child's transition from gestural pointing to the use of specific American Sign Language symbols for the pronouns "you" and "me." Despite the greater transparency of the pointing gesture's form (as opposed to that of spoken language), deaf toddlers made pronoun errors similar to those of hearing children of the same age. Pettito found her results "strongly suggestive of a universal process of personal pronoun acquisition ... despite radical differences in modality" (p. 47).

Similarly, Mayberry, Woodlinger-Cohen, and Goldin-Meadow (1987) conclude that "deafness does not interfere with the child's ability to develop and manipulate symbols" (p. 124). Deaf children who had the benefit of learning a sign language were able to develop symbolic understandings that enhanced their ability to read and to communicate.

Obviously, there is no analogy for the blind child of the sign system for the deaf child. However, the development of spoken language and communication competencies can be facilitated for these children in other ways. This is discussed in the concluding part of the chapter.

Reverberating effects of limited verbal skills. We began this section with a picture of the preschool-aged child, and mentioned the role that language has in fostering young children's skills. It is our belief that inadequate linguistic skills hamper the cognitive, social, and emotional growth of blind, deaf, and motorically impaired children that should take place during the preschool and school years. Admittedly, there is little research on these specific relationships, but there is every reason to suspect that trends found with nonhandicapped young children hold for those with handicaps. That is, communicative competence is explicitly tied to numerous cognitive and emotional achievements.

There are other implications, particularly for social-skill development. It is a fact that children with handicaps often experience problematic peer interactions (see Guralnick & Weinhouse, 1984; Hartup, 1983). This is due in part to attitudes of healthy children who make stringent requirements for peer groups (e.g., Hartup, 1983), and in part due to the difficulties handicapped children in general have in initiating and maintaining peer interactions. It is becoming increasingly obvious that a constellation of skills is involved, including the ability to communicate verbally when required, showing appropriate affect, and minimizing inappropriate or regressive behaviors (Kopp, Baker, & Brown, in preparation).

Equally important is the potential for adverse ramifications when children are isolated from everyday peer contacts (e.g., House, Landis, & Umberson, 1988; Parker & Asher, 1983; Parker & Asher, 1987). Recurrent loneliness, neglect, or rejection may lead to longer-term emotional and social problems.

In sum, it is our contention that a primary route to social interactions and skill is through communicative competency including verbal skills (for a description of the elements, see Hartup, 1983; Schaffer, 1984). There does not appear to be an alternative for conversational skills vis-a-vis social development.

Conclusions and implications for interventions

We have provided one view of the concept of multiple pathways. Our approach has been selective, with a concentration on infancy and early childhood. For both age groups, we focused on aspects of communication and social interactions.

We have suggested that the concept of multiple pathways has application to infancy, but also noted research findings that indicated there may be fewer alternatives available for developing competent social interactions even in this age period. In the language and social domains we explored for the preschool years, there seem to be few successful alternatives to language that would allow achievement in social skills.

It may be unrealistic – and even unwarranted – to suggest that there are numerous ways (sign language aside) to obtain the communicative and social skills that our culture generally seeks from its members. We do look for rather specialized skills in these domains from children at various ages. In fact, intervention programs for handicapped children are often designed with these skill goals in mind.

Given this specificity in pathways to social endpoints, are there solutions? We offer a strategy that may help infant and young child communication. For this, we turn to the developmental literature and studies of care giver–infant interactions.

It is clear from the literature that the developmental course of interactions between care givers and infants reflects different agendas and different communication emphases. Nicely summarized by Schaffer (1984), these developmental trends reflect *initial encounters*, in which care givers attempt to help the infants become responsive to the environment and to develop state organization; *face-to-face interactions*, in which care givers and infants work to maintain attention and interaction with each other; *topic sharing*, where care givers and infants maintain engagement with respect to an object of interest to both parties; and the beginning of *dialogues*, in which social interactions become more symmetrical, and the infants begin to perceive that they and their partners can each have needs, plans, and expectations. These are trends for the first year of life. Kopp (1987) has discussed some care-giver expectations for the second year involving standards for behavior.

It is our belief that it may be useful to try to capture these increasingly elaborate interactive trends with handicapped infants and their care givers, emphasizing whatever modes of communication are available. If each interactive step is developed with appropriate communicative competencies, it would seem to pave the way for the next step and more sophisticated communications and social interactions. Ultimately, the hope is that more efficient spoken language or use of signs will evolve. Clearly, our premises have yet to be tested.

However, the intervention literature suggests that alternative approaches may be warranted at this time. Recently, Stremel-Campbell and Rowland (1987) suggested that effective prelinguistic abilities may derive from intervention programs that are based on newer views of communicative and social competencies that have emerged in the past decade or so (e.g., from research of Elizabeth Bates, Inge Bretherton, Jerome Bruner, Roberta Golinkoff, and others). Stremel-Campbell and Rowland state that "... there is still a strong emphasis on vocal development, speech, or manual signs without prior consideration for development of reciprocal social interactions and preverbal communication" (p. 50). (These more developmentally oriented interventions have received impetus from the newly enacted Public Law 99–457, which provides additional financial support for infant programs.)

There are others who give increasing recognition to the role and importance of early interactions with primary care givers as a basis for subsequent language development (Fraser, 1986). Fraser's perspective can be summarized in this way. When the child's ability to interact is reduced in some way, an automatic limitation is imposed upon his or her environment. The effect of this limitation depends on a number of factors, not the least of which is a parent's expectations. Particularly reinforcing infant behaviors such as watching mother's face, responding to her vocalizations, or moving in a rhythmical way to her overtures are markedly absent within specific handicaps, and this absence may adversely affect the development of what Fraser refers to as "interactional synchrony." Parents and their handicapped infants are especially vulnerable to disruptions in the development of optimal attachment and communicative interaction.

Wood et al. (1986) make similar arguments. They see problems in communication between the child and the significant adults in the environment as likely to have far-reaching secondary consequences on cognitive development. Further, they state that the quality of the deaf child's process of communication, rather than the actual mode of communication, is the most important variable. Adults often expect deaf children to listen and speak, without considering whether the context of the communication is meaningful for the child.

Wood et al. (1986) underscore the significance of early interactive experiences as precursors to meaningful understanding of language. They point out that joint care giver–infant attention to objects results in a dual experience for infants. They can see the object and hear the language and language-related nuances used to describe it. Thus, the beginning acquisition of verbal meanings is embedded both in word sounds and in the personal, social, and emotional tone communicated by the adult.

Although effecting change in the quality of care giver and infant interactions is an important goal for achieving communicative and social competencies, it is not the only one. Eventually, interventions must focus on bringing about more effective social skills with peers. Although in many ways the peer social climate is often more egalitarian than that of care giver and child, it can also be less giving in terms of acceptance (Hartup, 1983). In addition, peers are frequently unable to compensate for a handicapped child's problems.

Guralnick and Bennett (1987) have issued a call for refinement of constructs and assessment tools so that emotional and social interventions can move forward. We would add that it may be reasonable to begin planned and systematic exposure (not teaching) of handicapped infants to peers (perhaps toward the end of the first year of life), with the aim of enhancing processes implicated in social skills (e.g., maintaining attention to another, providing contingent responses, acknowledging implicit "rules" for behavior such as empathy). Because handicapped preschoolers clearly demonstrate these problems (see Kopp, Baker, & Brown, in preparation; Strain, Guralnick, & Walker, 1986), infancy may be the time to begin to intervene.

Although we have offered a sobering view of the concept of multiple pathways for some ability domains, we firmly believe that interventions can be directed toward improving the functional use of communicative competencies for handicapped children. With this skill, perhaps social growth will move forward.

Finally, we emphasize that it is important to remember that even within the same diagnostic groups, children's handicaps are manifested in different ways. Not all blind, deaf, and motorically impaired children have the same level of difficulty with social communication. The nature of their experiences in the social world can differ. However, the development of competent social skills is facilitated by a supportive care-giving environment.

There is no question that efforts toward intervention must include provisions for helping parents promote child skills in a way that makes mothers and fathers feel competent and comfortable.

References

Andersen, E.S., Dunlea, A., & Kekelis, L.S. (1984). Blind children's language: Resolving some differences. *Journal of Child Language II*, 645–664.

Andersen, E.S., & Kekelis, L. (1986). The role of sibling input in the language socialization of younger blind children. In J. Connor-Linton, C.J. Hall, & M. McGinnes (Eds.), *Southern California occasional papers in linguistics: Social and cognitive perspectives on language*. Los Angeles: University of Southern California Press.

Bahrick, L.E., & Watson, J.S. (1985). Detection of intermodal proprioception and visual contingency as a potential basis of self-perception in infancy. *Developmental Psychology, 21*, 963–973.

Black, J., & Greenough, W. (1986). Induction of pattern in neural structure by experience: Implications for cognitive development. In M. Lamb, A. Brown, & B. Rogoff (Eds), *Advances in developmental psychology*, Vol. 4. Hillsdale, N.J.: Erlbaum.

Borke, H. (1975). Piaget's mountains revisited: Changes in the egocentric landscape. *Developmental Psychology, 11*, 240–243.

Bowlby, J. (1969). *Attachment and loss*. New York: Basic Books.

Brazelton, T.B., Koslowski, B., & Main, M. (1974). The origins of reciprocity: The early mother–infant interaction. In M. Lewis & L. Rosenblum (Eds.), *The effects of the infant on its caregiver*. New York: Wiley.

Bretherton, I., & Bates, E. (1979). The emergence of intentional communication. In I. Uzgiris (Ed.), *Social interaction and communication during infancy*. San Francisco: Jossey-Bass.

Brown, A.L., Bransford, J.D., Ferrara, R.A., & Campione, J.C. (1983). Learning, remembering, and understanding. In J.H. Flavell & F.M. Markman (Eds.), *Cognitive development*, Vol. 3. In P.H. Mussen (Ed.), *Handbook of child psychology* (4th ed.). New York: Wiley.

Clark, E.V. (1983). Meanings and concepts. In J.H. Flavell & E.M. Markman (Eds.), *Cognitive Development*, Vol. 3. In P.H. Mussen (Ed.), *Handbook of child psychology* (4th ed.). New York: Wiley.

Corsaro, W.A. (1979). "We're friends, right?": Children's use of access rituals in a nursery school. *Language in society*, 8, 315–336.

Corsaro, W.A. (1985) *Friendship and peer culture in the early years*. Norwood, NJ: Ablex.

Decarie, T.D. (1969). A study of the mental and emotional development of the Thalidomide child. In B.M. Foss (Ed.), *Determinants of infant behavior*, Vol. 4. London: Methuen.

Dennis, W. (1940). Infant reactions to restraint. *Transactions of the New York Academy of Science, 2*, 202–217.

Dunn, J., Bretherton, I., & Munn, P. (1987). Conversations about feeling states between mothers and their young children. *Developmental Psychology, 23*, 132–139.

Fewell, R. (1983). Working with sensorily impaired children. In S.G. Garwood (Ed.), *Educating young handicapped children: A developmental approach*. Rockville, MD: Aspen.

Fischer, K.W., Hand, H.H., Watson, M.W., van Parys, M.M., & Tucker, J.L. (1986). Putting the child into socialization: The development of social categories in preschool. In L. Katz (Ed.), *Current topics in early childhood, Vol. 5*. Norwood, NJ: Ablex.

Flavell, J.H. (1972). An analysis of cognitive-developmental sequences. *Genetic Psychology Monographs, 86*, 279–350.

Flavell, J.H. (1985). *Cognitive development* (2nd ed.). Englewood Cliffs, NJ: Prentice-Hall.

Fraiberg, S. (1971). Smiling and stranger reaction in blind infants. In J. Hellmuth (Ed.), *Exceptional infant*. New York: Brunner-Mazel.

Fraiberg, S. (1977). *Insights from the blind*. New York: Basic Books.

Fraser, B.C. (1986). Child impairment and parent/infant communication. *Child Care Health and Development, 12*(3), 141–50.

Garvey, C. (1974). Some properties of social play. *Merrill-Palmer Quarterly, 20*, 163–180.

Gelman, R., & Gallistel, C.R. (1978). *The child's understanding of number*. Cambridge: Harvard University Press.

Gesell, A. (1948). *Studies in child development*. New York: Harper.

Goldin-Meadow, S., & Mylander, C. (1983). Gestural communication in deaf children: The noneffects of parental input on language development. *Science, 221*, 372–274.

Goldin-Meadow, S., & Mylander, C. (1984). Gestural communication in deaf children: The effects and noneffects of parental input on early language development. *Monographs of the Society for Research in Child Development, 49*(3–4), Serial No. 207.

Goodenough, F.L. (1931). *Anger in young children*. Minneapolis: University of Minnesota Press.

Gottman, J.M., & Parker, J.G. (1986). *Conversations of friends: Speculations on affective development*. Cambridge: Cambridge University Press.

Gould, S.J. (1977). *Ontogeny and phylogeny*. Cambridge: Harvard University Press.

Guralnick, M.J., & Bennett, F.C. (1987). *The effectiveness of early intervention for at-risk and handicapped children*. Orlando, FL: Academic Press.

Guralnick, M.J., & Weinhouse, E. (1984). Peer-related social interactions of developmentally delayed young children: Development and characteristics. *Developmental Psychology*, 20(5), 815–827.

Harris, R.I. (1978). Impulse control in deaf children: Research and clinical issues. In L.S. Liben (Ed.), *Deaf Children: Developmental perspectives*. New York: Academic Press.

Hartup, W. (1983). Peer relations. In E.M. Hetherington (Ed.), *Socialization, personality, and social development*, Vol. 4. In P. Mussen (Ed.) *Handbook of Child Psychology*. New York: Wiley.

Horowitz, F.D. (1987). Targeting infant stimulation efforts: Theoretical challenges for research and intervention. In N. Gunzenhauser (Ed.), *Infant stimulation: For whom, what kind, when, and how much*. Stillman, NJ: Johnson & Johnson.

House, J.S., Landis, K.R., & Umberson, D. (1988). Social relationships and health. *Science*, 241, 540–545.

Jones, M.C., & Burks, B.S. (1936). Personality development in childhood. *Mongraphs of the Society for Research in Child Development*, Vol. 1, 4.

Kagan, J. (1971). *Change and continuity in infancy*. New York: Wiley.

Kagan, J. (1984). *Nature of the child*. New York: Basic Books.

Kaye, K., & Fogel, A. (1980). The temporal structure of face-to-face communication between mothers and infants. *Developmental Psychology, 16*, 454–464.

Kekelis, L.S., & Andersen, E.S. (1984). Family communication styles and language development. *Journal of Visual Impairment and Blindness*, 54–65.

Kopp, C.B. (in press). Regulation of distress and negative emotions: A developmental view. *Developmental Psychology*.

Kopp, C.B. (1987). The growth of self-regulation: Caregivers and children. In N. Eisenberg (Ed.), *Contemporary topics in developmental psychology*. New York: Wiley.

Kopp, C.B., Baker, K., & Brown, B. (in preparation). The social skills of developmentally delayed preschoolers.

Kopp, C.B., & Shaperman, J. (1973). Cognitive development in the absence of object manipulation during infancy. *Developmental Psychology, 9*, 3 (brief report).

Kuhl, P.K. (1987). Perception of speech and sound in early infancy. In P. Salapatek & L. Cohen (Eds.), *Handbook of infant perception: From perception to cognition*. New York: Academic Press.

Liben, L.S. (Ed.) (1978). *Deaf children: Developmental perspectives*. New York: Academic Press.

Mayberry, R., Wodlinger-Cohen, R., & Goldin-Meadow, S. (1987). Symbolic development in deaf children. In W. Damon (Ed.), *New directions for child development* (No. 36). San Francisco: Jossey-Bass.

Meadow, K.P. (1980). *Deafness and Child Development*. New York: Academic Press.

Millar, S. (1988). Models of sensory deprivation: The nature/nurture dichotomy and spatial representation in the blind. *International Journal of Behavioral Development, 11*, 69–88.

Mogford, K. (1977). The play of handicapped children. In B. Tizard & D. Harvey (Eds.), *The biology of play*. Philadelphia: Lippincott.

Murphy, L.B. (1956). *Personality in young children*. New York: Basic Books.

Parke, R., & Asher, S.R. (1983). Social and personality development. *Annual Review of Psychology*. Palo Alto: Stanford University Press.

Parker, J.G., & Asher, S.R. (1987). Peer relations and later personal adjustment: Are low-accepted children at risk? *Psychological Bulletin, 102*, 357–389.

Petitto, L.A. (1987). On the autonomy of language and gesture: Evidence from the acquisition of personal pronouns in American Sign Language. *Cognition, 27*(1): 1–52.

Piaget, J. (1970). Piaget's theory. In P.H. Mussen (Ed.), *Carmichael's manual of child psychology*, Vol. 1. New York: Wiley.

Rogers, S.J., & Puchalski, C.B. (1984). Development of symbolic play in visually impaired infants. *Topics in Early Childhood Special Education, 3*, 57–64.

Rogers, S.J., & Puchalski, C.B. (1988). Development of object permanence in visually impaired infants. *Journal of Visual Impairment & Blindness*, 137–142.

Rogoff, B., Sellers, M.J., Pirrotta, S., Fox, N., & White, S.M. (1975). Age assignment of roles and responsibilities to children. *Human Development, 18*, 353–369.

Scarr-Salapatek, S. (1976). An evolutionary perspective on infant intelligence: Species patterns and individual variations. In M. Lewis (Ed.), *Origins of intelligence*. New York: Plenum.

Schaffer, H.R. (1984). *The child's entry into a social world*. London: Academic Press.

Schlesinger, H., & Meadow, K. (1972). *Sound and sign, childhood deafness and mental health*. Berkeley: University of California Press.

Seidman, S., Allen, R., & Wasserman, G.A. (1986). Productive language of premature and physically handicapped two-year olds. *Journal of Communication Disorders, 19*(1): 49–61.

Siegler, R.S. (1978). The origins of scientific reasoning. In R.S. Siegler (Ed.), *Children's thinking: What develops?* Hillsdale, NJ: Erbaum.

Spelke, E.S. (1987). The development of intermodal perception. In P. Salapatek & L. Cohen (Eds.), *Handbook of infant perception: From perception to cognition*. New York: Academic Press.

Spelke, E.S. (1988). Where perceiving ends and thinking begins: The apprehension of objects in infancy. In A. Yonas (Ed.), *Perceptual development in infancy*. The Minnesota Symposia on Child Psychology, Vol. 20. Hillsdale, NJ: Erlbaum.

Stern, D.N. (1985). *The interpersonal world of the infant*. New York: Basic Books.

Strain, P., Guralnick, M.J., & Walker, H.M. (1986). *Children's social behavior: Development, assessment, and modification*. New York: Academic Press.

Stremel-Campbell, K., & Rowland, C. (1987). Prelinguistic communication intervention: Birth-to-2. *Topics in Early Childhood Special Education, 7*, 49–58.

Tronick, E.Z., Cohn, J., & Shea, E. (1986). The transfer of affect between mothers and infants. In T.B. Brazelton & M.W. Yogman (Eds.), *Affective development in infancy*. Norwood, NJ: Ablex.

Uzgiris, I.C. (1967). Ordinality in the development of Schemes for relating to objects. In J. Hellmuth (Ed.), *Exceptional infant, Vol. 1*. Seattle: Special Child Publications.

Wellman, H. (1985). The early development of memory strategies. In H. Weinert & M. Perlmutter (Eds.), *Memory development: Universal changes and individual differences*. Hillsdale, NJ: Erlbaum.

Wenar, C. (1982). On negativism. *Human Development, 25*, 1–23.

Wood, D., Wood, H., Griffiths, A., & Howarth, I. (1986). *Teaching and talking with deaf children*. Chichester, England: Wiley.

12 Summing up and going forward: New directions in the developmental approach to mental retardation

Robert M. Hodapp, Jacob A. Burack, and Edward Zigler

The contributors to this book were asked to perform a difficult task – to specify what has come to be known as the developmental approach to mental retardation. They were asked to delineate what general developmental theory, findings, and perspectives tell us about retarded development, and what mental retardation research tells us about general developmental processes. The hope is that by joining findings from these two areas we can gain a clearer understanding of both normal development and mental retardation.

The construction of a comprehensive developmental approach to mental retardation is difficult to accomplish because it encompasses two topics that many consider to be incompatible. On the one hand, developmental theorists have typically considered only nonhandicapped persons when discussing the nature of developmental processes. Even in debates concerning individual differences and the universality of development, little attention has been paid to the development of mentally retarded persons. Similarly, debates about sequences, structures, and environments have also been conducted without regard to evidence from retarded populations (see Inhelder, 1968, and Woodward, 1979, for notable exceptions).

On the other hand, researchers of mental retardation have had little use for general developmental theory. Mentally retarded persons have traditionally been viewed as different from other persons in that they suffer from one or a few specific defects; their functioning has therefore been judged to be incompatible with traditional developmental theory. The hegemony of defect theories shows this indifference to developmental theory in the majority of work in the mental retardation field.

In contrast to both these views, it has been our contention that the failure to enjoin an interplay between work on normal development and mental retardation has hindered our understanding of both these areas. As the contributors to this book have demonstrated, there is much that developmental theory can teach us about mental retardation and much that

294

mental retardation can teach us about general developmental processes. It is to issues in these two areas that we now turn.

Contributions of developmental work to the understanding of mental retardation

The two-group approach and beyond: How best to differentiate retarded individuals for research or intervention

During the past half century, most developmentally oriented researchers in mental retardation have been proponents of the two-group approach. These researchers have argued that mentally retarded persons can be divided into two groups. The first group consists of those persons whose retardation can be attributed to some specific organic damage (the organically retarded group). The second group consists of those individuals with no known organic insult (the familial retarded group). This distinction between two groups of retarded individuals has been thought to be helpful for purposes of both research and intervention.

During the past quarter century, Zigler and colleagues (Zigler, 1967, 1969; Zigler & Balla, 1982a; Zigler & Hodapp, 1986) have been the leading advocates of both the two-group approach and the application of developmental theory. In synthesizing these two ideas, these researchers have argued that the development of familial retarded persons does not differ from that of nonretarded individuals, except that it progresses at a slower rate and attains a lower asymptote (Zigler, 1967, 1969). Zigler suggests, however, that the development of organically retarded persons does not necessarily conform to typical developmental processes. He argues that "If the etiology of the phenotypic intelligence (as measured by an IQ) of two groups differs, it is far from logical to assert that the course of development is the same, or even that similar contents in the behaviors of two such differing individuals are mediated by exactly the same cognitive processes" (Zigler, 1969, p. 533).

Zigler's view has recently been called the conservative developmental approach (see Cicchetti & Pogge-Hesse, 1982) in that it considers only familial retarded persons within a developmental framework. In contrast, liberal developmentalists such as Cicchetti (e.g., Cicchetti & Pogge-Hesse, 1982) and Kopp (e.g., Kopp & McCall, 1982) have proposed an expanded developmental approach. These workers hypothesize that developmental theory can be applied to both familial and organically retarded persons. They assert that certain achievements occur in the same manner in all persons; even specific or severe organic insult might be unable to alter the universal course of such developments. Studies on developmental sequences in different etiological groups also help inform us about (1) the specific functioning of certain groups, (2) factors that can interfere with typical developmental processes, and (3) the limits to which developmental processes can be altered.

In order to gain a more precise understanding of developmental processes of mentally retarded persons, liberal developmentalists have emphasized the need to study specific etiological groups. Heretofore, the general consensus among researchers in mental retardation has been that etiological differences have little effect on maturational processes (Ellis & Cavalier, 1982; MacMillan, 1982; Zeaman & House, 1979). As a result, mentally retarded persons have generally been studied as a homogeneous group. Even advocates of the two-group approach, who distinguish organic from familial retardation, have not usually differentiated among the more than 200 types of organic retardation.

Despite these longstanding views, it is becoming increasingly evident that there are considerable differences in development among the various etiological groups of organically retarded persons (see Burack, Hodapp, & Zigler, 1988; also chapter 2). For this reason, any attempts to understand the developmental processes of mentally retarded persons must utilize fine-grained research strategies that consider etiology.

Indeed, in order to extract a maximum amount of information from a given study, investigators can utilize a hierarchical research strategy in which etiology serves as the beginning, not the end, of the classificatory process. Within such an approach, subjects are differentiated by specific etiology (e.g., Down syndrome) and, where appropriate, by etiological subgroups (e.g., trisomy 21, mosaic, and translocation subgroups within Down syndrome). If there are differences among these subgroups in the behavior being studied, this information would be preserved, and the groups would have to be considered independently. Certain subgroups could, however, be combined for statistical purposes if, and only if, no differences were found among them on the behaviors being measured.

Effects on rates of development in retarded individuals

A second contribution of the developmental approach to MR work involves analyses of those factors that change the rate of development within different etiological groups. The issue is whether changes in rate of development (e.g., IQ) are due more to the changing nature of the tasks facing the developing child or to maturational changes in neurological structure.

At present, it appears that with different etiological groups, different task or brain mechanisms are operative. For example, it is a common finding that Down syndrome children slow down in their rate of development over time; although these children continue to develop, their rate of development (as demonstrated by IQ scores) gradually decelerates with increasing age. This gradual deceleration seems to be due to the difficulties in making the qualitative mental leaps involved with each stage transition. In reviewing the development of Down syndrome children over the first 2 years of life, Kopp and McCall (1982) note that these infants fall further behind their nonretarded age mates at MAs of 2, 8, 13, and 21 months – the so-called transition points of infant intelligence (McCall, Eichorn, & Hogarty, 1977). "We speculate that these transitions may mark the time when infants with known central nervous system impairment begin to separate from their peers, not just in rate of developmental change, but also in respect to density, richness, and adaptability of sensorimotor repertoire" (Kopp & McCall, 1982, p. 55; see also Hodapp & Zigler, in press). For Down syndrome children, then, decelerating rates of development may be due to problems in mastering new and qualitatively different developmental tasks.

For males with fragile X syndrome, however, IQ changes may be more related to changes in neurological structure. As noted by Dykens and Leckman (chapter 9), males with fragile X syndrome demonstrate relatively steady IQs until the early teen years, when MAs plateau and IQ declines. As this decline in IQ seems related to the age of the child – not to difficulties in dealing with complex new tasks – neurological rather than task explanations seem appropriate. In this case, earlier-than-usual hormonal changes associated with puberty seem implicated, not particular difficulties in mastering new, high-level tasks of development (Dykens, Hodapp, Ort, Finucane, Shapiro, & Leckman, 1989). In contrast to Down syndrome children, where slowing rates of development come about as the child has difficulty in overcoming new, qualitatively different tasks, fragile X males show decelerating developments due to hormonal and other neurological changes associated with puberty.

Such differences between task versus brain factors are shown in Figures 12.1a and 12.1b. Comparing two children of different IQs (and thus progressing at differing rates over time), Figure 12.1a shows the effects of a task-related problem, such as that associated with the entrance into symbolic functioning for Down syndrome children. At whatever age the child reaches this task-related (or, in general, MA-related) "wall," further developments are slowed. The impediment will, however, arrive for two different children at different CAs, as it is a difficulty associated with the

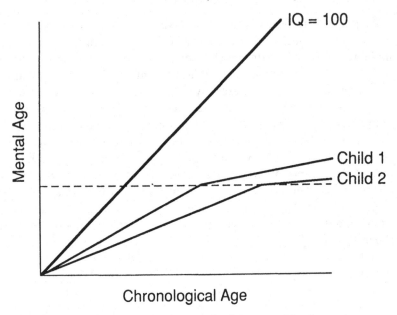

Figure 12.1a. Effects of changes in type of task on rate of development.

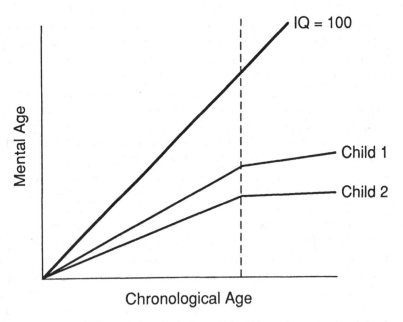

Figure 12.1b. Effects of changes in neurobiological structure on rate of development.

task, not with age. Conversely, Figure 12.1b shows two children of different IQs as they each encounter problems associated with brain maturation. In this case, developmental rates slow once the child reaches a particular CA, regardless of the MA level already achieved. This type of problem associated with brain maturation seems implicated in the slowing rates of development shown by males with fragile X syndrome as they enter the early teen years (Dykens et al., 1989).

Role of the environment in fostering or delaying development

A third contribution of developmental knowledge to our understanding of mental retardation involves the environment. Granted, the nature and effects of the environment continue to be only generally understood by workers in developmental psychology and related fields. Specifically, we know little about which particular aspects of the environment help children to develop in which areas, at which times. How different parts of the environment interact is also unclear, and the effects over time of a multi-layered environment are also generally unknown. In short, Kessen's statement that "we have no agreed upon theory of the environment" is as true today as when it was written in 1968.

There are, however, movements within the fields studying environments in nonretarded children that are beginning to be applicable to work with children who are retarded. In particular, Sameroff's (1975; Sameroff & Chandler, 1975) transactional model has informed work on input language (Rondal, 1985; Snow, 1972) and on mother–child interaction (Hodapp & Mueller, 1982; Kaye, 1982; Stern, 1985). These studies, in turn, have begun to delineate how mothers structure the linguistic and nonlinguistic environment to aid their children's development, especially in the earliest years. Similarly, Bronfenbrenner's (1979) focus on family systems has spurred much work on aspects of the family (e.g., family system itself – Minuchin, 1985; siblings – Dunn & Kendrick, 1982) and on the inter-relationships among the different environments that affect children (Cochran & Broussard, 1979). Although our knowledge of the nature and effects of the environment(s) might still be considered primitive, work on normally developing children has at least helped sketch the outlines of such a discipline. Indeed, most would now agree that the environment consists of social and nonsocial aspects, is changing and developing with the child, and is composed of multiple and interacting layers.

Although the outlines are in place, the specifics, especially concerning the environments of children with retardation, still are generally lacking. Mental retardation researchers are beginning to understand the nature of adult social and linguistic behaviors to retarded children (Marfo, 1988), but there remain huge gaps in our knowledge of the family systems of retarded children, of maternal reactions to and perceptions of their retarded children, and of the behaviors of nonretarded children to their retarded siblings. The feelings and behaviors of fathers of retarded children are almost completely unknown; indeed, it is the rare study that even includes fathers of retarded children.

The remaining job is to examine more specifically aspects of the environment and how they affect different domains of functioning for retarded children. Sameroff's identification of factors leading to lowered IQs for at-risk children (Chapter 5) is a step in this direction, but more specific examinations of the environment are needed. In addition, it is important to examine different environmental outcomes, not solely (or even predominantly) the child's IQ score (Zigler & Balla, 1982b).

There may also be no single "environment" for all types of retarded children. Just as Down syndrome, fragile X, autistic, and multiply handicapped children differ one from another, the reactions and behaviors of the care givers of each type of child may similarly be specific to particular etiologies, or at least to the specific disability as perceived by the parent (e.g., Goldberg, Marcovitch, MacGregor, & Lojkasek, 1986). Like the problems inherent in specifying the nature and effects of different levels of the environment, the difficulties involved in understanding the environment vis-a-vis different etiologies of mental retardation are also complicated.

There are, then, several contributions of developmental work to the understanding of mental retardation and development in retarded individuals. An increased emphasis on etiology, the causes of differing rates of development, and the understanding and application of knowledge of the environment should all help applied efforts with retarded individuals in the future, although much work remains to be accomplished.

Contributions of mental retardation work to the understanding of normal developmental processes

So far, both in this chapter and throughout the book, most discussion has focused on one aspect of the developmental approach to mental retardation – the ways in which normal development can be applied to retarded populations. These issues have included the idea of an active organism and behavior as reflective of underlying cognitive, linguistic, and motivational structures; the orthogenetic principle; the similar-sequence and similar-structure hypotheses; and the nature and effects of the environment. In all cases, the theories, findings, and methodologies used to understand nonretarded children have been applied to retarded individuals.

But the interplay of nonretarded and retarded development does not proceed in only one direction. Indeed, mental retardation in general, and different etiological groups in particular, can be thought of as "experiments of nature" that afford unique opportunities for the study of normal development. For instance, retarded individuals proceed at slower rates, allowing for a more precise examination of developmental sequences. Similarly, the nature of cross-domain relationships is open to a closer examination in different groups of retarded children than might be possible using only nonretarded children. Finally, the effects of inherent characteristics of the child on the surrounding environment are also more fully examined using retarded individuals. It is to these three ways that retarded functioning informs normal development – sequences, cross-domain relationships, and children's effects on their environment – that we now turn.

"Lock-step" orderings versus multiple pathways, or reconciling universal and individual sequences of development

Among interventionists, researchers, and others in the mental retardation field, it is commonplace to hear that not enough attention is paid to the individuality of retarded individuals. Workers decry the use of theories of development that focus on fixed or "lock-step" sequences – orderings of development that do not allow for other than one specific mandated sequence in the acquisition of behaviors. Even developmentally oriented workers such as von Bertalannfy (1968; see also Davidson, 1983) have occasionally decried an overly rigid developmental model, noting that there are many pathways to a single end.

At the same time, findings pertaining to the similar-sequence hypothesis indicate that there may often be only one ordering of development for a particular achievement. Weisz, Yeates, and Zigler (1982) have shown that at least in cognitive development, retarded children proceed through Piagetian stages in invariant order. These single, universal orderings are found for any number of Piagetian domains, leading one to espouse a lock-step ordering of development for achievements in these domains. Are there many pathways to development, or does development occur in a single, lock-step ordering?

The use of retarded children to study universal versus idiosyncratic sequences of development provides three answers to this question. The first emphasizes the difference between those domains that develop earlier and are more biologically based and those that are achieved later and are more social or cultural in origin. As noted by Hodapp in chapter 3, Piagetian sensorimotor developments might be thought of as both earlier and more biologically based; these skills are "highly canalized" to develop in the single, universal order in all humans (McCall, 1981; Scarr-Salapatek, 1975). In contrast, such areas as moral development, person perception, and even formal operational thought might be considered to be achievements that are more culturally based or that take place later in development. Such developments seem to occur in more idiosyncratic fashion from culture to culture, child to child, or across children with different types of disabilities.

A second answer to the lock-step versus multiple pathways question concerns the distinction between orderings of development and the modalities by which one interacts with the world. Blind children, deaf children, and children without limbs all interact with the world differently, using different sensory modalities. But as Kopp and Recchia note in chapter 11, even despite these major differences each group proceeds through universal sequences in the usual manner. They argue that such multimodal patterns of acquisition may be limited primarily to sensorimotor developments, but at least these achievements can be attained using any of several sensory modalities. It is almost as if for these hard-wired developments the organism is preprogrammed to proceed in this single, lock-step ordering, irrespective of the sensory modality with which the child interacts with the world.

A third answer to the lock-step/multiple pathway issue is that not all achievements that occur during childhood develop in a universal and invariant sequence in any group of children, even those without retardation or other developmental disabilities. Even within a single domain such as language development, aspects such as early semantic relations (Slobin, 1970) and English grammatical morphemes (Brown, 1973) develop in a set order, whereas pragmatic functions – the uses of language – do not seem to be so fixed in their orderings. In their earliest speech, some children use language to express functions that are predominantly social (e.g., greetings such as "hi mommy"), whereas others mainly produce object-related utterances (e.g., "want ball"; Dore, 1975; Halliday, 1975). No preferred ordering of social versus object-related functions seems evident in the early communication of nonretarded children.

In the mental retardation field, sequences within such "individualized" developments might be related to the etiology of the retarded child. For example, autistic children issue more demands and other object-related pragmatic functions in their early speech (Curcio, 1978; Wetherby & Prutting, 1984); only at higher levels of language do autistic children engage in quasisocial communication (i.e., language to get the adult's attention) or social communication (Wetherby, 1986). Indeed, Prizant (1988) has speculated that autistic children have their own, etiology-specific ordering of pragmatic functions. Such a movement from object-related to quasi-social to truly social uses of language is very different from patterns found in normally developing children. This pattern may also differ from sequences found in children with Down syndrome or other etiologies characterized by strengths in social skills; these children demonstrate social or quasisocial functions in their earliest communications (Leifer & Lewis, 1984). Most importantly, however, the interplay of behaviors showing more fixed orderings with those of more flexible orderings allows for a compromise between lock-step and idiosyncratic sequences of development, in both retarded and nonretarded children.

Interplay of developments across different domains: Is development organized or disorganized?

As Cicchetti and Ganiban note in chapter 8, we have come a long way from the view that retarded children are simply defective. Even if there are particular defects in some etiological groups – areas where, when matched on MA, retarded children of particular etiologies perform worse than nonretarded individuals – there may still be some "organization" within development.

The examination of behavioral functioning in different etiological groups offers a unique opportunity to specify such relationships. Because behavioral characteristics are often specific to a particular etiological group (Burack, Hodapp, & Zigler, 1988), any commonalities found across all groups would seem to indicate a true relationship between two domains. Thus, Down syndrome children may have dampened affect and problems in language, but relatively high levels of social skills (see chapter 8). Fragile X boys, on the other hand, may have sequential-processing problems and attention deficit disorders (see Dykens and Leckman, chapter 9), whereas extreme social deficits and echolalic and gestalt-like language seem to characterize functioning in autistic children (Volkmar, Burack, & Cohen, chapter 10). But if each of these groups shows similar cross-domain relationships, it seems likely that such relationships indicate necessary connections across development between two or more domains.

The analogy of a signal-to-noise ratio – of common signals that come through despite large amounts of etiology-specific noise – might be one way to think of this approach. If several types of retarded children show identical relationships across two domains, one can more confidently assert that there is a real relationship between these domains. In fact, several specific cross-domain relationships do seem to hold across different types of retarded and nonretarded children. The presence of sensorimotor means–ends abilities (the use of one object as a means to retrieve another) seems to be related to the earliest of communicative behaviors, both for nonretarded children (Bates, Benigni, Bretherton, Camaioni, & Volterra, 1979) and for autistic children (Curcio, 1978). Cicchetti and Ganiban (chapter 8) note that as with nonretarded children (McCune-Nicholich & Bruskin, 1982), different levels of symbolic play seem related to levels of early language in Down syndrome children (Beeghly & Cicchetti, 1987) and, possibly, in autistic children as well (Mundy, Sigman, Ungerer, & Sherman, 1987). In each of these groups, prelinguistic children generally mouth or handle objects, children in the one-word stage engage only in single-schemed play (e.g., using a toy cup to "drink"), and children beginning two-word sentences (early stage I; Brown, 1973) combine simple schemes such as feeding a doll, then grooming it. If such relationships are also seen in fragile X syndrome children, or in children with other disorders, one might reasonably conclude that a true relationship exists between levels of functioning in these two areas. This use of cross-domain relationships that are identical across different etiological groups would seem to be a powerful demonstration of those behaviors that must go together in development.

Similarly the examination of diverse areas of functioning in children with a particular defect can show the extent to which behaviors in many areas are affected by a single deficit. Dykens and Leckman (chapter 9) note that the sequential-processing deficits identified in fragile X syndrome boys (Dykens, Hodapp, & Leckman, 1987) seem to be implicated in their cognitive, linguistic, and adaptive functioning, as well as in the type of psychopathology sometimes shown by these children. Such pervasive effects of a single disability help identify which behaviors require which component skills, and how and to what degree children with a particular deficit can overcome these difficulties. In addition, as noted in chapter 9, workers can construct intervention strategies that capitalize on the strengths that these children possess.

A final issue, mentioned in chapters 4 and 7, concerns the relationship between molar and molecular behaviors. Developmental theory has, incorrectly in our view, been considered a molar theory, focused only on Piagetian stages and other "grosser" areas of development. In constrast, defect theorists (see Hodapp, Burack, & Zigler, chapter 1) have championed various individual defects that supposedly account for the impaired functioning of all retarded children, regardless of etiology. Several workers (e.g., Detterman, 1987) have gone on to claim that the delay–difference debate is therefore simply one of different levels of analysis, that retarded children are delayed on the larger, more molar behaviors, but defective compared with MA-matched individuals on the smaller, more molecular aspects of functioning.

This hypothesis leads to several implications that are both untested and, at first glance, untrue. First, as the chapters of this book demonstrate, etiology matters. Down syndrome children do seem different from autistic children, who in turn differ from cerebral palsy or fragile X syndrome individuals (Burack, chapter 2; Burack, Hodapp, & Zigler, 1988). Although not every etiological group is unique in each area of functioning, there are enough differences to make suspect any global pronouncements about "retarded functioning."

Second, there must be some relationship between molar and molecular functioning. Molar functioning is, after all, comprised of a host of molecular skills. One cannot uncover an object in an object-permanence test without being able to follow objects in space, to remember where the object was hidden, and to coordinate motor schemes to remove the cover. Still, Mundy and Kasari (chapter 4) argue that there may be some distinction between a child's functioning on information-processing and Piagetian tasks, as "individuals may vary on rate related cognitive phenomena [i.e., information-processing tasks], while not varying on stage-dependent logical operations or problem-solving skills [Piagetian tasks]." Alternatively, Weisz's argument (chapter 7) that nonorganically retarded children perform worse on information-processing tasks because these tasks are less ecologically valid, may also be true. In short, much more work is necessary on the relationship between molar and molecular behaviors. The specification of this relationship will, in turn, tell us much about the organization of intelligence in nonretarded children, nonorganically retarded children, and in children within each of the many etiological groups.

From this discussion, then, we note that development is organized within retarded individuals, but that the issue of how this organization works is still unclear. The possible uses of different etiological groups to specify necessary cross-domain relationships, the manifestation of single defects across domains, and the specification of the relationship between molecular and molar behaviors are all open to study using mentally retarded populations.

Effects of the handicapped child on the environment

A third area in which evidence from mentally retarded children can inform theories of nonretarded development involves the environment. In particular, the retarded child helps elucidate how environments react and, ideally, how the environment itself is organized.

To date, such work is in its earliest stages, but a few themes are beginning to emerge. Parallel with the work on mother–nonretarded child interactions, there is a burgeoning interest in the perceptions and emotions of the mother. Whereas mother–child interaction had previously been focused solely on the behaviors of each partner, studies of both retarded and nonretarded children are currently focusing on how each person conceptualizes the other (Hodapp, 1988). In studies of nonretarded children, recent topics have included the nature of mother–child interactions with depressed mothers (Tronick & Field, 1986); the mother's knowledge and perceptions of the infant (Sigel, 1985; Young, 1988); the infant's perceptions of the mother (Klinnert, Emde, Butterfield, & Campos, 1986); and even the infant's emerging sense of self (Stern, 1985). Each of these studies indicates the importance of the perceptions and emotions of both participants in mother–child interaction.

In work with retarded populations as well, such a focus on the perceptions and emotions of each partner is becoming evident. Take, first, the finding that mothers of Down syndrome children are appropriate in the level of language they provide for their retarded children (Rondal, 1977), but are much more controlling and didactic than are mothers of MA-matched nonretarded children (Cardoso-Martins & Mervis, 1985; Jones, 1977). Recent work has suggested that aspects of *both* the child and the mother may produce such findings. Retarded children, especially those with Down syndrome, may be more difficult to "read" correctly (Cicchetti & Sroufe, 1976). Therefore, mothers may have a more difficult time understanding when these children are themselves initiating interaction. Second, it may also be the case that, due to their dampened affect (Cicchetti & Ganiban, chapter 9), Down syndrome children require interactions that are more "parent centered" (Schneider & Pelland, 1987). Third, mothers of retarded children may differ from mothers of nonretarded children; specifically, mothers of retarded children are thought to go through a process of "mourning the birth of the defective child" (Blacher, 1984; Solnit & Stark, 1961). These mothers might therefore at times be comparable to the depressed mothers examined by Tronick and Field (1986) and others. Finally, there might be differences in how the mother of a handicapped child perceives the nature and function of interactions; if she is worried about her child's being delayed in cognitive abilities, she might attempt to take every opportunity to teach the child. Hence, a more didactic style. Although work in this area is only beginning (and indeed, hypotheses are not mutually exclusive), it does seem the case that an increased attention to the perceptions and emotions of mother and child will be necessary to understand fully the interactions between mothers and their retarded children.

At the same time that retarded children affect their environment, they are in turn affected by that environment. In addition to the personality and motivational factors explored by Zigler and his colleagues (Merighi, Edison, & Zigler, chapter 6), we have recently become interested in environmental effects that are more cultural in nature. One such area is the place of age-appropriate behavior in the lives of retarded children. Nonretarded children engage in a series of age-appropriate roles – toddlers play in sandboxes, children in the early school years participate in clubs and organized sports, and early and late adolescents engage in their own specific age-appropriate behaviors and interests. Studies of retarded children – children who are older in CA than in MA – allow for a more fine-grained examination of the determinants of such CA-role behavior. Our preliminary results indicate that at early CAs, mildly and moderately retarded children behave equal to their MAs, not their CAs. It is only in the late teen years – from 16 to 18 – that retarded children begin to behave somewhere between their CAs and MAs (Evans, Hodapp, & Zigler, 1988). In essence, the realization that one should try to "act one's age" is only felt by retarded children in the late teen years; younger retarded children behave much more like their MAs than their CAs on these everyday behaviors and interests. Such attention to the interplay between aspects of the child and of the culture is only beginning to occur in developmental work with retarded individuals.

Conclusion

As a major theoretical orientation in the field of mental retardation (Baumeister, 1987), the developmental approach is a varied perspective with a rich history. Begun in the late 1960s, the developmental approach was originally concerned with similar sequences and structures in non-organically retarded populations. As this book has shown, however, the perspective is currently being expanded to apply to groups with specific organic etiologies, and the issues of cross-domain relationships, sequences of development, and the nature and effects of the environment have been assimilated into the developmental approach in new and complex ways. This is not to say that there is agreement about what nonretarded development tells us about retarded development, or vice versa, but the issues have become more elaborated and refined over time.

Indeed, in examining the history of the developmental approach to mental retardation, one could argue that the approach is only beginning to be effectively applied to retarded individuals, that the interplay of nonretarded and retarded development continues to be underexplored. For example, the number of cross-domain relationships found in both retarded and nonretarded groups is very small at present, and the information about specific environmental effects remains distressingly sparse. From the opposite perspective, we still know very little about the psychological functioning of many etiological groups, making intervention efforts less precise and less likely to be effective.

Just as our understanding of how to employ the developmental perspective is expanding, so too is the theory upon which that perspective is based. Influential workers in developmental psychology are today questioning many of the field's basic tenets – ideas such as unified stages of cognitive development, sequential development in every area, and context-free theories of development (Bronfenbrenner, Kessel, Kessen & White, 1986; Wertsch & Youniss, 1987). This rethinking of developmental theory has made its application to retarded populations a challenging venture, somewhat akin to building a house on shifting sands. At the same time, these challenges have broadened the focus of developmental work with retarded groups. For example, changes in theories of how nonretarded children develop have made much more prominent the work on families of retarded children, the various contexts of development, cross-domain relationships, and relationships between retarded children and the culture in which those children develop. Even the issue of molar versus molecular aspects of cognition in retarded individuals is partly an application of post-Piagetian views of cognitive development (e.g., Case, 1984). All of these areas, while hinted at in earlier times, were not nearly so prominent as they are today. In short, although the developmental approach will probably always be in flux, that flux provides new directions, new research ideas, and new ways to help retarded individuals.

We are left with a field that is in many ways at its most exciting time. As the contributors to this book have shown, the general outlines of the developmental approach to mental retardation now exist, but the picture remains to be filled in, to be explored in ways that tell us about functioning in both retarded and nonretarded children. Such is the challenge of those interested in the developmental approach to mental retardation in the years to come.

References

Bates, E., Benigni, L., Bretherton, I., Camaioni, I., & Volterra, V. (1979). *The emergence of symbols: Cognition and communication in infancy.* New York: Academic Press.

Baumeister, A. (1987). Mental retardation: Some conceptions and dilemmas. *American Psychologist, 42,* 796–800.

Beeghly, M., & Cicchetti, D. (1987). An organizational approach to symbolic development in children with Down Syndrome. In D. Cicchetti & M. Beeghly (Eds.), *Symbolic development in atypical children. New directions for child development* (No. 36). San Francisco: Jossey-Bass.

Bertalannfy, L. von (1968). *General systems theory.* New York: Braziller.

Blacher, J. (1984). Sequential stages of parental adjustment to the birth of a child with handicaps: Fact or artifact? *Mental Retardation, 22,* 55–68.

Bronfenbrenner, U. (1979). *The ecology of human development.* Cambridge: Harvard University Press.

Bronfenbrenner, U., Kessel, F., Kessen, W., & White, S. (1986). Toward a critical social history of developmental psychology: A propaedeutic discussion. *American Psychologist, 41,* 1218–1230.

Brown, R. (1973). *A first language.* Cambridge: Harvard University Press.

Burack, J.A. (this volume). Differentiating mental retardation: The two-group approach and beyond. Chapter 2.

Burack, J.A., Hodapp, R.M., & Zigler, E. (1988). Issues in the classification of mental retardation: Differentiating among organic etiologies. *Journal of Child Psychology and Psychiatry, 29,* 765–769.

Cardoso-Martins, C., & Mervis C. (1985). Maternal speech to prelinguistic children with Down syndrome. *American Journal of Mental Deficiency, 89,* 451–458.

Case, R. (1984). The process of stage transition: A neo-Piagetian view. In R. Sternberg (Ed.), *Mechanisms of cognitive development.* New York: Freeman.

Cicchetti, D., & Ganiban, J. (this volume). The organization and coherence of developmental processes in infants and children with Down syndrome. Chapter 7.

Cicchetti, D., & Pogge-Hesse, P. (1982). Possible contributions of the study of organically retarded persons to developmental theory. In E. Zigler & D. Balla (Eds.), *Mental retardation: The developmental-difference controversy.* Hillsdale, NJ: Erlbaum.

Cicchetti, D., & Sroufe, L.A. (1976). The relationship between affective and cognitive development in Down syndrome infants. *Child Development, 47,* 920–929.

Cochran, M., & Broussard, J. (1979). Child development and personal social networks. *Child Development, 50,* 601–616.

Curcio, F. (1978). Sensorimotor functioning and communication in mute autistic children. *Journal of Autism and Childhood Schizophrenia, 12,* 264–287.

Davidson, M. (1983). *Uncommon sense: The life and thought of Ludwig von Bertalannfy, father of General Systems Theory.* Los Angeles: Tarcher.

Detterman, D. (1978). Theoretical notions of intelligence and mental retardation. *American Journal of Mental Deficiency, 92,* 2–11.

Dore, J. (1975). Holophrases, speech acts, and language universals. *Journal of Child Language, 2,* 21–40.

Dunn, J., & Kendrick, C. (1982). *Siblings: Love, envy, and understanding.* Cambridge: Harvard University Press.

Dykens, E.M., Hodapp, R.M., & Leckman, J. (1987). Strengths and weaknesses in the intellectual functioning of males with fragile X syndrome. *American Journal of Mental Deficiency, 92,* 234–236.

Dykens, E., Hodapp, R.M., Ort, S., Finucane, B., Shapiro, L., & Leckman, J. The trajectory of cognitive development in males with fragile X syndrome. *Journal of the American Academy of Child and Adolescent Psychiatry*, 28(3), 422–426.

Dykens, E., & Leckman, J. (this volume). Developmental issues in fragile X syndrome. Chapter 9.

Ellis, N., & Cavalier, A.R. (1982). Research perspectives in mental retardation. In E. Zigler & D. Balla (Eds.), *Mental retardation: The developmental–difference controversy*. Hillsdale, NJ: Erlbaum.

Evans, D.W., Hodapp, R.M., & Zigler, E. (1988). *Age-role behavior in the leisure activities of children with mental retardation*. Presentation to the meetings of the Society for Research in Child Development, April 1989.

Goldberg, S., Marcovitch, S., MacGregor, D., & Lojkasek, M. (1986). Family responses to developmentally delayed preschoolers: Etiology and the father's role. *American Journal of Mental Deficiency*, 90(6), 610–617.

Halliday, M.A.K. (1975). Learning how to mean. In E. Lenneberg & E. Lenneberg (Eds.), *Foundations of language development: A multi-disciplinary approach*, Vol. 1. New York: Academic Press.

Hodapp, R.M. (1988). The role of maternal emotions and perceptions in interactions with young handicapped children. In K. Marfo (Ed.), *Parent–child interaction and developmental disabilities: Theory, research, and intervention*. New York: Praeger.

Hodapp, R.M. (this volume). One road or many? Issues in the similar sequence hypothesis. Chapter 3.

Hodapp, R.M., Burack, J.A., & Zigler, E. (this volume). The developmental perspective in the field of mental retardation. Chapter 1.

Hodapp, R.M., & Mueller, E. (1982). Early social development. In B. Wolman (Ed.), *Handbook of developmental psychology*. Englewood Cliffs, NJ: Prentice-Hall.

Hodapp, R.M., & Zigler, E. (in press). Applying the developmental perspective to individuals with Down syndrome. In D. Cicchetti & M. Beeghly (Eds.), *Children with Down syndrome: A developmental perspective*. New York: Cambridge University Press.

Inhelder, B. (1968). *The diagnosis of reasoning in the mentally retarded*. New York: Day.

Jones, O. (1977). Mother–child communication with prelinguistic Down syndrome and normal infants. In H.R. Schaffer (Ed.), *Studies in mother–infant interaction*. New York: Academic Press.

Kaye, K. (1982). *The mental and social life of babies: How parents create persons*. Chicago: University of Chicago Press.

Kessen, W. (1968). The construction and selection of environments: Discussion of Richard H. Walters' paper on social isolation and social interaction. In D.C. Glass (Ed.), *Environmental influences*. New York: Rockefeller University Press and Russell Sage Foundation.

Klinnert, M., Emde, R., Butterfield, P., & Campos, J. (1986). Social referencing: The infant's use of emotional signals from a friendly adult with mother present. *Developmental Psychology*, 22, 427–432.

Kopp, C., & McCall, R.B. (1982). Predicting later mental performance for normal, at-risk, and handicapped infants. In P. Baltes & O. Brim (Eds.), *Lifespan development and behavior*. New York: Academic Press.

Kopp, C., & Recchia, S.L. (this volume). The issue of multiple pathways in the development of handicapped children. Chapter 10.

Leifer, J., & Lewis, M. (1984). Acquisition of conversational response skills by young Down syndrome and nonretarded young children. *American Journal of Mental Deficiency*, 88, 610–618.

MacMillan, D.L. (1982). *Mental retardation in school and society*. Boston: Little, Brown.

Marfo, K. (Ed.) (1988). *Parent–child interaction and developmental disabilities: Theory, research, and intervention*. New York: Praeger.

McCall, R.B. (1981). Nature–nurture and the two realms of development: A proposed integration with respect to mental development. *Child Development, 52*, 1–12.

McCall, R.B., Eichorn, D., & Hogarty, P. (1977). Transitions in early mental development. *Monographs of the Society for Research in Child Development, 42*.

McCune-Nicholich, L., & Bruskin, C. (1982). Combinatorial competency in symbolic play and language. In D. Pepler & K. Rubin (Eds.), *The play of children*. New York: Karger.

Merighi, J., Edison, M., & Zigler, E. (this volume). The role of motivational factors in the functioning of retarded individuals. Chapter 6.

Minuchin, P. (1985). Families and individual development: Provocations from the field of family therapy. *Child Development, 56*, 289–302.

Mundy, P., & Kasari, C. (this volume). The similar-structure hypothesis and differential rate of development in mental retardation. Chapter 4.

Mundy, P., Sigman, M., Ungerer, J., & Sherman, T. (1987). Nonverbal communication and play correlates of language development in autistic children. *Journal of Autism and Developmental Disorders, 17*, 349–364.

Prizant, B. (1988). *Communication and communicative intentions in autism: Mechanisms underlying the clinical syndrome*. Presentation to the Yale Child Study Center, New Haven.

Rondal, J. (1977). Maternal speech in normal and Down's syndrome children. In P. Mittler (Ed.), *Research to practice in mental retardation*, Vol. 2. Baltimore: University Park Press.

Rondal, J. (1985). *Adult–child interactions and the process of language acquisition*. New York: Praeger.

Sameroff, A. (this volume). Neo-environmental perspectives on developmental theory. Chapter 5.

Sameroff, A. (1975). Early influences on development: Fact or fancy? *Merrill-Palmer Quarterly, 21*, 267–294.

Sameroff, A., & Chandler, M. (1975). Reproductive risk and the continuum of caretaking casualty. In F.D. Horowitz, M. Hetherington, S. Scarr-Salapatek, & G. Siegel (Eds.), *Review of child development research*, Vol. 4. Chicago: University of Chicago Press.

Scarr-Salapatek, S. (1975). An evolutionary perspective on infant intelligence: Species patterns and individual variations. In M. Lewis (Ed.), *Origins of intelligence*. New York: Plenum.

Schneider, P., & Pelland, M. (1987). *Relationship between maternal and child behaviors in interactions involving developmentally delayed preschoolers and their mothers*. Paper presented at the biannual meetings of the Society for Research in Child Development, Baltimore, April 1987.

Sigel, I. (Ed.). (1985). *Parental belief systems*. Hillsdale, NJ: Erlbaum.

Slobin, D. (1970). Universals of grammatical development in children. In G.B. Flores d'Arcais & W.J.M. Levelt (Eds.), *Advances in psycholinguistics*. New York: American Elsevier.

Snow, C. (1972). Mother's speech to children learning language. *Child Development, 43*, 549–565.

Solnit, A., & Stark, M. (1961). Mourning and the birth of a defective infant. *The Psychoanalytic Study of the Child, 16*, 523–537.

Stern, D. (1985). *The interpersonal world of the infant: A view from psychoanalysis and developmental psychology*. New York: Basic Books.

Tronick, E., & Field, T. (Eds.). (1986). *Maternal depression and infant disturbance: New directions for child development*. No. 34. San Francisco: Jossey-Bass.

Volkmar, F., Burack, J.A., & Cohen, D. (this volume). Deviance and developmental approaches in the study of autism. Chapter 11.

Weisz, J. (this volume). Cultural–familial mental retardation: A developmental perspective on cognitive performance and "helpless" behavior. Chapter 7.

Weisz, J., Yeates, K., & Zigler, E. (1982). Piagetian evidence and the developmental-difference controversy. In E. Zigler & D. Balla (Eds.), *Mental retardation: The developmental-difference controversy.* Hillsdale, NJ: Erlbaum.

Wertsch, J., & Youniss, J. (1987). Contextualizing the investigator: The case of developmental psychology. *Human Development, 30,* 18–31.

Wetherby, A.M. (1986). Ontogeny of communicative functions in autism. *Journal of Autism and Developmental Disorders, 16,* 295–316.

Wetherby, A.M., & Prutting, C. (1984). Profiles of communicative and cognitive-social abilities in autistic children. *Journal of Speech and Hearing Research, 27,* 364–377.

Woodward, W. (1979). Piaget's theory and the study of mental retardation. In N.R. Ellis (Ed.), *Handbook of mental deficiency research* (2nd ed.). Hillsdale, NJ: Erlbaum.

Young, K. (1988). *An analysis of parental and expert beliefs about infant development.* Unpublished doctoral dissertation, Yale University, New Haven, CT.

Zeaman, D., & House, B. (1979). A review of attention theory. In N.R. Ellis (Ed.), *Handbook of mental deficiency, psychological theory, and research* (2nd ed.). Hillsdale, NJ: Erlbaum.

Zigler, E. (1967). Familial mental retardation: A continuing dilemma. *Science, 155,* 292–298.

Zigler, E. (1969). Developmental versus difference theories of mental retardation and the problem of motivation. *American Journal of Mental Deficiency, 73,* 536–556.

Zigler, E., & Balla, D. (Eds.) (1982a). *Mental retardation: The developmental–difference controversy.* Hillsdale, NJ: Erlbaum.

Zigler, E., & Balla, D. (1982b). Selecting outcome variables in evaluations of early childhood special education programs. *Topics in Early Childhood Special Education, 1,* 11–22.

Zigler, E., & Hodapp, R.M. (1986). *Understanding mental retardation.* New York: Cambridge University Press.

Author index

Abel, T. M., 143
Abichandani, F., 250
Abrams, M., 240
Abramson, L. Y., 159
Achenbach, T., 76, 80, 124, 125, 143
Ahmad, R., 240
Ainsworth, M. D. S., 186, 187
Allen, J., 256
Allen, R., 282, 284, 285
Alpern, G. D., 249, 256
Altshul-Stark, D., 231
American Psychiatric Association (APA),
    28, 73, 252, 254
Andersen, E. S., 285
Anderson, G. M., 250
Anderson, M., 30, 80, 87
Anderson, N. B., 260
Andrews, R., 174–6, 187, 258
Arend, R., 184
Armstrong, D., 178
Aronfreed, J., 144
Asher, S. R., 287
Aslin, R., 274n
Atwood, A., 254
Auger, M., 233
August, G. J., 250
Aumeras, C., 233
Axelrod, J., 177
Aylsworth, A., 238

Baer, D., 5
Bahrick, L. E., 276
Baikie, A., 43
Baker, B., 66, 236
Baker, J. A., 129
Baker, K., 287, 290
Baker, L., 249
Baldwin, A. L., 102
Baldwin, C., 102
Balla, D., 11, 13, 28, 36t, 79, 116, 117–18,
    119, 123, 124, 125, 126, 140, 150, 154,
    156, 161, 170, 234, 235, 264, 295, 300

Baller, W., 235
Barocas, R., 97, 99, 100f, 101t
Bartak, K., 249
Bartak, L., 259
Barton, S., 256
Bates, E., 18, 19, 51, 208, 281, 288, 304
Bateson, G., 240
Baumeister, A., 30, 71, 76, 89, 307
Bayley, N., 174, 183, 192
Beck, H. S., 14, 37
Becker, L., 178
Beckman, P., 21
Beckwith, L., 80, 86
Bedrosian, J., 63
Beeghly, M., 20, 41, 57, 169–70, 171, 184,
    185, 189–90, 199, 200, 206–7, 208, 210,
    214, 217, 304
Beethoven, L., 277
Begab, M. J., 127, 238
Bell, R. Q., 207, 211
Bell, T., 143
Belsky, J., 104, 186, 199, 200
Benigni, L., 18, 19, 208, 304
Bennett, F. C., 289–90
Berger, J., 191, 200, 205–6, 207, 211, 218
Bergman, A., 188
Berry, A., 230
Berry, P., 174–6, 187, 258
Bertalannfy, L. von, 19, 301
Bettleheim, B., 248, 260
Bever, T. G., 3
Bice, H., 238
Bierman, J. M., 98
Bijou, S., 5
Binder, A., 148
Birch, H., 41
Birns, B., 98
Blacher, J., 306
Black, F., 176
Black, J., 274–6, 275t, 281
Blackwell, J., 157
Blehar, M. C., 186, 187

313

Subject index

ability profiles, 20
abnormality, 97
abstract reasoning, 41
accidental mental retardation, 27
accommodation, 73n1, 82, 86
activity (quality), 173
adaptation, 127, 172; in attachment, 186
adaptive behavior/functioning, 19, 66, 115;
  in autism, 264; in fragile X syndrome,
  226, 234–7, 239, 241–2; impairments of,
  28; regulatory systems in, 103–4
adopted children studies, 139–40
adrenalin, 178
adult–child interaction, 116–17; in development, 11, 54, 55; see also parent–child
  interaction
affect: dampened (Down syndrome children), 207, 303, 306; organization of,
  184–5
affect/cognition relationship, 212; in Down
  syndrome children, 174, 175, 180–1, 182–
  6, 190
affiliation, 187, 213
age-appropriate behavior, 277, 307
agency, 282
amaurotic family idiocy, 31
amentia, 31
American Association on Mental Deficiency, 137, 138
American Sign Language, 286
Anxiety Disorder, 234
approach: in Down syndrome children,
  173, 176, 177, 179, 180
arithmetic skills, 277
arousal modulation, 207
assessment techniques, 128, 253
assimilation, 73n1, 82, 86
ataxic type (cerebral palsy), 42, 43
athetoid type (cerebral palsy), 42, 43
attachment: in Down syndrome children,
  186–7, 213; and outerdirectedness, 123,
  124–5

attachment behavior: development of, 278,
  280
attention, 81, 86; in Down syndrome children, 191–5, 212
Attention Deficit Disorder with Hyperactivity, 234, 237
attention fixation, 181
attention–retention capabilities, 30
attention span, 191, 237
attentional control, 84, 86
attentional focus, shifting of, 30
attentional needs, 117
attentional problems, 234, 237
attributional overextension, 162
atypical development/behavior, 49; study
  of, 246–7
atypical populations: opportunities presented by study of, 4, 21, 74–5, 240, 246,
  261, 263, 264–5, 300–7
auditory attention, 193–4
autism, 20, 44; behavioral features and developmental level in, 259–61; cognitive
  development in, 256–8; deviance and developmental approaches in study of, 246–
  71; diagnosis and definition of, 251–4; as
  diagnostic concept, 247–54; historical
  background of, 248; language and communication in, 259; onset of, 254–5, 255f;
  organic factors in, 249–51; similar-
  sequence hypothesis and, 261–3; similar-
  structure hypotheses and, 263–5; social
  development in, 258–9; subtypes of, 253–
  4; see also infantile autism
autistic children, 300, 304, 305; language
  development in, 302–3; pragmatic skills
  of, 209
autonomy: toddler, 188
avoidance, 129

basal ganglia, 43
Bayley Scales of Infant Development, 174,
  183, 184

323

Printed in the United States
By Bookmasters